P9-DWZ-603

DATE DUE

DEMCO 38-296

MOVING
VIOLATIONS

12

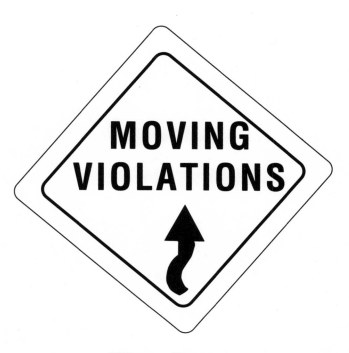

MOVING VIOLATIONS

*War Zones,
Wheelchairs,
and
Declarations
of Independence*

John Hockenberry

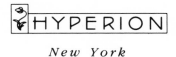

New York

Library of Congress Cataloging-In-Publication Data

Hockenberry, John.
    Moving violations : war zones, wheelchairs, and declarations of
independence / by John Hockenberry.
        p.   cm.
    ISBN 0-7868-6078-2
    1. Hockenberry, John.   2. Paraplegics—United States—Biography.
3. Journalists—United States—Biography.   I. Title.
RC406.P3H57   1995
362.4'3'092—dc20
    [B]   94-37190
                                                                        CIP

Text Design: Levavi & Levavi, Inc.

FIRST EDITION

10 9 8 7 6 5 4 3

Margaret (Peggy) Zinn gave her life for this book. I thank
Richard Rutkowski for saving my life, Tom Hockenberry
for pushing, and Charlie (Peter) Slagle for having lived a
life after all.

Contents

1 ➤ WALKING WITH THE KURDS   1

2 ➤ GRAVITY'S CHILD   15

3 ➤ A FAREWELL TO ARMS   28

4 ➤ THE CUTTING BOARD   42

5 ➤ TYING KNOTS   57

6 ➤ 'BYE, BIKE   70

7 ➤ FEAR OF BEES   87

8 ➤ LOOSE SCREWS   103

9 ➤ CRIP JOB   115

10 ➤ THE STARING   126

11 ➤ ROLL MODEL   135

12 ➤ REACHING THE PEDALS   145

13 ➤ REAL JOB   160

14 ➤ LIVE AT FIVE · 171

15 ➤ LOST CAUSES · 183

16 ➤ THE POINT OF NO COMMENT · 207

17 ➤ BEAT REPORTER · 215

18 ➤ GETTING PAST SECURITY · 229

19 ➤ CHEATING · 245

20 ➤ FOOTNOTES AND CHECKPOINTS · 264

21 ➤ RADWAN · 275

22 ➤ KHOMEINI'S REVENGE · 283

23 ➤ PUBLIC TRANSIT · 296

24 ➤ SEALED ROOMS · 311

25 ➤ CHARLES PETER SLAGLE · 334

26 ➤ SOMALIA · 354

ACKNOWLEDGMENTS · 369

America
Centre of equal daughters, equal sons,
All, all alike endear'd, grown, ungrown, young or old,
Strong, ample, fair, enduring, capable, rich,
Perennial with the Earth, with Freedom, Law, and Love,
A grand, sane, towering, seated Mother,
Chair'd in the adamant of Time.

—Walt Whitman,
"Leaves of Grass," 1888

MOVING
VIOLATIONS

Walking with the Kurds

*T*here were legs below. Stilts of bone and fur picking around mud and easing up the side of a mountain near the Turkish border with Iraq. Two other legs slapped the sides of the donkey at each step like denim-lined saddlebags. They contained my own leg and hip bones, long the passengers of my body's journeys, and for just as long a theme of my mind's wanderings.

I was on the back of a donkey plodding through the slow, stunned bleed of the Gulf War's grand mal violence. The war was over. It remained only for Desert Storm's aftermath to mop up the historical details wrung out of Iraq. The Kurds were one such detail. It had taken another war, Desert Storm, for the Kurds to unexpectedly emerge from the obscurity they had received as a reward for helping the Allies during the First World War, nearly eight decades before. The Kurds had helped the Allies again this time, but this was just another detail.

In the calculus of victory and defeat echoing through world capitals and in global headlines, in the first moments of Iraq's surrender there were few details, and fewer human faces. The first pictures of the war were taken by weapons; Baghdad, a city of five million, rendered in fuzzy, gun-camera gray. Snapshots of hangars, bridges, roads, and buildings. No people.

We had won.

They had lost.

The winners were well known: they were the faces on billboards. The smiling, enticing face of the West, its prosperity and its busy president, Bush, were known to the youngest schoolchild in the Middle East. In the West only one Middle Eastern face was as prominent, the face of the demon who became the vanquished, the singular, ever-present Saddam Hussein. The other losers were invisible. As time went on the war began to bleed the faces of its true victims.

Here on the Turkish border it was an open artery of Kurdish faces, streaming out of Iraq and down mountainsides in Turkey and Iran as the world's latest refugee population. Under cover of surrender and Western backslapping, Saddam Hussein had uprooted the mutinous Kurds and sent them packing under helicopter gunship fire north and east into nations that are neighbors only on the most recent of maps. To the Kurds, the region from northern Iraq to eastern Syria, southeastern Turkey, and western Iran is all one land: Kurdistan. It has been this way for more than one thousand years of warfare and map drawing. So for these Kurdish refugees, border checkpoint traffic jams were just old insults lost in the latest slaughter.

My fists held tight to the saddle and up we went toward the final ridge on the edge of Iraqi Kurdistan. A village called Üzümlü on the Turkish side was the destination. It lay three or more valleys beyond. There, the horizon contained the spilled wreckage of the refugee exodus from inside northern Iraq. Here it was just mountains against the brisk, gray, clouded sky punched through with brilliant patches of blue. Deep below in the valley roared the Zab River, muddy with the melting snowpack's promise of spring.

In March of 1991 the spectacular sky and the brisk air rimmed with intermittent hot alpine sun was a welcome escape from the visa lines and news briefings, SCUD missile attacks and second guessing of Saddam, Bush, and Schwarzkopf that so dominated the business of covering Desert Storm. I watched the sky while everyone else stared at their own feet. Ahead and behind, Kurdish men in black slacks walked with enormous sacks of bread on their backs. Like a line of migrating ants, a parade of white bundles snaked up the mountain on black legs.

Neither the heroic foot-borne relief efforts, anticipation of the horrors ahead, nor the brilliance of the scenery around me struck home as much as the rhythm of the donkey's forelegs beneath my hips. It was walking, that feeling of groping and climbing and floating on stilts that I had not felt for fifteen years. It was a feeling no wheelchair could convey. I had long ago grown to love my own wheels and their special physical grace, and so this clumsy leg walk was not something I missed until the sensation came rushing back through my body from the shoulders of a donkey. Mehmet, a local Kurd and the owner of the donkey, walked ahead holding a harness. I had rented the donkey for the day. I insisted that Mehmet give me a receipt. He was glad to oblige. I submitted it in my expense report to National Public Radio. The first steps I had taken since February 28, 1976, cost thirty American dollars.

It was a personal headline lost in the swirl of news and refugees. I had been in such places before. In my wheelchair I have piled onto trucks and jeeps, hauled myself up and down steps and steep hillsides to use good and bad telephones, to observe riots, a volcano, street fighting in Romania, to interview Yasir Arafat, to spend the night in walk-up apartments on every floor from one to five, to wait out curfews with civilian families, to explore New York's subway, to learn about the first temple of the Israelites, to observe the shelling of Kabul Afghanistan, to witness the dying children of Somalia. For more than a decade I have experienced harrowing moments of physical intensity in pursuit of a deadline, always keeping pace with the rest of the press corps despite being unable to walk. It is the rule of this particular game that it be conducted without a word of acknowledgment on my part. To call attention to the wheelchair now by writing about it violates that rule. My mind and soul fight any effort to comment or complain, even now, years after the events I write about.

This quiet, slow donkey ride was easily the farthest I had gone, out onto a ledge that was never far from my mind during the fifteen years I had used a wheelchair. It was a frightening edge where physical risks loomed like the echoes of loose stones falling into a bottomless canyon, and the place where I discovered how completely I had lost all memory of the sensation, the rhythm, even the possibility of walking. I held onto the saddle or the donkey's neck. The locking of donkey knees and the heavily damped strokes of each donkey leg finding a cushioned foothold in the cold, soft mud of the Iraqi hillside rippled up my hanging limbs and drove into the bones of my arms. My arms were the sentries holding me in place, doing the job of arms and legs once again, as they had for a decade and a half. Though this was the closest to walking that I had felt in all of that time, the job of my arms could not change. FIRST STEPS IN FIFTEEN YEARS. It was a headline composed and discarded, footnote without essay, ridiculous, like the young blond man on the donkey on the mountain. And it was all perfectly true.

In March 1991 I found myself climbing a hillside where civilization was bulldozing a whole people up onto the mud and snow of a place

called "no man's land" on maps. It was the end of a very long journey;
I had arrived in a place that I could not have imagined. In this soupy
outpost, the trucks seemed to have arrived long before the roads. As I
watched out taxi windows, I could see that there would come a point
where the wheelchair would have to be left behind if I was to make it
to the place where early reports said hundreds of thousands of civilians
were fleeing Saddam Hussein's terror. Wheels of any kind were out in
this terrain. Saddam Hussein had chased the Kurds to the edge of pavement and well beyond. In the pockets of snow, starvation, rock and mud,
only legs could travel.

The story of the Kurds had drawn me from a hotel room in Ankara,
onto a plane to Istanbul, then on a charter flight to Van, an old Kurdish
city once part of the Armenian empire, on a long, boring drive to the
village of Hakkari and then a plunge through the boulder strewn mountain trails to the border town of Çukurca. I left my wheelchair with the
driver from Van beside the road to Çukurca and climbed onto a tawny-
colored, medium-size donkey who accepted without a sound what was
a more than ample load. Before we began the steep ascent, I had only
the time it took to cross a rope and plank bridge in a perilous state of
disrepair to figure out how to keep my mostly paralyzed body on the
animal's back. We crossed over the raging waters of the Zab River in the
first weeks of the spring thaw and began the slow, steep climb toward
Üzümlü.

The bare facts of what had happened in Iraq and Kuwait in the initial
aftermath of Desert Storm read like a random shooting in America:
"World outraged as crazed father attacks neighbor then turns guns on
family and self." The truth was not as simple. For one thing, Saddam
took great pains to make sure that he would not get hurt. Others were
neither so lucky, nor did they have much in the way of control over
their destiny. The civilians in Baghdad, the Shia of southern Iraq, and
the Kurds of the north were all innocent bystanders, caught in the forty
day drive-by shooting that was Desert Storm. Unlike the Kurds, I had
some control over my destiny, but in pursuit of this slice of Saddam's
long, brutal story I took none of his pains to avoid harm. I would get
into northern Iraq any way possible. Whatever difficulties I might encounter in being separated from my wheelchair in the open mountainous country across the border, I would deal with then. I had made this
calculation many times before in covering the Middle East, or in deciding to do anything out in a world not known for its wheelchair-friendly
terrain.

I had often thought of riding a donkey in the mountains of western

America as recreation but had never found the time to orchestrate such a break in space and time. As a vacation it had seemed like a lot of bother, but here, for the sake of a story, the impulse to toss my own wheelchair to the wind was as natural as carrying a notebook is to other journalists. Still, that I would find myself here, holding on for dear life, with no sense of what lay ahead and certainly no way to control events from the top of a donkey, was unsettling. Was I supposed to be here, or was I in the way? To Mehmet the donkey man, I was just another paying customer.

Feeling out of place was an old sensation, almost as old as the paralysis in my legs. It was a feeling I had among friends, among strangers, and just as often when completely alone. I worried when I held up a check-out line at the supermarket. I smiled sheepishly at restaurant patrons as I made my way through the narrow spaces between the tables to my own place. My anonymity torn from me, I interrupted conversations, intruding on peaceful diners. Was it their eyes or mine that said I was in the way until proven otherwise? I could go away or push ahead. Where wheelchairs could not venture, people working together inevitably could. Still, the choice of pushing ahead through the obstacles or just going away was always a matter of selecting the lesser of two evils. Going away was always a defeat. Pushing ahead was never a victory, and asking for help always reduced the score.

The staring began with the trickle of refugees near the village. They walked slowly, mostly downhill now, toward Turkey. They looked up from their feet at the passenger on the donkey. The incongruity suggested neither disability nor pity. The first refugees we met were the least affected by their week-long trek and a harrowing three days in the mud and snowy cold of the mountainous border region. They carried sacks and misshapen crates of clothing and provisions looted from their own hastily departed neighborhoods in Mosul, Sulaimaniya, Zakho, Kirkuk, and Erbil. Some of the women raised their eyes, wondering why a perfectly good donkey should be wasted on a blond Westerner who seemed to be so well-fed. One man suggested to the guide that the donkey would be better suited to carrying a sack of bread, or perhaps a dead or sick person. In Arabic and Kurdish, Mehmet told them that I was a reporter come to see Üzümlü, and that I was unable to walk.

I had been anonymous for a moment; now I was unmasked. The faces of these Kurdish refugees became faces of familiar worry and pity, faces that I had spent so much time thanking. Their concern was appreciated, I told them, but misguided in my case. The men and women gathered around and started to warn me of the dangers ahead. "If you cannot walk, why are you here?" they asked. "There is only death here. People are dying everywhere in Üzümlü. Saddam is killing everyone. Why did America not help us?" they asked. "There is no food. You could die."

I responded just as I did when people wanted to push my chair, or hold a door, or hand me something they thought I was looking at on a supermarket shelf. With a workable, relaxed face of self-assured confidence I could dismiss all of these people politely or rudely, but dismiss them I did. "No need to be concerned." I said. "I've got the door. I am fine. I can make it across the street. No problem. I'm not sick. I don't need a push. I'm not with anyone, no." It was habit, not arrogance that caused me to insist: "I'm just fine here on the donkey in the middle of one hundred and fifty thousand starving, war-terrified refugees."

In Üzümlü, flimsy shelters made of sticks and plastic sheets covered people forced to sleep on crusted mud. A dirty graveyard contained the twenty to fifty people who died each night. The yellow, bloodless, milky-eyed corpse of a child lay next to a partially dug grave. Perhaps two hundred thousand people would pass through here on their way to official Turkish refugee camps. The first had come across minefields, and among the initial group to gather around me and Mehmet and the donkey were a man and the gray-skinned unconscious companion on his back. He had an ugly blackened bandage around his waist, and one of his legs was merely a stump. This man would not make it to the Zab River, let alone the medical facility in Hakkari three hours away by car and already overflowing with casualties. His back and leg had absorbed a mine explosion that had halved his brother. The man carrying him looked at me with authority, pointed at his wounded friend, and said: "There is danger here. He cannot walk . . . we have here many who cannot walk. We have enough," he said with muted anger. "Why are you here?"

I got down off the donkey, sat on the ground, and assembled my tape recorder and microphone. The Kurdish refugees wanted to know why I couldn't walk and if the Iraqis had shot me. Gradually they began to talk.

"The helicopters came and we had to leave. I am a teacher," said one. "I am an engineer," said another.

To an outsider, they were only the sick and the well. Otherwise they were differentiated by the time of day they had decided to flee for the border. Those who fled at night were wearing pajamas under overcoats. Those caught during the day had time to don what looked like their entire wardrobes, especially the children, who stood staring and bundled up like overstuffed cloth dolls. Occasionally someone would walk by in just a thin jacket and torn slacks. Such shivering people explained that they were caught away from home running errands when the gunships came.

Mostly they wanted to talk about "Bush." It was in the bitterest of terms that the leader of Desert Storm was evoked on those cold muddy hills. "Bush is liar. Why he not help us?" "We fight Saddam, but why Bush let Saddam fly helicopters?" They said the word "helicopter" with the accent on the third syllable, and spit it out like an expletive. I sat cross-legged beneath a circle of anger, aiming the microphone to catch the shouting voices.

At that moment, much of the world I knew was reveling in victory. Two days earlier in a conversation with someone from Washington I had learned of the stellar approval ratings for President Bush. Historic peaks in the nineties, enshrining in statistics the apparently unshakable kingship behind the second sacking of Baghdad in a thousand years. As the Kurds might have said, "The warlord Tamerlane did a better job the first time," in 1253. The wind picked up and rattled the plastic sheeting anchored to stubborn mountain shrubs. The plastic made blurry apparitions of the blank young and very old faces inside. A large man stepped up and grabbed my microphone and began to speak in a hoarse, exhausted voice.

"Why is Saddam alive and we are dead? What is for America democracy? Bush is speaking of freedom and here we are free? You see us. They send you to us. You, who cannot stand? You are American, what is America now? Why are you here?" His words echoed out from the hill and mixed with the sobs and squeals of the refugees. To him my presence was an unsightly metaphor of America itself: able to arrive but unable to stand. I could not escape his metaphor any more than I could get off that mountain by myself. These were the questions. And so they remain.

The day was beginning to fade. It was a four-hour ride back down the mountain and at least another hour to file stories to Washington. It was time to go. Mehmet and I hoisted me up onto the donkey and we started our descent. The Turkish army had begun to airlift soldiers by helicopter to the mountaintop to urge the refugees down from Üzümlü and into a camp at a lower elevation. Later the Kurds would discover that this new camp was actually inside Iraq by a couple of hundred yards, a fact Secretary of State James Baker would learn in a photo op visit to the camp three days later. With its own far less headline-grabbing program of Kurdish oppression in southeastern Turkey, the Turkish government made it clear that it did not want the Iraqi Kurds.

Until the biblical scale of the catastrophe was apparent, the U.S. government was inclined to agree with Turkey. James Baker and George Bush spoke of territorial integrity in regards to the Kurdish issue. There would be no partitioning of Iraq, they said. The Kurds would have to move . . . again. The Turkish soldiers on the mountain pass fired their automatic weapons into the air, herding people like cattle. The narrow trail down to a spit of Iraqi border territory near the Turkish town of Çukurca was soon clogged with Kurds.

Donkey riding was a slow business. Without any abdominal muscles, my spine twisted and folded with each step. To sit up straight was to get a brief respite from the sharp back pains, but it could only be sustained for a few moments. I held the entire weight of my upper body in my wrists, rubbery and cramped from hours of gripping. They collapsed with each stumble and downward slide of the donkey, pressing my face helplessly into the mane of my tireless friend.

I hadn't figured that the trip down the mountain would be so much harder than the trip up. With the donkey angled upward during the ascent, my weight was pulled back, and holding on had been a simple clinging maneuver. With the donkey descending and angled downward in something of a controlled slide, I had to maintain my weight on my hands, balancing my shifting hips with sheer arm and wrist muscle. The alternative was to tumble down onto the rocks or into one of the many ravines. The crush of refugees narrowed the options for my sure-footed companion and had the effect of periodically spooking him. Mehmet had begun to tire of the earlier novel challenge of escorting the paraplegic on the donkey, and was dragging on the harness. He was also aware that the trail was in considerable danger of jamming into a pedestrian gridlock of desperate refugees.

The sounds of Turkish gunfire caused the donkey to lurch, and me to hold tighter. The rhythm of the donkey's forelegs was intoxicating; it vibrated mechanically up my arms. My whole frame was suspended like a scarecrow on two sticks locked at the elbows. Beneath me walked people clutching their belongings and hurrying to get to shelter before the sun set. Their heads wound along the trail stretching to the horizon.

All around me children stopped to relieve themselves in an agony of diarrhea. In the very same soil, the muddy foot tracks of people and animals filled with snowmelt and rainwater, and children stooped to drink from the puddles. They stood up, and their lips were ringed with brown mud like the remains of a chocolate milk shake. I had drunk nothing all day and had eaten nothing either.

If I was different from other reporters it was in the hydrogen peroxide I carried along with microphones, notebooks, audio tapes, cassette recorders, and cash. Peroxide was the most important item, especially here. In this remote area soaked in mud and surrounded by human waste, there were limits to sanitation. While the closest most reporters came to contaminating their own bodies was by eating a piece of local bread with unwashed hands, for me it was quite different. I use a catheter. Every four hours, every day, for the past fifteen years I have had to insert a tube to empty my bladder. It is a detail which can remain fairly discreetly hidden in most situations. While the processes demanding filling and emptying remained just as urgent here, this environment was hardly optimal for maintaining the near-sterile conditions necessary for using a catheter safely. To expose the catheter to the elements for even a few seconds was to risk infection as definitively as using a contaminated hypodermic syringe risked introducing hepatitis, or worse, into the blood.

After two days my hands had become utterly filthy, and my tattered gloves were soaked through with every local soil. At a certain point one can feel the collective momentum of a human tragedy. With overwhelming power, biological forces penetrate skin, culture, geography, careers, and deadlines. The Kurdish refugees clawed through the mountain foliage, plowing up a rich loam of conquered humanity. I did not want to become fertilizer.

It was not the first time I had encountered potentially lethal mud in the course of covering a story. To prevent infections in such situations, I adopted a simple if crude strategy of self-denial that had served me well in the past. I would go into something of an emergency-induced body shutdown. Nothing in; nothing out. No food meant no waste. No water meant no parasites and therefore no infection.

In an environment without anything resembling a toilet, the inability to stand, squat, or balance above the ground meant that the simplest of bodily functions was impossible to perform without making a mess well outside the specifications of a person's normal notions of human dignity. In this place, human dignity was hard to fathom and beside the point.

But to lose control meant certain contamination. Aside from preventive deprivation, I could ration the peroxide carefully, avoid food and water, and pop vitamin C tablets to keep the acid content and therefore the antibacterial chemistry of my urine high. There was no room for error out here. The weakness that came with intense thirst and having starved for three days, along with being an equal number of travel days from any kind of hospital, would give infection an absolutely lethal head start.

So whatever my face conveyed to the concerned refugees coming down the mountain, I was no more fine than they were, and I was about as confused as to why I was here in this barely inhabitable edge of two warring nations. The accumulated delirium of the war, the Kurdish refugees, and my own deprivation made a dirgelike dream of the donkey ride. From this perch I was again as tall as I used to be. I could see the tops of heads and the shoulders all around me laden with leather straps tied to overstuffed suitcases. In this position my knees seemed farther away from my face. My feet were fully out of view. I had to strain to see them below the flanks of Mehmet's donkey. My abdomen was stretched by my extended and hanging leg bones. It gave me the impression that my lungs had grown larger. None of these details would have mattered to anyone else sitting on a donkey. To me they were a richly hued garment of memory and sensation long lost. In this wondrous garment I was invisible.

The joy of these sensations stood out in surroundings overrun with terror and death. I was unknown and unseen here. There were no presumptions about my body. All that people could tell, unless they were told otherwise, was that I was well-fed and blond. Beyond this, nothing was given away. As time went on I ceased even to look like an American journalist. Anonymity intensified the feeling of who I was, where I had come from, and how my own body worked, or didn't. As an American I had no right to be afraid here, I thought. I was safe and distinct from this horror. As a human being I had no way to separate myself from the river of Kurdish flesh making its way toward the valley. In my own invisible way, I was as close to death as they were. As a paraplegic, I was inside a membrane of unspoken physical adversity. There was no reason to expect bodies to function in such conditions, and each additional moment of life required a precise physical calculation. Durability of flesh pitted against the external elements. Each transaction final. The limits fully real. There was no room for mistakes.

I was not alone in contemplating those limits. Each dying person knew who he or she was. Each struggling refugee could see how much they had left to wager. The chill of circumstance made the crowd and myself quiet. Energy was conserved. The well-fed Turkish conscripts ahead and behind swaggered and fired their weapons, breaking the collective silence of one hundred thousand people.

Why was I there? It is an imperative of journalists to get the story. It was an imperative of those civilians to make their way off the mountain. There were others. The global imperatives of America to confront Saddam. The imperative of America to go home and beat the drum or lick its wounds. In victory, the United States lifted off from Iraq just as it did from the embassy roof in Saigon in 1975 following defeat in Vietnam. Some Vietnamese clung to the chopper back then. They imagined that despite the circumstances of defeat, the promises of America might be honored elsewhere.

In 1991 those promises seemed hollow and frozen, archived for un-born historians. The Kurds wondered why in victory the Americans would leave them to the wolves more swiftly and surely than the Cam-bodians and South Vietnamese were abandoned following America's hu-miliating defeat in Indochina. Aside from the few colorless platitudes thrown their way from Washington, the Kurds had little to do with the business at hand for a triumphant president and his new world. In the anger of the Kurds there was no expectation that America would find their cause worthy, no expectation that their cries would be heard. They had given up on this America without a message and no interest in moving hearts and minds in Iraq. This time when the American chopper lifted off, no one would bother to hold on. Walking in the mud seemed the surer course now.

Fifteen years after lying in an intensive care unit in Pennsylvania I was near the summit of a mountain on the Iraqi border. If this was another event in the struggle for independence and triumph over physical adver-sity, what about the people who were dying all around me? Was I here to do something for them, or was it for me?

On a donkey among the Kurds at the end of a dreadful back-lot surgi-cal abortion of a war, the paths of truth and physical independence seemed to diverge. I had no good answer for the Kurdish man who insisted that there were already too many people who could not walk in Üzümlü. Why I had gone to Kurdistan was as complicated a question as why George Bush's army did not in the first weeks after the war. What seemed an unquestionable virtue had become an excuse for doing something in my case, nothing in the president's.

During the Gulf War, President Bush spoke a lot about how America could regain its sense of mission, its confidence as a world leader, and declare independence from a burden of history. But in a war against historical burdens, the wider battlefield is blocked from view. There is no place for the identity of the people who are simply fighting to save their own miserable lives, the lives that never made it onto the American gun-camera videos, the lives of those we called the enemy, or the Kurd-ish friends in Iraq we never even knew we had until many thousands of them were dead.

I was fighting my own burdens. Holding on to the flimsy saddle and feeling each donkey step in my back and in my cramped and throbbing fingers, I could see that my entire existence had become a mission of never saying no to the physical challenges the world presented to a wheelchair. It was this that had gotten me through a fiery accident and would provide me with a mission upon which I could hang the rest of my life. I had made the decision to get on that donkey when I had gotten out of a hospital bed years before and vowed never to allow the world to push me. I would pull it instead. In Kurdistan I discovered that the world is a much larger place than can be filled by the mission of one man and his wheelchair.

If the Kurds had truly left me alone and gone about the business of only saving themselves, I would just have died right there, holding my tape recorder. They did not. "I'm fine," I said. There on the mountains between Turkey and Iraq, I had lost my way. It was up to Mehmet, the donkey, and me to find my way back.

In the last valley before the river, the steep trail was teeming with refugees. Just eight hours before it had been deserted and tinged with early spring grass; now each bend had been churned into slippery mud. The donkey was having trouble keeping its footing; Mehmet pulled on the harness as the beast locked knees next to a family pushing a wheelbarrow piled with clothes, utensils, a cassette player, and some toys. The animal would not budge, and Mehmet angrily shoved it and yanked on its tail. The donkey made a spitting noise, moaned, and bolted down a steep slope toward the grass. I held on and twisted as the animal half-tumbled off the trail.

Trail was a generous description for the steep, narrow switchback that folded three times along the gravelly slope. With tens of thousands of refugees clogging the trail, the hillside began to look like a rickety shelf of old books shaking in a earthquake. Every few minutes rocks from the upper trail would be dislodged by someone's feet and tumble down on people one and two tiers below. Shouts and screams would greet the stones. A shower of debris was kicked up by the feet of my fleeing donkey. He landed in a hillock of grass at the river's bank and began to munch and graze with a resolve that suggested that his paraplegic reporter carrying duties had ended.

I had slipped off the donkey's back farther up the hill. With an exhausted smile, I rolled onto my back, clutched my bag of equipment, and stared up at the sky. The refugees made a moving silhouette against the fiery dusk sky, and the rope bridge over the river was now in darkness. The only sounds were the roar of the river and the shouts of refugees who argued with Turkish soldiers attempting to control access to the bridge.

The crowd was trying to storm a flimsy bridge that could withstand perhaps twenty people at a time without collapsing. The sound of Turkish weapons fired into the air peppered the din. My arms and cramped fingers ached. It felt good to lie down in the cold, wet grass. But I needed to cross that bridge to have any chance at all of filing a story. Without a donkey there seemed to be no way to even approach it from my repose on the river's bank. I turned my head and saw the muddy water raging in frosty darkness. There was no chance of swimming the Zab. The water churned its way around the canyon toward the Tigris, Baghdad, and the Persian Gulf hundreds of miles away. The opposite bank was a traffic jam of relief trucks and makeshift camps, as flimsy shelters from Üzümlü were erected once again along the road to Çukurca. Flickering fires and headlights made shadows on the rocks. Prone and unable to walk on the bank of an unswimmable river with a runaway donkey lost in a crowd of one hundred thousand refugees seemed to be as good an excuse as any for missing a deadline.

Mehmet was taking my predicament much more seriously than I was. He had brought back three men, and insisted on carrying me up to the bridge on a blanket. On the boggy riverbank the blanket quickly became saturated, making it difficult to hold with a body inside. They dropped me half a dozen times and eventually gave up. I laughed. Mehmet's crew went back to attend to their own places in the line to cross the bridge.

I lay there reveling in being invisible. My sore arms were stiff. There was a certain joy in just lying quietly in the grass while the river and the people swirled around me. For two years, more or less, I had been a correspondent in the Middle East. For all that time I had stood out as an American or as a journalist with a microphone; for fifteen years I had been scrutinized continuously because of my wheelchair. But for that moment in Kurdistan surrounded by thousands of refugees, covered with mud, without a chair, and lying in the grass, I was utterly, completely anonymous.

Mehmet's attempts to move me had brought us closer to the bridge, and the confusion of the mob was almost overhead. Sheep grazed near my head in the growing darkness. Up on the bridge some members of the international press corps had arrived and were shooting pictures. I recognized two faces, though I couldn't remember which newspaper they worked for. But they looked at the man with the backpack and after a moment recognized me. They must have recalled that I used a wheelchair. They looked around with some alarm. No wheelchair to be seen. I shrugged my shoulders at them. I mouthed the words "I'm fine." I chuckled out loud, and said, "I could use a donkey right about now." Like the slow movement of the moon over the sun during an eclipse, my moment of anonymity was passing.

In the end, Mehmet himself, a cigarette in his mouth, carried me on his back up the slope to the bridge. After a screaming argument with the Turkish officer, he carried me across and put me down next to a family with their belongings spread out by the road.

"I am American," I said when asked by a young Kurdish boy.

"Do you know Chicago?" he asked. "I have a brother in Chicago."

I nodded and tried out some broken Arabic on him to pass the time. As darkness fell, the Kurdish taxi driver from Van who had been taking care of my chair for twelve hours found me in the crowd and joyfully hugged me. He had watched the exodus of his Kurdish compatriots with tears in his eyes, and with alarm had watched all day for me to appear in the crowd. He brought my wheelchair over and I hoisted myself into it: it felt so good to move and to feel its support beneath my sore shoulders. There were my feet, just below my knees and my lap, right there below my face. Creased since 1976, my six-foot frame folded itself back into a sitting position once again. After only a day I had forgotten what it felt and looked like.

I took a breath and paused for a moment before I rolled toward where the driver had parked his cab. I looked around. There around me, the noise of the refugees quieted. I saw all eyes watching. In their staring gazes I was home. I waved good-bye. I made the deadline.

Gravity's Child

I am haunted by leap years. In February 1976 I lost a day. That year and day are frozen in time now.

There is a place on an interstate in Pennsylvania where an abandoned gas station holds sentry for a pile of gravel. Across a field, a graying barn is powerless to prevent the mid-afternoon February sun from streaming through the holes in its roof. The air is filled with the musty smell of spring, and the sadness that its premature birth will not survive the next snowstorm. There have been a few days of unseasonable heat. It has stopped time.

The gravel pile defies two nineteen-year-old boys to take its summit. In a simian run-crawl they race to the top. "King of the hill," one of them shouts. Laughs and curses echo off the back wall of the gas station, and after a moment one boy stands alone atop the pile. Brushing off, he tightens the muscles in his buttocks and locks his heels in a motion that stretches the long tendons that run the length of his legs. He pulls himself up to full height. The blood rushes to his head and he is dizzy. His hips thrust forward in puppylike ardor, and with arms thrown wide he yawns the length of the solar system.

Like a hardened Polaroid pinned in a closed scrapbook I retain only that artifact of walking. There is a place in my mind where I stand, arms forever thrown wide, feeling those tendons, looking down at my friend

Ricky who walks back toward the waiting car. A statue of memory. The color long aged past recognition: it has been nineteen years as I write these words.

The picture I took that day was not a Polaroid. It was not a picture of myself standing on my legs, or the gas station, or Richard Rutkowski, my college roommate, or the Chevrolet in the parking lot, or the two girls from a college in St. Louis we were driving with. These things were deemed unimportant. Instead, I aimed my camera at the barn in the trees and the low winter sun finding a crack between two clouds. I pressed the shutter, knowing that the picture was another one of those sappy pastoral scenes that barely justified the inch of film exposed to record it and never justified the work in the darkroom to produce a print.

"Let's go now," Ricky called from the small car parked by the gravel pile. We were the very best of friends. We had brought our guitars with us on this unwise and unscheduled break during the winter quarter at the University of Chicago. On more than guitars, we played a music entirely of our own making. Ours was a powerful bond born in the smoldering first moments of manhood. We had each never imagined having someone like the other as a friend. We were as different as two young college boys could be. What we did best together was play music.

Ricky had brought a mahogany steel-string acoustic instrument that was his second love. His first love was the unfinished Fender Stratocaster he would rig with strings so light that for a time you could bend and stretch one string across the path of two others without breaking it. After a while, they would break. Rick broke a lot of strings.

I played a classical guitar with nylon strings. While I had studied classical piano and could read music, my guitar skills were better described as inspired and well-executed bad habits, playable in just a few keys, generally A minor. Rick could not read music, and like me, his habits were bad, but his playing was brilliant. It was a fully developed personal style. He paid appropriate homage to the guitar legends of the sixties and seventies, but thought of himself as a contemporary of Hendrix and Jeff Beck, carrying on their work as artists. This, to me, was dazzling. I just played the guitar.

I was outwardly brash, public-school educated, fearless, and without decorum. Ricky was educated at The Lawrenceville School. When I first saw him play the guitar, I said that he was the best player I had ever seen close up. He responded with a modest chuckle that also suggested that I must be something of a backwater hick. "Then you should hear Clapton play," Rick said. "He came to Lawrenceville one time." While I watched Ricky's fingers he talked to the other prep school students in his group of friends. They were from another world. Douglas was going to run a multinational corporation. Patrick would found a record company or run some entertainment conglomerate. Ricky said nothing about what he would do. It was understood that if Patrick was lucky, Ricky might sign with his record label. Ricky said little about the future. "I *am* a poet," he would announce.

Rick called himself a poet without any permission from anyone. This was an act of boldness and courage beyond any of the pranks and schemes that I could imagine. Outwardly, I was the crazy rebel. I stole city buses to joyride up and down the South Side of Chicago. I sold psychedelic mushrooms to double my quarterly student loan check and pay the expensive tuition at the University of Chicago. I studied mathematics, but among the Nobel prize winners on the university faculty I dared not imagine ever being a mathematician. I had thought I was among the smartest people in my high school. Here I was an overloud, barely literate fool with a lousy collection of record albums and an embarrassing stereo in my dorm room.

Rick and I took a single class together. In it we read Goethe's *Faust*. I found it obscure. He acted as though it had been written by a classmate at Lawrenceville. He spoke of his favorite lines in Faust: "the little Gods of earth." It best described how I looked at Ricky. I never knew it, but it was how he came to think of me.

"Let's go now," Ricky calls from the car, and I descend slowly from the top of the sandpile behind the gas station that marked the last place I would ever stretch my legs. After the others are firmly in their seats, I reluctantly fold myself into the backseat of a Chevy Nova, assuming, once again, the fetal position that American automotive engineers are so fond of proscribing to backseat passengers. I had stood up on the bones of my legs for the last time. This would take a lifetime to comprehend.

People always ask whose fault it was. It seems such an odd question, and yet for me the answer is just a shrug. I was hitchhiking from Chicago to Massachusetts with my college roommate. We got into a car in Pennsylvania on a sunny February day. I fell asleep in the backseat. The driver and her college roommate fell asleep in the front seat.

When I awoke our car had snapped the thread holding it to earth. We hurtled over a flimsy guardrail and down an embankment. The steel of the roof crumpled on first impact, and the car's subsequent rolls and bounces rammed the frame of the passenger compartment into my back again and again. Four times, I counted, and then it came to rest. I sat pinned in that car for a long time, feeling the life bleed out of me in a warm puddle that made my hands slippery, that covered my face with the dripping, sticky confirmation that I was very seriously injured.

I made a solitary attempt to leave the car, placing my hands on my knees in an effort to push off and straighten up. My hands felt my knees but the sensation was not returned. The knees were warm and clearly mine, yet I could no longer feel them. It is that exact moment and that precise memory that divides my life into the time when my legs carried me and the time I have spent carrying those same legs. As these words are written, the moment falls at the exact midpoint of my life, nineteen years on either side. Upon touching those knees and feeling the sensation only in my hands, I knew. My spinal cord had been severed. Whatever else was wrong with me, I would not walk again. The most powerful sensation I have ever felt is of no sensation at all.

Breath was short and painful. The sunlight glinted off the fresh blood on my hands, chest, and lap. The forces that had torn me nearly in half had done their work quickly and had moved on. They had crushed the Chevy and killed the driver. Blue sky and yellow afternoon sun were still visible through the crack of the crumpled car roof. There was plenty of daylight left. It was still a beautiful day.

I thought of three things: I guess we're fucked. I suppose I'll never walk again. Where was the center of mass in a rotating and falling subcompact vehicle?

In a delirium vivid and silly I imagined how I might, in theory, calculate the precise forces that had wrought all of this damage. Center of mass was one of my college physics problems. I had been working nonstop on the weekly problem sets since starting school in the fall. I was deeply worried about my grade.

I thought of asking Rick his estimate of the distance from the road so as to calculate the momentum of the car at the point of impact. But when I called to him, he seemed to be crying. I was still alive, but I could tell that I was not okay. I said something to that effect to Ricky. He went for help.

"It's going to be all right," he said. "Don't worry, man. You're going to make it, man."

I told him one other thing: "I don't think I am ever going to walk again, Rick. I think my back is broken. I cannot feel my knees." I was absolutely certain of this. Ricky didn't argue with me. In a voice thickly laden with fear, he told me to hold on, that the police were on the way.

My legs were hidden, pinned crudely into the backseat. The whole passenger compartment was smashed. The roof was collapsed, the back-seat crushed into the front seat, the dashboard twisted and deformed like a discarded toy. Gasoline leaked from a open tank just behind my fractured back. There were flames in front. I could smell the fumes. The same forces that mingled benzene with my nostrils would join oxygen and carbon in a flaming footnote of elementary chemistry. Ricky went to find someone to put out the fire. I tried not to think about chemistry. I preferred physics.

Gravity tugs. The illusion of legs and arms that lift and pull and hold objects against the will of gravity is that gravity might be resisted, things that would just as soon go down can be made to go up . . . on a shelf . . . on the counter. A pedal pushed to the floor sends 2 tons of metal and plastic with a core of fleshy awareness up a hill. Every foot up a hill is another foot to be reclaimed by gravity coming down. For me, a lifetime of ascent was reclaimed in one brutal transaction. It was a run on the bank. It took only a moment for us to slip the bonds of gravity, carom off the hard, still, frozen earth, and come to rest 200 feet below.

We live in the thin crust of things we can count and describe. Boundaries press in, flattening faces with fear. Ghosts lurk all around. When darkness would fall in the woods of my childhood, shadows became the sinister lurking of wolves. The wolves in my imagination didn't care if I was a good boy or about any of the other little-kid cliffhangers of grades and chores and the judgments of grown-ups. A wolf would presumably find me just as nutritious if I said my please's and thank you's as if I had omitted them. This hypothesis caused me to run swiftly back home to the warm lights of the kitchen, the messy room, and the angry admonishments of adults. At least I had eluded the wolves, one more time. I have always been haunted by their shadows.

The forces that write the history of objects like planets, stars, and their atoms are calculable, countable, and describable. They are also unfathomably primitive. They act in an instant, carving up the surface with a heavy steel blade. We feel only their tug. Gravity merely has to tap us on the shoulder in an elevator and we feel it deep in our stomachs. The truly primitive things have no interest in humanity's good intentions, manners, or legible penmanship.

When the car lost its perch on the pavement and sailed into space, I became a bag of water in a can of steel, and there were three other bags in that can with me. It is what I remember most vividly about the accident. The forces beyond the clearing were there. I could not elude them this time. At least real wolves would have had the decency to eat me. The forces that propelled that car had no knowledge of me; my good intentions were not redeemable here. We were all strangers in that car, but we locked gazes, and together understood that the only way back to the world we knew was to hurtle through space and be stopped by something bigger than we were. We were so very small at that moment. It would be the last time I would ever see two of those faces. Ricky would see them once more.

Driver Margaret (Peggy) Zinn and her friend Barbara Byrne had been on the road for eighteen hours when they picked us up in Pennsylvania. They were also college roommates taking an unscheduled vacation, driving to Port Chester, New York, from their school in Missouri. It had been a grueling trip. We had stopped at the gas station because everyone was drowsy. Barbara was attractive and instantly charmed by Rick. His wire-rimmed glasses, RAF aviator jacket, and curly dark hair made him look like someone you had stood in line for tickets to see. It was as it was supposed to be. I was misshapen and brash like Margaret the driver. We sat on the left side of the car while Barbara and Ricky talked and flirted on the right. We were the handlers. They were the stars. I said nothing to Margaret, but saw her face in the rearview mirror as I drifted off in the backseat. Sleep came easily for all of us in the springlike warmth.

When I awoke, the car had swerved across two lanes of traffic. Margaret seemed to have awakened at the same moment. She saw the car aimed straight for a rock wall left of the highway, and she screamed. Barbara, in the front seat, reached over to grab the wheel. She pulled it hard to the right. I remember the look on her face. Partly it was sheer horror, but there was also a banal, rehearsed look of disapproval, a hint of what their relationship at school must have been. Her friend had done something goofy again, or needed protection. The hierarchy of friendship, true to the end. She had probably nagged her friend often for saying the wrong thing or playing the wrong music. I had the impulse to be sympathetic to Margaret, to say, "Gee, she just fell asleep. It wasn't her fault."

From the passenger seat Barbara now pulled on the steering wheel to keep us from slamming into the rock wall on the left. She put all of her weight into it. We missed the rock wall and swerved severely to the right. At the moment the car hit the guardrail I could feel the whole car and all of its occupants as a single object. We were top-heavy. The guardrail would trip us like a lumbering giant. I could feel its flimsiness in my stomach as we became airborne. The rear wheels left the ground. We were going over.

On the way down, at some point before the first crunching bounce, Margaret opened her door and was thrown out of the car. The rest of us remained inside. Ricky and Barbara were able to crawl out of the crumpled car. I could not. Ricky seemed to have received no injury. I looked at him from inside the car. It made sense that I was hurt and he was not. If someone had to die, it would best be me, I thought. Barbara had been injured but not too seriously. I never saw her again.

Ricky walked up the hill, back toward the interstate. The drivers who had watched the Chevy leave the road were getting out of their cars and coming toward him. Ricky walked over to where Margaret had landed. It was only the sound that came from the face of her mortally wounded head that Ricky could recall years later. He got no closer than a few feet. He stopped and turned away, understanding that he could not help her.

"When I try to remember her, I can't see her," he said the only time we ever talked about it. "It was just something so awful. But I have never forgotten the sound she made." As he started to explain, his face darkened, and he could speak no more of it. Margaret Zinn died of massive head wounds a few hours after her car left Interstate 80.

I learned Margaret's name long after that, when an insurance policy taken out by her parents began paying a twenty-year claim. Each month a check for $420.80 arrives in the mail. There are two names on the check, mine and Margaret Zinn's. I am the beneficiary. My relationship with her began after she died. Of her life I know only the contorted last image of her face and the sounds of her dying. Like the hum of life support in a darkened hospital room, the monthly checks have a somber, relentless rhythm. They drift in the background like dry leaves blown from a tree during a long-ago tornado. I never asked for anything from her, but for the past two decades she has made her payments without fail. She has never let me down.

People are always surprised to learn that the accident was in the middle of the day, on dry pavement, under brilliant sun, with no traffic. Perhaps such stories always begin with dark stormy nights, but a blizzard would have kept us all from sleeping. The warm sun of an unseasonable February made the world dreamy. College students on a cross-country road trip. I could see the remains of the road trip through the deformed sliver of a car window.

I could hear the harsh sound of my own breathing. Each breath was a labored climb, hand over hand, along a thread of oxygen and powerful gasoline fumes. The pain was beginning to slip away. Time began to pool around me. I was caught upstream of my life, slowly breathing. Events began to move by me in the current. The moment spread out flat and deep, and I floated there just above the surface.

Next to me in the car, where Ricky had been sitting, were our sleeping bags and soft suitcases full of clothes. I turned my head back and saw the fractured stump of a guitar neck. The steel strings dangled off the tuning pegs and I read the words "steel reinforced neck". My face had snapped the neck in two. It was Ricky's mahogany Guild acoustic guitar. I made weak little fists. My hands still worked. The break in my spine had not affected my hands. I looked at the pieces of Ricky's guitar. At least my neck wasn't broken.

My own guitar was also crushed and splintered. Its softer gut strings and Spanish wood had spilled like a box of toothpicks from its torn black case. My body was the hammer that had destroyed all of these things. I chuckled. Ricky could still walk around because he had sat with the soft things. I was broken and bleeding because I had sat with the hard ones. The camera at my chest was in two pieces, a telephoto lens ripped from the camera body. It all made sense, I thought: I had thrown myself in the path of an assassin's bullet. I was the bodyguard assigned to protect Ricky. The assassin had failed. Ricky hadn't received a scratch. I watched the destruction like a bystander. It was mesmerizing, as though I was witnessing a real car wreck. I laughed. My sternum ached. Calmly, I pieced together the points of force and waited.

A truck driver who had seen us leave the road ran down the hill with a fire extinguisher. I heard the hissing of the spray off in the distance. I had no sense of an impending fire. The commotion outside seemed to be far away, downstream. It all seemed to have nothing to do with me. I watched Ricky outside, running around. He seemed so alone and afraid. He seemed vulnerable to me for the first time. I wanted to get out of the car and embrace him and tell him everything was all right, and again I felt my knees. They were still numb. I watched quietly.

Up to that point it had already been the worst hitchhiking trip we could have imagined. We had missed rides. We had been let off in the wrong places. It had rained. We had fallen asleep in a blue van that had dropped us somewhere far from the main highway. We had had to walk to a McDonald's to convince someone to drive us back to the interstate. They got us further lost. We ended up walking three miles loaded down with guitars and backpacks. To get from Illinois to the East Coast we had to go through the nightmare of Indiana, where state troopers were legendary for their eagerness to arrest hitchhikers.

An RV picked us up at one point and offered to take us all the way to Massachusetts, until the fuel pump broke and we had to get out. We had gotten off I-90 and were stuck on I-80 because of bad rides. When we got into the last car we were a few miles from Highway 81, which would have taken us north and back to 90. I had wanted to be let off there, but

Margaret had told Rick that they were going all the way to Port Chester, New York. We had had no ride longer than an hour on this whole trip. We got in.

Rick and I had been making jokes about all of the things that had gone wrong. Anything that went right we noted in the nasal voice of a high school basketball play-by-play announcer who has to make the best of a forty-game losing streak: "Let's take a minute to recognize the fact that we have not been robbed once. This ball club, whatever you want to say about it, has not been contaminated with deadly plutonium. These shoes are giving 110 percent. An extraordinary effort; the shoes have remained on the feet."

I knew we were in Pennsylvania. I knew Ricky was alive. I knew they were sawing the car in half. I could hear the commotion of paramedics and police. I could feel myself drifting, my face pressed into the back of the front seat. I remember smiling. I would turn my head to look at the crack of sun outside. The shadows on the grass were long. The day was ending. I wondered what time it was. I wondered what day it was. I knew it was leap year. Every once in a while I placed my hands on my knees. They were still numb. I chuckled. It seemed that I had never before stopped to appreciate how good it was to be able to play music. I looked at my fingers, and in my mind someone was giving a speech honoring my fingers. The crowd applauded long and enthusiastically.

Behind the speaker there was a screen. On that screen were pictures of places I had been. I sat in the audience thinking how unusual it was that all of those pictures were places I knew very well. I turned to look at the faces around me. They were focused on the podium, smiling and clapping. I looked back at the pictures and realized that it was my life on the screen. I blinked hard. I recalled what my mother would always say about death: "Your whole life passes before your eyes."

The pictures were arranged according to those things I had worried about most. The candy I had stolen at age six. With tears streaming down my face, I was in the office of the store manager of the A & P, giving him back a nickel. Or the time I ripped off all of the library books from the high school and had to work for three years in the library as compensation. I thought of how much I had enjoyed working there: would they be angry if they knew how much I had liked that punishment? And there I was dead drunk on the debate team. At a dinner in front of the whole state tournament I had passed out in my salad. For that I was kicked out of high school. It was a movie shot on a long stairway, and each discrete anxiety went by like some rounded antique banister. There was a powerful sense of relief that I didn't have to worry about any of that now. I finally stopped worrying about my breathing. I listened to it. The pain had slipped away.

Simply, and without fear, it all seemed to be ending. My life's worries had shrunk to a handful of trinkets. I laughed at them and blinked slowly. All around me was light and the soft colors of green and blue. I saw the trees and roadway and the commotion far away that was the scene of the accident. I felt sorry for Ricky and the girl I felt was already dead. I felt sorry for the young man trapped in the car. I had forgotten his name.

The forces that had torn the car and the bodies inside suddenly seemed benign. Life was just a box. The infinite was the toy surprise, and every box had one inside. I felt it all and wanted to cry. I felt so alive just wondering these things. In point of fact, I was dying, but that seemed a detail. The essential transaction of conscious beings with the cosmos is to wonder about it. All creatures are permitted to look up into the sky, or under the rock at their feet, to wonder for the sheer joy of it. We spend so much of our lives wondering how things are going to come out for ourselves.

Until the car accident that day in 1976 I understood the world only as an evolving landscape of clockwork challenges and gradual change. I would grow up. I would graduate. I would have a career. I would be happy. The upheavals of radical change and quantum unpredictability were taught to me as aberrations, deviations from the essential orderliness of the system, failures. As surely as the accident tore my body, altering and ending its function, the experience planted seeds and etched riddles that have been my companions ever since. I can be back in that car in my mind even today. It is a gift to learn the fabric of unpredictability. We are taught to see the world as a big machine. On the fringe, chance intervenes like a lottery ticket. There are fabulous winners and the horrible losers. In the middle is everyone else, the hopeful players. The demoralizing effect of this worldview is everywhere.

Physics is full of the riddles of fractured orderliness. There is no lottery, just levels of accident filled with new truth and the chance to remake the world. Only at the surface is dreary continuity maintained. The old Newtonian view of the universe states that disability is like a brake on the wheel of life that runs you down with friction. If a force is opposed to you, you are opposed to it. In the struggle you either collapse from exhaustion or explode in triumph; in either case you retain the feeling that something has been subtracted, that you have been cheated.

The quantum view of disability allows you to dare to think that you can have lived two lives, two bodies occupying two places at once. Suddenly, in an instant, radical change: I was different, yet I was still the same person. I knew that was possible then. It would take a lifetime to be sure.

In a quantum era we creep along a crumbling ledge made by Descartes, a ledge where the unknown is just the writing on the pages we haven't turned. All knowledge and experience are bound together in a handsome volume. Humans still need to believe that there is a sea of stuff out there in which everything bobs. We are just beginning to confront the lack of order in the world.

The modern age and its emblematic chaos has left us without luggage at a junction of human thought. In the beginning, Isaac Newton's imagined and unseen force of gravity was just a phantom that dared to demote the idea of God first to king, then to a pantheon of ubiquitous phantoms, to benign eighteenth-century clock maker, to incompetent nineteenth-century clock maker, to twentieth-century ghost with no headstone. In the twenty-first century we have lost the clock altogether and sit blinking, once again, at the phantoms in the forest. In that simple act we are more like our earliest human siblings than any archeology could ever bind us. The capacity to wonder is the gift itself. It is all we really had, even during all of those moments of human history when we thought we knew everything. All else is fine print, scrubbed clean by history and available for viewing in museums.

It was the inklings of these thoughts that coursed through my bleeding head that afternoon in 1976. I began to feel more and more tired, and that some end was near. But as the light began to dim, there was noise and activity centered around me. I became aware of being pulled in some way. I took a deep breath and can still recall the tingle as the oxygen landed on the starved griddle of my injured lungs. I suddenly understood that I would return to the car. In the place where I was I wanted to ask if I could take all of these feelings back with me. There was no one or nothing to ask, but I knew the answer was no. The feelings had no meaning outside the place I was in. I would just be laughed at.

The car's roof was the only metal pliable enough to force an opening a body might fit through. It was also the only part of the car that could be moved without tearing me apart. They finally cut through the car and pried its twisted metal up enough to allow the paramedics to try and lift me. I was pulled from the rear window like a baby from a womb. The sun was still shining. I could hear the sounds of birds. I looked for Ricky and joked in our nasal play-by-play voice, "Isn't it great that these birds come down here like this? They don't get paid. They really deserve a lot of credit. What a job they are doing."

There was a foggy ride in an ambulance. I remember screaming about punching someone named Miegsfield. The only Miegs Field I knew was the airport in downtown Chicago. It was dark when we arrived at the hospital in Clearfield, Pennsylvania. I had a fractured skull, a broken shoulder and collarbone. My eyesight was dim and cloudy. The shock of the guitar to my face, along with the impact on the seat, had blackened my cheeks, nose, eyes, and forehead. My eyeballs had bled under the surface, replacing the whites and my blue irises with a bright red. My scalp was sliced open, and several ribs were broken.

It appeared that the nerve damage was severe, but no one could say if it was permanent. I recall one doctor with cold hands pulling a sharp object from his pocket and poking it into my chest. I could feel one nipple and only half of the other. Below—nothing. The doctors sewed me up and hoped for improvement. The only regional hospital with a spinal cord rehabilitation facility was hours away in Williamsport, Pennsylvania, where a decompression laminectomy was performed. Doctors observed three crushed vertebrae. There was a three-inch lesion on the dura, the circulatory lining of the spinal cord. It was not severed, but as dead as an earthworm pinched in the middle by a rolling bicycle tire.

I had stayed awake for everything except for a few moments of unconsciousness after the car had hit the ground, and during the first examination. On the ambulance cart, unable to speak or sit up, I looked at Ricky and lifted my hands. I made the motions of someone playing the guitar. I tried with my face to convey to him that it was all right. I could still play. It could have been worse. A tear rolled down his face. I dropped my arms, exhausted. I finally slept on the long ambulance ride to Williamsport.

Although he has never said it to me, Ricky has told family and friends that at some point very early on I told him that I thought it was better that I was paralyzed, not him. That he could never have dealt with it. I certainly have not lived to believe that I, better than anyone else, can "handle" being paralyzed. I can believe that I might have said it to Ricky then. He was the poet. He was the rock star. In protecting him I would now live in a way that required no one's permission. I could not know what that would be. I could understand only that it would involve a life's work.

I woke up in intensive care in Williamsport. There were tubes everywhere. Around me machines were beeping and humming. I was in severe pain. I tried to reconstruct what had happened. I knew that I was pretty badly injured, but I felt unmistakably that I would live. I asked the nurse if I was in serious or fair condition. She said, "Critical." I immediately looked over at the screen with my heartbeat on it. I decided I would keep an eye on this just in case. I tried to figure out what time it was. In the whispering darkness and chill of the ICU there was no sense of time.

I knew that it had been the twenty-seventh of February when we left Chicago. We had spent one night on the road. So it must be the twenty-eighth. I remembered that it was leap year, so it was either very late on the twenty-eighth or some time on the twenty-ninth. I motioned to the nurse once again. "Is it the twenty-eighth or the twenty-ninth?"

"It's March first," she said, "late in the evening."

I had lost a day; leap-year day, the twenty-ninth of February, 1976. I had also lost the use of much of my body. For the rest of my life I would find ways of using what was left of my body to make up for the loss of bones, muscles, and nerves. There was nothing I could do about the lost day. Every February 28 I remember the accident and the hard work and painstaking efforts taken over the past nineteen years to relearn a physical life. I live in the leap-year days now; my life is a piece of that ancient anomaly. The leap-year day claims lineage from a familiar month of every fourth year; it is also an outcast, its number unlucky and prime, indivisible. Leap-year day corrects for the imperfect synchrony between the rotation of the earth and its orbit of the sun; it is the single visible sign of the calendar's disability.

In the same way, my lineage is split. My birth is claimed by a day in June 1956, in the city of Dayton, Ohio. My survival is claimed by leap-year day 1976 on an interstate highway in Pennsylvania near the town of Clearfield. I am from the same orphanage where all of the twenty-ninth days of all of the misfit Februarys live. Every leap year I remember the lost day. I am always chasing it, determined to win it back.

A Farewell
to Arms

*M*y life began in one body and will end in another. At the halfway point between my birth and the present moment lies an intermediate ending and beginning. My life is bisected between its end points. It contains two beginnings, and when death finally comes it will have a pair of ends. In geometry, one and only one line is determined by two points. Between any two points on that line lies infinity. The beginnings and ends of days, moments, thoughts, dreams. First inspection suggests that I am living in the second of two lives. Perhaps on closer inspection there are many more.

I have a permanent irreversible spinal-cord injury at the chest level. In medical terminology it is an incomplete dural lesion at the T4–6 level, which refers to the fourth, fifth, and sixth thoracic vertebrae. If you break your back at the chest level, the sensation stops at about the same place. For me, just below the nipples there is a three-quarter-inch band of an odd receding sensation, and then complete numbness. There are two places on my back where sensation divides into constituent spectra. Temperature without pressure in one spot. Pressure without temperature in another. There is a place just under my right scapula where nerves are rerouted. The point is numb to the touch, but a finger pressed down there produces a sensation about eight inches away. On the other side of my spine I feel a finger pressing down where no such finger exists. Slipped wires, sensory illusions, and the map of the body is confused.

There is nothing visible about my border of feeling and numbness. It is all the same skin and the same bones, but somewhere between the eighth and ninth rib you pass Checkpoint Charlie. It is a border that snakes around my torso, higher in the front, lower in the back, following the contours of the ribs and nerve endings that flare from the sternum like gentle wings. In the summer the border is easier to notice. Only my upper body sweats. Below the spinal cord break the nerves have been yanked from the thermostat. Heat stays bottled up inside like an old office building, stuffy, no air-conditioning, plenty of closed windows.

I spent much of 1976 in two hospitals. The first was in Pennsylvania near where the accident took place. The second was in Grand Rapids, Michigan, where my parents lived. The Michigan hospital was housed in an old brick building and was originally about as wheelchair-accessible as the Tower of London. It had noisy, hesitant elevators and lots of steps that had been sledgehammered into ramps to make way for wheelchairs. It is no longer in the same building today, but it has the same name: Mary Free Bed Rehabilitation Hospital.

A rehabilitation hospital is like a prep school where they serve really awful food and talk about toilet training more than history or algebra. Rehab is also like boot camp. Mary Free Bed had some quasi-religious connotation aside from sounding like someone I would have liked to date in high school. Almost immediately, any strangeness in the name was lost in the strangeness of the cast of characters rolling around the halls, myself among them.

There was smiling Nurse O'Leary with the red tube, the rubber glove, and the K-Y jelly. On my first day at Mary Free Bed, she whipped the sheet back and jammed a long rubber tube inside me. I knew there was only one place she could have put it. But I couldn't feel a thing. There it was. When I wasn't worried about the ugly red acne on my face, this bit of my body had been the focus of most of the last eight teenage years. Now my forlorn little appendage looked like something that had escaped from the circus. The Amazing Hose-swallowing Penis. She kept pushing the tube inside. No sensation. This was a five-alarm fire intruder alert, and I could feel nothing. She kept pushing. She knew what she was doing. I knew what she was doing. I expected the tube to emerge from my mouth or ear. I couldn't decide which was more disturbing, the fact that I couldn't feel any of this, or the smile that never left this nurse's face.

"How do you know when it's inside enough?" No response. Suddenly a yellow fluid began pouring from the tube into the steel bowl.

"How am I doing that?" I wasn't pushing out. I couldn't push out even if I had wanted to.

The nurse took her eyes off the business for an instant and said, "Poke a hole in a bag of urine and it drains, honey. I don't need you to do anything."

Finding a personal concept of normal in a place where nurses patrolled your urethra was the main task in the hospital. What you imagined being able to do was one thing; what you could actually accomplish was something else again. You could imagine the tragedy of never being able to do things, only to discover that there was a way to do them after all. The concept of what is normal became quite foggy and obscure once you figured out the normal response to such an overwhelming physical change. Normal was hard to see through. There were lots of things to bump into, lots of ways to improvise.

Normal for the people in the rehabilitation hospital along with me was something else altogether. We were all fucked-up in some way. We hated the food, and we were all trying to beat the system. Days were spent finding ways to sleep in, slip out, obtain contraband, obtain privacy, simply gain a few moments of freedom. It was us versus them. We had the most fun. The staff held all of the cards. We did all of the work. They were paid minimum wage. We kept things lively. They always won.

My fellow inmates would identify themselves with the only details they could remember about their accidents. One younger man whose body was scarred and looked as though it had been scraped with a paring knife was "motorcycle collided with a station wagon." Often, he would add, "Went through two windshields." A strong burly mechanic with big, hairy arms named Larry was "put the Dodge Power Wagon into the trees." Thin, chain-smoking Harry was "end over end down the ravine." Walter was "diving." Hilda was "crazy person ran into me with a green pickup truck and ruined my life . . . we never found out who it was." There were more than a few "I was drunk. Then I woke up in the hospital."

The nurses had more succinct if far less dramatic clinical medical names for all of us. I was a para. There were quads and hemis (hemiplegic), or CP's (cerebral palsy), BS's (brain stem strokes), or CVA's. Ron was a TBI, which meant traumatic brain injury. Ron could not tell you what had happened to him. It was on his chart that he had bled profusely from the ears at the scene of his accident and had gone into a coma. Ron's misshapen skull was a welcome explanation for why he constantly stared at the ceiling, drooled, and had periodic uncontrollable seizures. Ron never spoke and never argued. Ron laughed a lot. He was the floor psychologist's favorite, which seemed to say more about the psychologist than it did about Ron.

Roger had been injured very high in the neck in a car accident. He was a "high quad." Only his head moved. He was sixteen years old. Roger had a crew cut and a round head that recalled one of those freckled and overly jolly faces in magazine ads from the fifties and early sixties. Roger operated his chair by using a joystick with his mouth. His hands sat, pink and motionless, palms down on a tray in front of him. His neck bore the pink scar of the tracheal tube inserted in neck fracture patients whose respiration fails as a matter of course. The tube is placed in the base of the neck by paramedics and is only removed many days later when they can breathe on their own.

Roger and I would devise ways of disrupting the schedule. He would roll into my bedroom while I was still asleep and wake me up, saying, "You can't be asleep." Roger's schedule was determined by the attendants who woke him, dressed him, washed him, fed him, and plugged in his batteries. He was on their schedule. I could dress myself, barely. So I could sleep in.

Roger would crash his heavy electric chair into my bedside rail. On his tray table was a Styrofoam cup with a long straw. His mouth could go from joystick to straw in an instant. He would give his joystick a sudden, perfectly precise movement and ram his chair into my bed just enough to disturb me but not to be heard by any of the white coats in the hall. When I would peek out from the covers he would be smiling, his mouth peacefully drinking from the straw. I would drag my reluctant body upright and blink at him. He was always perfectly groomed and dressed in the morning, like a doll from a horror movie.

"Is it fun to get up this early?" I knew the answer to that question. Roger was the highest quad on the floor: C-1, the first vertebra in the neck. The nurses who worked the hall would do him first since he involved the most labor. He was the big item on the daily to-do list. If the nurses did Roger first, they could expect to take their break at ten sharp. It was the peculiar tyranny of being someone else's task.

In his former life Roger had been a regular teenager. He stayed up late and hugged the pillow until well past noon. Now he only indulged vicariously in the slovenly yawns of sleeping late by witnessing my unkempt hair and tardiness. "I'm going to steal your breakfast," he said. I blinked at his face and watched him stare at my untouched tray of cornflakes, milk, and cranberry juice. I knew my breakfast wasn't going anywhere.

"John, would it still count as stealing if you fed me your breakfast?" Roger wasn't hungry, he was starved for volition. He told me that he used to steal cars for fun. Now he couldn't make a pencil roll off his tray table.

Roger would get his life back on the night shift. The nurses on nights would put him down last, sometimes waiting until after the eleven o'clock shift change so they could watch Johnny Carson while they stripped and washed him. I would hear his comments out in the hall. He described his body as a collection of mischievous boys, himself the pack leader. His legs would be spastic, his body difficult to move; he would make an embarrassing noise. Each difficulty Roger would claim as his own intended sabotage of the nurses. He orchestrated the campaign of resistance from his moving, animated head. It was good fun, but Roger had nothing to do with it. His body did what it wanted. Roger simply claimed the credit. The nurses played along.

Any choice denied the nurses, we would try to claim for ourselves. We wondered if Roger could sleep in if we unhooked the battery to his electric wheelchair. One night after the "Tonight Show" I went in and at Roger's suggestion removed a condenser, which shut the chair down without betraying its malfunction right away.

The next morning Roger was there in my room at the same ungodly hour ramming my bed and talking about stealing my breakfast. "They got the custodian to fix the chair," he said. "He has a drawer full of condensers. I had to tell him you stole the first one. I couldn't just say I did it." Roger grinned at me and wiggled his head with a "no jury would convict" expression on his face. It was just the look you could imagine seeing from Roger in the middle of an empty bank vault surrounded by crime lab police looking for stolen cash.

"If I have to pay the day shift to all call in sick, I swear, Roger, one of these days you are going to sleep in so I can." "You're a paraplegic, John," Roger would say. "You can do anything you want . . . what's the problem?" For Roger, paraplegia was about as serious a disability as an untied shoe. To complain about it was whining, and Roger would have none of it.

Roger and I usually went to PT (physical therapy) at the same time in the morning. There he would sit and do shoulder lifts and head moves with sandbags weighing him down for resistance. Roger also used the blow bottle to exercise his lung capacity. The more muscles you had, the harder you worked in PT. I had to lift weights and do sit-ups and transfers and push-ups. Roger would provide the commentary, noting with glee any struggle, strain, or sweat on my part, and especially any stains on my shorts. The obsession for all of us in PT was to not have an accident on the floor mats. The therapists didn't care. The entire room could be hosed down in case of an attack of dysentery. The transformation from physically strong, self-assured adults to pathetic, marginally toilet-trained wretches meant that the slightest exertion would put us back to personal hygiene's square one. It was to live in fear of grunting.

As time went on we managed to find the humor in all of this. Or someone would find it for us. Usually it was Roger. Whenever anyone would slip behind the count, or fade and stop before the allotted time or number of push-ups, Roger would note it immediately and call out. Roger sat comfortably doing his shoulder lifts while the rest of us sweated like pigs. He watched covetously as we went through our pitiful motions like a chorus line from some telethon. Roger was the choreographer. Mostly we just ignored Roger or threatened to move the straw on his evening milk shake away from his mouth as revenge. But Roger had one good motivator. If he saw any of us frustrated and angry he would call out, "Hey, look over there, it's one of Jerry's kids." To be identified with the young poster people in wheelchairs dressing the set on the Jerry Lewis muscular dystrophy telethon each year was the lowest of the low.

Roger's custom-crafted insult fused two powerful and contradictory themes in American life: sympathy and self-reliance. In rehab we were taught never to allow people to push our chairs. We were taught to do things ourselves and never ask for help. We were proud crips who were going to play basketball and win races and triumph over our disabilities. Outside rehab, self-reliance was a high-risk proposition. To people raised on telethons, it looked suspiciously like a chip on the shoulder. Somewhere between bitterness and anger and Jerry's kids, we would all have to live. After listening to Roger, we all knew which pole we wanted to stay closest to.

Doubtless, Jerry Lewis had no clue that his telethon provided a useful low-end benchmark for disability empowerment. For that reason alone it is useful far beyond the millions of dollars it raises for research and cures. Much of Jerry's money goes into investigating genetic screening to prevent people with MDA from even coming into the world. Jerry's kids are people in wheelchairs on television raising money to find a way to prevent their ever having been born. When crips watch the telethon, the words "bravery" and "courage" and "heroism" do not come to mind.

The telethon looks like some kind of interminable Eastern European Politburo meeting where obscure regional collectivized farm managers give little speeches long into the night. The party chairman is the hero and master of ceremonies. He struts across the stage, interrupting the low-level ministers grabbing the microphone and shouting slogans to the masses. Every once in a while he gives a tearful melodramatic pep talk, extolling the virtues of the grand national vision. The grand national vision of Jerry in Vegas with the crips is that seven or eight digit number flashing on the stage every hour to the accompaniment of Ed McMahon.

More even than finding cures, America's health-care system loves to come up with genetic tests to prevent anyone from having to drag their useless limbs across the stage. Most crips would need more than an hour to drag themselves any distance anyway. No one would think of having a telethon to raise money to build accessible housing for wheel-chair consumers or to find jobs for them. But look for a way to eradicate their experience, or even the possibility of their existence, and you can qualify for the big bucks. Society must be utterly convinced that those lives are not worth living. Of course, one can never truly be convinced of such a thing. Life does not convey its value in price tags or tote boards accompanied by studio orchestras in Las Vegas.

Long before anyone worried about the health-care system in America, we could see its bizarre priorities and patterns of care at the Mary Free Bed hospital. If we had another identity besides our injury it was the label of our insurance policy. So much was determined by the patterns of insurance coverage. The most confident fully covered folks were the ones injured in car accidents. With the pool of all licensed drivers in America paying for it, insurance companies could afford to be generous. Car accident injuries could expect almost complete medical coverage, with wheelchairs provided for the rest of patients' lives in many cases.

People injured in public places such as playgrounds or swimming pools, where liability was a question, came next. They usually benefited from the payout of some insurance policy on the facility where they were injured. They also generally could count on some kind of legal settlement if they sued the facility. The next group were those injured at work, who came under workers' compensation. Coverage here was less than for auto accidents, but fairly complete nonetheless. Medical bills were paid, but the purchase of wheelchairs was more problematic.

In considerably worse shape were those people with degenerative conditions that came on suddenly. These people often exhausted their insurance in the first weeks of acute care and had little or nothing left for rehab. Such people could count on charity to buy less than state-of-the-art wheelchairs and accessories. They were the recipients of a kind of medical rationing. One chair would have to last a long time. It could not be used or abused too much. If it broke down, the Easter Seals donors did not have the resources simply to replace it.

This set of medical priorities meant that a drunk driver who lost control of a vehicle, someone whose injury was nearly self-inflicted, received a full ride from the health-care system. But someone whose disability was the result of disease and had occurred through no fault of his own was left out in the cold.

The absolutely worst off were the people with the rare degenerative diseases that no one had ever heard of. They had no insurance, no treatment, and the most expensive care. A six-year-old covered with oozing bandages roamed our halls in a little electric cart. His name was Roger, so we called him Little Roger. He had a disease I never heard called by any name other than "his skin is falling off." The adhesive that was supposed to bind his layers of skin together was defective, and the slightest touch to his skin caused it to fall off. Little Roger's disease had no treatment, its rarity meant that it was not considered by insurance companies, and it had little chance of finding its own telethon. Roger would never be able to live outside the hospital because no one could afford to pay for his support.

Insurance also determined what life would be like outside the hospital. In particular, it determined whether you would get a car paid for or modified to the special needs of a disability. Everyone hoped for a car. The biggest prize was to score a van. In the van world, the quadriplegics ruled. Paraplegics would be able to get out of their chairs and sit behind the wheel of a regular car with hand controls, but quadriplegics would need to roll aboard their vehicles.

This required electric doors and chain-operated lifts and other advanced technology. And there was plenty of technology applied to the problem of getting a car to move when most of a driver's body couldn't. Driving was an option for even the highest quads. Vehicles could be outfitted with electronic devices that connected the steering brakes and throttle to motion sensors worn on the head. Some of the most advanced vans could be driven solely by moving the head or eyes. Some had no regular steering wheel at all.

Of the cast of white-coated physical therapists, shrinks, nurses, and professional nurturers (social workers), the most popular staff person in the hospital was Doug, the driver's training instructor. While most everyone else was either measuring out urine or running around monitoring who was in denial and who was in remorse, Doug at least had a real job. He had none of the rehab speak or the black humor of the nurses. Doug said things like, "If you push this, it's your brake. Pull this, it's your gas. When the chain on the wheelchair lift gets stuck, put a little grease on it like this." Here were problems we could all solidly put our minds to solving.

As much as anything else, rehab was committed to getting broken bodies back behind the wheel of a car. Everyone wanted to get back on the road. Technology was the cure-all. We loved to watch the machines work. But it was the same old twentieth-century con: the gadgets will save you. Technology will make you free. This was ironic, principally because cars were responsible for putting most of the people in this place here to begin with.

Bob was the van expert in our group. He was a C-4 quadriplegic, and would explain his injury by saying that he had been hunting trees. His car had left the road, and he was discovered by paramedics, drunk and near death. He had found a tree. But, as he used to say, the tree had bagged him. He knew he had been drunk. He could remember nothing else.

Bob could use his arms and had some use of his hands. He was a funny man who wore thick Coke bottle glasses and had red hair. At night in the ward where four of us slept, he would talk about the van he was going to get. His van was going to be the place where he would get away from it all. Being in a wheelchair, he said, was his big break. He could barely see as it was. His thick glasses suggested a profound vision impairment even when Bob wasn't hitting the beer. He used to say, "John, I'm so fucked-up now, the license people will never notice my bad eyes. If I can make a right turn with these arms, they'll hand me the license right then and there. I could be drunk and blind." He was right.

Back in the seventies, Dodge made the longest, biggest van. Bob wanted it; he assured us that Dodge vans were the best. Bob had all of the brochures. We looked at the brochures and came to the same conclusion. We all wanted the big, long Dodge. Bob's was to have a water bed in the back. His stereo and fishing equipment would be in the van, ready to go at all times. "You can't bait a hook, Bob," we would say. "You can't turn over in bed by yourself."

"I'll get myself a woman who can slide a crawler on to a fishhook, and herself down on my big pink hook. She can turn me over if she wants. She can do everything; I'll just lie there with a smile on my face."

When he talked like this, I would blush like the teenager I was. I had never had such close contact with adults. Even at the steel factory where I had worked as a welder the previous summer, we had all gone home after work. Here we slept, ate, and wet the bed together. Adults made everything real. Their tragedies were real, like their mortgage payments; the sense of change was far more real for them than for me. I was just a kid; my life was still ahead of me. They had spent their lives doing things they would no longer be able to do. But for as long as we were in rehab, we shared the same questions and predicaments.

Adults had wives, husbands, and families. They told the most disturbing off-color jokes; they had been teenagers long ago and had done it all. We pried into the details of each others' lives like nosy mothers. Having the output of your intestines and kidneys known by everyone around you generates a certain familiarity impossible to achieve in normal, everyday interactions.

The charts next to our beds indicated how many cc's of urine we had produced in the past twenty-four hours. A large amount of output immediately created the suspicion that you had been drinking somewhere away from the nurses. When the output on any one chart rose, you were immediately suspected of holding out on the others. Larry, in the bed next to me, watched my chart. With a straight face, some nights I would return to my room and try to fill two jugs without my roommates noticing. They always did.

"Where's the beer, John?" Bob would say. "John had a party and didn't invite us." Bob would point the straw he always kept near him for drinking right at me.

When someone went home on a family or friend visit, upon their return everyone gathered around to see the kidney's verdict on the outing. If the output was high, everyone remarked that it must have been a good time. Low output meant you had been forced to attend church or something. Five hundred cc's was a good result. A thousand was a tribute to the floor. Anything over 1,400 was outstanding and would dominate the conversation during physical therapy the next day.

"Larry had a fourteen hundred-cc party last night," Bob would say. "I think we may have to call Larry's insurance company and tell them to get Larry a tanker truck instead of just a van. I figure he might just explode one night at the bars and injure an innocent person."

Bob had a certain charm. He fell in love with his physical therapist, who eventually moved in with him. She seemed like someone who could bait Bob's hooks. Harry's and Larry's marriages crumbled in the hospital, and the ward where we slept was often closed while Harry and his wife had emotional discussions that ended with Harry red-faced and his wife tearful, running out the door with a child in tow. Larry said he was going to ditch his wife before she ditched him. He lost that race. She filed for divorce one afternoon while we were in physical therapy and Roger was calling somebody a Jerry's kid and somebody else had had an accident on the exercise mat. Larry didn't talk much after that. Mostly he worked to master his crutches and leg braces. He checked himself out of the hospital the next week.

Roger and I were single teenagers with no romances to lose or gain. We watched the trials of Larry and Harry and Bob with sympathy and befuddlement. We cared more about finding a way to shut down physical therapy so we could sleep in at least one morning before we were discharged. With two wheelchairs, no legs, no sharp objects, and only a pair of arms between us, we had our work cut out for us. "I've got my shoulders," Roger said. "Great, Roger, you can be in charge of dialing the phone or wrestling intruders to the ground."

The elevator operator needed a key to stop and start the car to load people on board with their chairs and walkers and stretchers. Roger came up with the idea of removing the control panel and ripping out a wire. Roger rolled down to the far end of the hall with me, and motioned with his head for me to look in the pocket on the back of his chair. "I got Doug to give me a Phillips head screwdriver from the driver's education room." Roger's voice was soaked with larceny and vandalism. He could make thoughts seem like crimes. In Roger's case, they were all he had. "The trouble with ripping out a wire, Roger, is that we will have to spend the night in the elevator after it breaks." We needed some slow-acting sabotage short of a bomb.

We found some white carpenter's glue and some epoxy in one of the therapy rooms. If we could pour enough glue inside the keyhole on the elevator panel, by morning it would be stuck solid. The plan was clever enough, but it lacked a certain dramatic flourish. If we were going to commit small-time terrorism, then we teenaged boys needed a way to claim responsibility for the terrorist attack.

Before getting on the elevator to return to the upper floors where the wards were, we stopped by the main office, which was open. I told Roger to hold the door and watch for nurses in the hall. One office contained the building-wide public address system with a big, old-fashioned taxi dispatcher microphone. I called to Roger.

"Go and call the elevator, and hold it with your chair."

"What are you doing?"

"I'm mixing the glue, and when I'm finished I'm going to make an announcement on the public-address system."

Roger left his post in the hallway and came into the office. Using the force of his electric chair, he noisily bludgeoned the doors open. "Let me make the announcement. Let me talk on the microphone," he said flatly.

"It was my idea, Roger." I wanted to make a final statement of protest before we left Mary Free Bed for good. Taking over the public-address system had the quality of history about it, echoing the Attica prison uprising, or prefiguring the Romanian revolution.

"I'll read whatever announcement you write. Just let me read it. If they hear my voice, it will really freak them out." Roger certainly had a point. Putting me on the PA was just a straightforward prank. The thought of the voice from Roger's bobbing head and motionless body commanding the nurses and doctors who decided when he got up and when he got down was a truly inspired protest. I quickly jotted down some notes. Roger jammed himself through the door and planted himself in front of the microphone table, knocking down a couple of chairs in the process.

He was still a few feet away. I placed the paper on his lap table. "Can you read it?" I asked. "Yes, put the microphone up to my mouth." I squeezed the Talk button, held the mike out, and said, "Go!" I could hear the clicking over the hall speakers. We were on the air.

"This is Roger Duncan speaking. Unfortunately, physical therapy will be canceled tomorrow so that we may present a movie for your enjoyment."

He whispered at me, "Is it on?"

"Yes, yes. Continue."

"This is Roger Duncan again. The title of the movie will be *A Farewell to Arms*. The story of a family of amputees during World War One."

We grabbed the glue and raced down the hall to the elevator. Roger held it open while I dumped two kinds of glue, epoxy and white, down inside the keyhole. As I worked, Roger said, "I always wondered what that book was about." I wiped the keyhole clean so that dripping glue could not be detected, then said to Roger, "Get in." We rode back to the second floor.

Physical therapy was canceled on my last day at the hospital. Nurse O'Leary found the two kinds of glue in the bag on Roger's chair. There in the morning, banging against my bed asking about my breakfast, was Roger; he had not slept in. He had his sandbag weights on his shoulders. They had brought physical therapy upstairs. But Roger was smiling. "I'm a hero this morning, John. Even drooling Ron was laughing when I went to bed. Of course, the nurses want to kill you."

"Thank you for letting me know, Roger." I called out from under the covers.

"You haven't packed yet," he said.

"I was sleeping, Roger."

When I sat up I could see that Roger wasn't smiling. It was the last time I would ever see him or any of the other characters in this rehab class of 1976: Roger, Harry, Larry, Ron, Hilda, Bob, and Little Roger. "What's going to happen to me?" Roger asked quietly, and I could see that he was afraid. I was fully awake now. But I had no answer. There was a nine-and-a-half-inch difference in where his spine was broken and where mine had been injured permanently. The difference in our lives could not be measured. I felt the distance between us. I would miss Roger. "The nurses said my voice sounded good on the loudspeaker. Maybe I could get a job in radio? Do you think I could do that, John?"

I nodded. "There's an idea, Roger."

Harry and Larry both got divorced and returned to the hospital with serious complications of their original injuries. Bob got his van and married his physical therapist. They had a child. Years later, Bob's body was found in his van. He had asphyxiated in a closed garage with the motor running. Some people suggested that he had been unable to reach the ignition key and get out of the vehicle. He had very poor eyesight, they said, and as it was dark in the garage he might have been a little drunk and couldn't get the seat belt off. Only with a quadriplegic crip would people assume that you could turn your own garage into Dachau by simply fumbling with your car keys.

There was no proof that Bob had killed himself, but many of us understood. Bob was a quadriplegic, but he needed no Kevorkian. The tree he had been hunting had finally found him and finished the job. Bob did get away from it all in his big, long Dodge van. I have no doubt that he was thinking about fishing at the end.

I left the hospital three months after arriving there from the intensive care unit in Pennsylvania. It was the training for the outside world. I came in weak, scared, and sick. I departed in a coral-red wheelchair that reflected my intention of aggressively taking on the world, wheelchairs be damned. I got a blue General Motors van with a lift that got fourteen miles to the gallon back when gasoline was just beginning to cost more than a dollar a gallon. It had seemed like a good idea at the time, but a coral-red vinyl chair and a blue gas guzzler were not going to work in my new real world. My second wheelchair was black, as was every chair I have since owned. I eventually got rid of the blue van. I got tired of the crowds who gathered to watch the electric lift work and tell me they had seen the same van on "Ironside," the TV show. I learned how to toss my chair into the backseat of a normal passenger car.

We imagine one life and live another. We trace our lives on a map of places we will never visit and landmarks we wish we had missed. Each journey alters the map. Our signatures are written in possibilities, the ink dries as the indelible mark of change. Roger went off to live in a nursing home. I went back to Chicago to college, where I dropped out, moved out west, and eventually ended up riding a donkey in Kurdistan.

Life's end points come in pairs; all else defies counting. Down long corridors, possibilities beckon and vanish at the horizon. It is with the pain and resentment preceding wisdom that we gradually discover the doors that have closed behind us and how the straight path ahead is not ours, though we may claim it as our own dream. Life removes possibilities one by one from the pillows beneath our sleeping heads. The dreams are not stolen; they just go quietly by themselves, passing like time, replaced by real events beyond imagining. I lost touch with Roger. It was me who, years later, ended up with the job in radio.

The Cutting
Board

*N*umbness is a distinct feeling. Just as zero gives meaning to all numbers, numbness is a placeholder of the flesh, the boundary where consciousness and body divide, where life becomes the inanimate vessel we live in. Our lives are played out under an inanimate universe. Sensation is the sideshow, a spotlight inside a tent of darkness. We step in and out of the white circle. It blinds us if we look directly at it. We are just as sightless in the dark.

We worship sensation, longing to make its impressions real. We endow our awareness with the divinity of the creator. We scour our pleasures for a sign that good feelings mean that the universe actually likes us. We make excuses for our pain, insisting that others acknowledge its seriousness. Or we push into our pain, seeking the actual mechanical limits of our bodies. We yearn to equate sense with reality. We discover, every time, that sensation is just the playpen where we have been put. The odd toys handed down to us are all we have to work with. Like a baby, we can throw toys away, but we cannot get any more.

To honor sensation is to honor an illusion. To honor what has none is humanity's original act of faith. My legs have no sensation. Neither does my abdomen or much of my chest. With heart and lungs inside, my chest and abdomen retain their function despite numbness. My legs have lost even that. They are culs-de-sac of blood and bone that carry no weight, must themselves be carried, and justify their existence on the slimmest of pretexts: that regardless of all that, they are still my legs.

Occasionally they will jerk with a spastic, repeating rhythm. The accidental poke of a pen point, the drops of scalding water dribbled from a teapot, an ice cube landing in my lap are sometimes answered by a muscle's spastic movement. Their connection to the spinal cord, if not to the brain above it, is still intact. My legs move by themselves. I feel nothing, but my legs must still feel something akin to pain or pleasure. They remain connected; their nerves do what they have always done. They call home. The phone has been ringing off the hook for nineteen years.

The loss of sensation takes some getting used to. On my left thigh, midway between my knee and my hip, is a scar about six inches long and two to three inches wide. It looks like Madagascar. It also precisely resembles the shape that the bottom of a large Corning Ware baking dish makes when pressed into soft dough, or the soft spongy tissue that used to lie between my lap and my left femur. In 1977 I was cooking stuffing for a Thanksgiving turkey on an electric stove in an apartment in Springfield, Oregon. The Corning Ware dish was taken from the refrigerator first. Its ceramic handles were quite cold, a sensation they conveyed even after several minutes on the hot burner of an electric range.

If this had been a metal pot, a few minutes on the burner would have conducted heat all over its surface and into the air around it. A metal pot would have broadcast its temperature, conveying immediately that it was an object to keep well away from the skin. On any other body but mine, if the pot had made accidental contact, pain would have made sure the pot was swiftly moved. But ceramic is not a conductor of heat. Just a few minutes out of the refrigerator, the dish was cold to the touch everywhere but underneath, where the burner of the stove was beginning to cook the bread cubes, spices, and melting butter. On the bottom of the dish, next to the burner, it was probably three hundred degrees. It was certainly close to that temperature when I picked up the dish, and holding its still-cold handles set it down absently and squarely on my lap.

With a wooden spoon, I mixed the crumbs and spices and butter while I held the dish steady. The aroma of cooking rose from inside the dish. I felt nothing. With no saucepan resting on its element, the electric burner I had taken the dish from moments before began to glow red. Its heat hit my face. I continued to stir. I added a little milk and heard a sizzling sound as the liquid contacted the hot bottom of the plate. I still felt nothing and continued stirring and adding spices, and talking to whoever else was in the room.

When I removed the dish, my left leg trembled. The spasticity was odd. Normally my legs had coarse, slow movements when they were spastic. This time their motions were tiny and very fast. There was no sensation, but a slight queasiness passed over me. Something was wrong, but the idea that I had actually set a hot pan on my lap and had been calmly stirring its contents for several minutes was so absurd that even then I did not think I had burned my leg severely. It seemed impossible that such a thing could have happened.

It was only after I could see a slight outline of fluid on my pants leg that I suspected something terrible might have happened. I looked at the leg. Its motions now were more pronounced, erratic, and unknown to me. I had not seen this kind of motion before. From my detached position, looking down, it was as though I was watching a horror movie. My legs appeared to be in agony. It was clear even without sensation that the legs were now trying to account for an act of the creator above that seemed senseless and cruel. I felt embarrassed and foolish. Then, as the stain on my thigh became more apparent, I felt scared.

Removing my trousers revealed the place where the hot dish had sat for perhaps two full minutes. It was something to see, and even more shocking to watch, without feeling the slightest pain. The skin was gathered into a leathery, shrunken depression on the top of my thigh. The hairs had all been cooked into a blistered white wound. The root of each hair was a raised dot where the glands beneath the skin had simply exploded from the heat. There was no blood, for reasons that would become apparent later. The wound looked unearthly. It was just as unusual to the doctors at the local hospital who examined it and concluded that it was only a second-degree burn.

If I had any sensation about this whole affair, it was embarrassment. To go to the hospital over something that didn't hurt at all seemed like complaining. I laughed about it with the doctors. I was ashamed to have done such a stupid thing. I was trying to be a good paraplegic and not make silly mistakes. I felt sorry for wasting the doctors' time. That I felt nothing, and was so apologetic about what appeared to be a pretty serious burn, made the doctors suspicious. They began to ask about my life at home. Perhaps there was some more sinister explanation for the burn. "Did anyone get mad at you this morning?" a nurse asked. They asked about drugs or some angry relative who might have wanted to punish me. I told them I lived alone. They called my house to make sure it was so. One of the doctors asked if this burn might have been self-inflicted. "Yes," I said, "I told you it was." He looked at me again. "Is there anything you want to tell me?"

The burn no longer scared me. This emergency room intern who thought I might have tried to kill myself with a Corning Ware dish filled with bread cubes and butter pats was suddenly making me very nervous. He was so convinced that this was a plausible explanation for my leg burn that for a moment I thought I might be in shock, and that someone had actually tried to cook me that morning but that I was just blocking it out. "Look, I just made a stupid mistake with the dish. It felt cold on the top. I couldn't feel that it was hot on the bottom. I set it on my lap for a minute. I won't do it again. Can I go now?"

In their haste to establish some explanation for the burn other than that I had accidentally cooked my thigh while preparing a turkey, they missed just how serious a burn it was. The numbness in my legs threw them off. A third-degree burn is rarely the result of a moderate amount of heat applied over a period of minutes. More commonly, it is an extremely high temperature contacting the skin for a short period of time. A slowly cooked leg is not a textbook injury. It suggests torture, an unusual malady in Springfield, Oregon, in 1977. The doctors did what they normally would for a second-degree burn—they gave me a large bandage, some iodine, and sent me home.

The wound did not heal for months. For a while it shed large chunks of dead tissue and a brown fluid totally unlike anything I had ever seen emerge from my body. I tried to get it to scab over, or heal under a bandage. It simply got worse. Each morning and night I would look at a wound that, if I could feel it, would have been infinitely more painful than anything that had happened in my accident. I stared down at it from above as though I were on some leisurely balloon ride. I had no sensation, yet I worried about the leg. I felt sorry for its pain. It could not tell me how it felt, it could not do anything for me. I became sentimental about all of the times my legs had helped me. I wanted to help them. But I was also fascinated by the invulnerability of numbness. There was no urgency about this wound because I felt no pain. I slept normally. I ate normally. I had to bandage the leg before going out to prevent it from staining my pants, but otherwise I could go about my life without much concern that my thigh was dangerously infected.

This was still the case three months later, so I went to the only doctor I knew by name in Oregon. Dr. Ellison was a urologist who handled all of the local crips' catheter problems and said he would be glad to look at this burn trouble I was having. He told me to remove my pants. He eyed the size of the bandage as I started to untape it from the skin around the wound. When he saw the wound, he stopped cold. He told his nurses to shut all of the doors to the examination rooms and to scrub him for surgery. He declared the room I was in in quarantine and began spraying the air with antiseptic. When the nurse asked if he needed anesthetic, he nodded and then caught himself. "No, I guess I won't be needing it this time."

Without anesthesia, and for nearly an hour while I calmly watched, Dr. Ellison poked and scrubbed and pulled away dead skin. For the first time since Thanksgiving, my leg began to bleed profusely. When he was finished, he wrapped my leg in gauze and removed a surgical mask he had put on. "You would have lost your leg if you had waited much longer." He shook his head as he took my temperature. "If you had started to run a fever, you could have died."

All of this had happened with me as a spectator feeling no pain. I did feel guilty that I might have put my legs through a nearly fatal ordeal. With the wound cleaned and its dead tissue removed, my leg began to heal. The circulation came back. My thigh returned to its normal pink color. In a matter of weeks, the wound was fully closed. All that remained of the trauma was a spectacular scar. On my last visit to the doctor he noted that while the wound had healed well, the nerves in the thigh were probably damaged beyond repair. "There will be no feeling here ever again," he said gravely as he probed the scar with his finger.

It was odd to think that my legs and I shared numbness now. Two degrees of sensation: my own loss of feeling in the parts of me below the break in my spinal cord, and the loss of nerves in the skin on my thigh. With my fingers I could feel the cold, leathery numbness of the scar surrounded by warm, healthy skin. Numbness has a feeling and a texture. Doctor Ellison suddenly realized his mistake. "I'm sorry, I forgot for a moment that you can't feel anyway. I guess it doesn't really matter," he said.

This incident with the burn happened in the first two years after my accident, when those close to me were unconvinced that I might be able to survive on my own in a wheelchair. The burn shook my own confidence. When I finally told my family what had happened, which I did long after my leg had healed, they were almost as alarmed about this burn as they had been about my accident. My one living grandfather at the time, Grandpa Slagle, could not get it out of his mind. He spoke with me over the phone.

"What you need, Johnny, is something to put in your lap while you're in the kitchen," he said. "I've got an idea." When a package arrived from

Newark, New York, a few weeks later, I knew it contained Grandpa's solution to my problem. It was something he had conjured up from the magical workshop where he spent so many of his days fixing antique clocks. The package had brown wrapping. Inside was a box covered with newspaper padding. Inside the box was a cutting board exactly the size of my lap.

He had taken two pieces of oak and glued them together. He had sanded them and had carefully affixed to the back some green paper of the sort you might find lining kitchen drawers. The paper was rough, like coarse felt, so it would not slide on my legs. Finally, a sturdy metal handle was drilled into one edge of the board, for hanging. It was a simple thing, but each part had been made especially for the purpose of protecting my lap. The wood was cut to odd, narrow lengths; it was of half-inch stock, not the full inch or more of easily available butcher block wood. Grandpa wanted the board to be light enough to use from a sitting position so that I could lift it with a pan from my lap to the kitchen counter.

The board's metal handle had been fabricated by him, not pulled from the bin of screws and washers at the hardware store. There was not a nail or a fastener of any kind on this board. The oak boards had been glued like fine furniture. Each seam was a perfectly straight line, clamped and sanded to the tolerance of machine metal. Underneath the cutting board was a note in Grandfather's hurried, poor handwriting. The suggestion in his note was direct. "I thought you might need this for the kitchen. Your grandmother and I want you to be careful from now on, when you use the stove."

In all of my life I had never received a gift from my grandfather that had not been picked out by my very practical grandmother. Grandpa's participation had always been in the margin. The birthday, Christmas cards, and thank-you notes were signed "Grandma and Grandpa" but always in Grandma's handwriting on her elegant stationary. This package arrived with Grandpa's meticulous wrapping, and the enclosed note was torn from an oil-smudged legal pad. He had had to ask my grandmother for my address. The front of the package was in Grandma's careful block lettering.

The oak board sat perfectly on my lap. It covered the eight-inch scar on my left thigh with plenty of room to spare. From far away, with his leathery woodworker's hands, Grandfather sought to protect my numb legs from the lapses of a young, headstrong boy in the kitchen. My legs could not thank him; I could not feel them, but he could. Every time I set the cutting board down, I see Grandfather looking up at me.

What is the point of paralyzed legs which demand a third of the heart's energy and blood and do nothing but dissipate a fifth of the body's heat? Shortly after my accident, one of my parents' friends suggested that I cut my legs off to spare myself from the chore of carrying them around. I heard about this suggestion from my mother. It seemed like a perfectly rational idea. It also scared me to death.

I remember staring and straining to feel my newly paralyzed feet. I would close my eyes, think really hard about toes and ankles, knees and calves. When I opened them—nothing. Quite aside from the suggestions of voluntary dismemberment from helpful neighbors, numbness was frightening. It wasn't the loss of my legs that was tragic, it was their numbness that made the possibility of losing them real. Without sensation, they seemed vulnerable. I might forget that my legs were mine and accidentally chop them off one day. All kinds of horrors occurred to me. That I might burn my legs by accident did not enter my mind until it happened. I worried that one day my legs might find themselves in the way and I would just remove them in a fit of careless impatience. Without the possibility of pain, I could imagine it. Being able to imagine it made it infinitely more likely to happen.

"John should have his legs removed," the neighbor lady suggested. She had read about this being done for some paraplegics, as well as other ways doctors had for rendering the entire spinal cord dead below a break. The technique involved injecting a locally toxic solution into the spine that killed all of the nerve tissue and made any involuntary leg motion impossible. "It will prevent the spasticity," she would say. "If he keeps his legs, he might as well not have them moving unexpectedly." Without sensation, the argument for keeping my legs attached to me became chillingly abstract, like a debate over euthanasia, except it was my body that was the focus of the discussion. Without the possibility of pain to restrain me, I could suddenly see both sides of the "question". "Well, you know, if they don't work anyway . . ." You could make the case that keeping my legs even seemed a bit of an indulgence. Why would I even want to keep them? Just to show off?

The truth is, I love my legs, not for what they can do for me anymore, but simply because they are my legs. I look at my feet and see in their little spastic twitches an attempt to resolve the mystery of a nineteen-year-old trauma. They must see my body above the lesion as in a similar predicament. Calling down to them twitching and thrashing about. Every time I get on a plane and heave my legs into an airline seat I can see my feet and knees puzzling about the actions of the man upstairs. They must wonder about my life, just as I stare mystified at their sudden jerky movements. Are they in pain?

Sometimes my legs will jerk, and someone will notice and ask, "Does that hurt?" "I don't know," is the answer. I feel them trying to tell me something. I am two personalities inhabiting one body, Siamese twins connected at the soul. There is no surgery possible to separate us and have both of us live, there is no surgery possible to connect us. Can my legs know I am still up here? They must. Whether they do or not, they are still mine. I wonder if they are lonely.

The area below my spinal cord is not the only severed connection in my life. In 1936, twenty years before I came into this world, my uncle, Charles Peter Slagle, was born to my grandparents, Doris and John, in upstate New York. He was their second child, their first and only son. They called him Peter. My grandfather called him Petey. Their first child was my mother, Nancy, born five years earlier. Their third child, my aunt Susan, would not be born for another nine years.

In that time, my uncle's ties to his family would be severed in a manner more final, irreversible, and permanent than any injury of the spinal cord. He has lived most of his life without a family. His family has gone on without him. His existence is acknowledged in the faded black and white photos in which he is pictured with his parents long ago, the few pictures where he can be seen playing with his older sister, my mother. In a white knitted outfit, a chubby little boy sits in the sun. In another picture he is standing next to a tricycle. There is a picture of him sitting at the piano with his mother. A little boy and his sister play in a field near a swimming hole.

Three of the pictures in this photo album at my grandmother's house are particularly haunting. One is a picture of the little boy being held by his father, my grandfather, the man who made my cutting board. Both father and son are staring into the camera. My grandfather has been dead for more than a decade, yet his face is far more alive for me than the face of the little boy, who is alive and is today older than his father was in the picture. The second snapshot is of that same little boy lying on a blanket in the grass. He must be about three or four years old in this picture. His eyes are slightly splayed, their focus just missing the camera's lens. His arms and legs are bent oddly, as though he can't sit up by himself, which seems odd for a four-year-old. It is the last picture my grandmother has of her son. After 1941 he doesn't appear again.

The pictures in the photo album continue. My mother grows up, my grandparents are at parties with friends in overcoats that have come in and out of fashion since they were young. Their oldest daughter, my mother, goes off to college. Their second daughter, my aunt, is born and is seen playing with the same tricycle as in the earlier pictures. In these pictures, my aunt Susan has no older brother. Then, a page after, my mother brings my father home and they are shown holding hands in my grandparents' living room. The third haunting picture is on the very next page. It is of my grandfather holding a little baby boy, their first grandchild. His fat infant face has found the camera and staring out from the photo album his gaze finds me.

Grandfather looks barely aged in this picture. It is only the tones of the photographic paper that indicate it was taken in the fifties. Otherwise, this picture of a man holding a baby boy is just the same as the picture taken in 1940 of the same man holding another little boy, his son, a few pages and an eternity back in the photo album. The little baby boy from the fifties is me.

The toddler knows nothing of what came before, or what is to come. My grandfather's hand is cradling my knees, puffy with baby fat. When the picture was taken, the little boy could feel the skin of his grandfather's hand on his leg. The little boy's legs work although they cannot yet walk. There are no wheelchairs here. I know nothing of any Uncle Peter. Yet, there I am, affixed to the black pages of Grandmother's photo album, having lived most of my life just less than an inch away from the uncle I have never known.

Like some parallel civilization living underground in a science fiction movie, disabled people are discovered suddenly in childhood. Their discovery is one of the minor footnotes in the process through which we learn that the world is not what it seems at first glance. As a curious child, I too noticed the strange new people in public, and gleaned the little information I could obtain from my parents and other adults.

It had been explained to me that some people had to be in wheelchairs because their legs were paralyzed. To a little kid that meant they were stiff, like Frankenstein's monster. When I saw some guy in a wheelchair get into a car, what I had imagined about paralyzed people did not match what I saw. Instead of behaving like stiff boards, this young man's legs dangled unexpectedly when he moved from his chair to the car seat. They hung there for an instant, limp, like a puppet's dangling limbs, retaining only the form of walking.

It was a vivid, unimaginable surprise. That legs could be unconnected and connected at the same time was frightening and wondrous. It was also the true meaning of paralyzed, a meaning that seemed to have been concealed by the language my parents used to describe this man and others like him. He had dangling jelly legs, I thought, why didn't they say that about him? I started to say something—"Mommy, that man has—" but the sentence was aborted. I was shushed, all eyes averted. The mystery deepened.

Memories like these flooded back vividly in the hospital years later, after my accident, as I began to sort out the news that I wasn't going to be walking anymore. A sudden inability to walk was among the most unforeseen of circumstances, but notwithstanding my own childish horror at seeing cripples, there was considerable evidence that the parallel civilization of disabled people was alive and well. As I lay in the hospital wondering about the future, I could see that I had grown up with some of them. I had not thought of that jelly-legged man since I was a little child, yet the memory rushed forth, along with all of the other times I had tried to stare at someone and been sternly cautioned against it by some helpful adult.

I had spent a lot of time staring at my other grandfather, William T. (Tom) Hockenberry. As a young man he had lost an arm in an on-the-job accident. He had a fleshy stump with a crook in it where his elbow would have been. My one-armed grandpa was part of the family. His stump was something you didn't talk about much, but Grandpa made no effort to hide it in our home or around his house when we would visit him in Ohio. Grandpa Hockenberry was completely comfortable around us. I assumed the whole world was the same way.

I remembered the neighbor boy in Rochester, New York, where we lived when I was just two or three. He had a deformed ear that fascinated me. His head was normal, but his ear was just a little flap hanging near the hole in his head normally concealed and protected by the ear. He seemed so radically different from me, even frightening, yet his deformed ear seemed not to affect his hearing, which was the strangest thing of all. My parents said he had been born like that.

There was a paralyzed man with wrist crutches who spoke with my parents at a concert one time. They knew him from college or somewhere. While they all laughed and talked briefly, I stared at his feet in the oversized black shoes that were bolted to his metal braces. His metal crutches seemed so much more permanent than the forgiving wooden ones you could find in school clinics for sprained ankles and broken legs. When he hobbled away, I watched his legs swing.

He had polio, my parents told me, something I had been vaccinated against. Like his black prescription shoes, his disease was as obsolete as the seventy-eight RPM Glenn Miller records in my parents' closets. It made him seem even more like a dinosaur. Once he was out of earshot my parents both shook their heads and sighed in a kind of well-intentioned sympathy that they apparently would not have wanted him to see. "He's such a nice guy," one of them said. After a pause my mother wondered aloud if he would ever find someone who could handle marrying him. I wondered what this had to do with the crutches and legs I was staring at. My parents shook their heads and concluded that it would be the longest of long shots.

Lake Michigan, the summer between high school and college. As I walked on the beach alone, a young blond girl floated happily on an inner tube. Her smile invited me into a trance and I sat and watched. The spell was broken when she opened her mouth and tried to speak. Instead of mouthing words, she honked an unearthly laughter and spread her spastic arms and legs to be carried back to the beach by a companion. The spell was replaced by curiosity. I might have discovered why she was different, but instead I averted my eyes without a cue. I had learned my lessons well by then. She can now be recalled only in a fuzzy, indistinct memory of mental retardation or cerebral palsy, neither correct nor wrong. It was just enough information to say excuse me, and move on quickly.

In 1976, from a hospital bed in Pennsylvania, these random pictures of disability all came back without prompting. It was as though they had been quietly preserved in a glass case under a sign that said IN CASE OF PARAPLEGIA BREAK GLASS. I did. The pictures spilled out. There were lots of fuzzy pictures but pitiably little information about what it meant to undergo such an extraordinary change. I lay there wishing that I had just gone ahead and stared all those times when I came upon people in wheelchairs. Instead, their faces stared back at me from little windows of memory, high up, out of reach, and behind bars.

One face that did not stare back was the face of my uncle, Charles Peter Slagle. His connection to me was too remote, far too utterly broken by time and circumstances I was only dimly aware of back then. Yet in the very moments I was just beginning to imagine what life would be like in a wheelchair, he had already lived most of his life in one. At the moment I was in a bed surrounded by nurses monitoring my bodily functions and forcing me to eat bad hospital food, he was an old hand at both. The moment that I was wondering how I would be able to get into my parents' home with its stairs in the front and the back, he was the one member of my family who lived in a completely wheelchair accessible place and I didn't even know him.

The only thing about him I had ever been told was that he had been born with some disease, and that he had been sent away from home as a child. There was a single, faded portrait of him on my mother's dresser. His face looked just like her face. The fate of Charles Peter Slagle was a subject that I knew from an early age could produce tears in my mother's eyes. She would occasionally mention her brother, in passing. But there were few details of his existence for me to learn.

One time, an adult told me that I had an uncle who was a "total vegetable." The words "total" and "vegetable" were opaque, unrevealing, and terrifying. Surely other explanations were quietly and occasionally made, but what I fixed on was total vegetable. Locked away back in my mind with no face but the disembodied head shot my mother kept in her dresser, my uncle, the person my mother called Peter, simply could not hold on. As there was apparently no place set aside for him in the family, there was no place for him to live in my young mind.

In my mind he died. In my thirty-sixth year, during a casual conversation, I asked my mother for the year that my uncle Peter had passed away. She looked at me with a puzzled expression and said, "Who told you he was dead?" "Isn't he?" I asked. "He's still alive," she said. "He lives in a nursing home in the town of Phelps in Upstate New York." As though a large stone had been rolled away from the mouth of a deep cave, I looked at the address on an envelope from the nursing home. "No one visited him for so long they stopped calling him Peter. At the home they call him Charlie now," my mother said. "They always have." After a moment she looked up with a puzzled smile. "What made you think he was dead?"

Numbness is many feelings. As easily as I placed a hot pot in my lap, I had absently removed my uncle's existence from my own mind. In some unconscious house-cleaning impulse, my brain had thrown him away, declared him dead. In Uncle Charlie's case there was no muscle spasm to remind me that even though he was cut off and frozen in some paralyzed memory, he was still very much alive. Unlike my own legs, I could not feel him trying to tell me something. Whatever his capacities, he could not know of my existence because he had never been allowed to know me. Nevertheless, he was still my uncle, and he was still alive. I imagined him looking out a window somewhere. I wondered if he was lonely.

As I write this I will soon have lived most of my life in a wheelchair. It is this one single aspect of being paralyzed that I have never been able to fathom. All of the physical implications have been clear: the impressive clever wheelchair tricks, all learnable with enough practice, all of the social problems thorny but comprehensible, the medical questions straightforward. But what of the idea that one would live nineteen years in one body and then the rest of one's life in quite another? What could it possibly mean to be paralyzed for the rest of a life? I do not know. I only know what it has meant since 1976.

I had spent those years imagining that I was the only one in my family to be disabled. I was the pioneer blazing the trail back from near death, a path that stretched from Pennsylvania to Kurdistan. I imagined that I owned that path, which I guarded jealously, permitting no trespass. But I did not. I shared it with at least two others. There are two images of disability in my family. My grandfather, who lost his arm when he was a young man. My uncle, who might have lived in a beautiful red house in Newark, New York, but because of the time he was born into and the singular decisions of his parents, had a much different fate.

The story of Grandfather William and Uncle Peter are opposite poles of a moral compass. I have navigated alone for most of my life, but as time has passed those poles have grown stronger, each tugging at different parts of my soul. I have come to know the force that would declare me "in the way" and shut me off from the world as it did my uncle. I have also come to know the force that brought my grandfather back from the loss of an arm, the force that compelled him to invent and demand a full life, the force that convinced him to try and tie his own shoes with one hand. Far from shutting me away from the world, this force, in an almost demonic way, would have me instead fight back, invent my own world, and lead it.

My father's father, Mr. William T. Hockenberry, grew up in Ohio. I knew only the scantiest details about the circumstances surrounding the accident in which he lost a limb. My mother's younger brother, Charles Peter Slagle, grew up in central New York State. From the time he was a little boy my uncle Peter lived in a state-run institution where they called him Charlie. Tom's and Peter's lives share some common points in time, but little else.

If he had been born today or even forty years ago, my uncle would probably have lived a perfectly normal life. But in 1936 the condition he was born with, phenylketonuria, or PKU, was unknown and untreatable. This genetic disorder would not be identified for another ten years. A treatment was thirty years away. In 1936 phenylketonuria meant that a seemingly normal child would deteriorate over a period of about three years to become profoundly, and permanently, mentally retarded. In 1936 parents of PKU babies could only watch their children slowly develop the ability to say a few words, walk clumsily, and then see even those abilities slip away. In 1936 parents of PKU babies could only wonder what they had done wrong, and keep their horrible theories about injured babies, bad parenting, incompetent doctors, and dirty doorknobs to themselves. After watching their son learn to walk, barely feed himself, sing along with his mother at the piano, point at the night sky and say the word "moon," my grandparents watched as Charles Peter Slagle's sparkles of consciousness slipped away. Two months before his sixth birthday, about the time he would have entered the first grade, my grandparents sent their son, whom they called Petey, to a facility for the retarded and insane in Upstate New York. He has been institutionalized since the 1940s, referred to in the laconic medical language of the time as an "idiot" or "imbecile." He grew up a few minutes' walk from the house and the bedroom that would have been his.

But quite apart from measures of distance, Charles Peter Slagle's exile from his family, and me, was unfathomable. For reasons that will perhaps never be fully understood, a few years after he was sent away my uncle was also nearly erased, his existence denied by the family that had brought him into the world. He became something forbidden, a scandal never to be spoken of.

The person who was most responsible for Charles Peter Slagle's exile was his father, my grandfather. The man who had with his hands made the wooden cutting board shield to protect my numb legs from the harsh accidents of a world they couldn't control, had more than thirty years before sent his own son away and ordered that he be forgotten. This contradiction I see in the seams of the oak boards in my lap. It is unresolvable. I never spoke of my uncle with my grandfather. I learned everything about him after Grandpa died.

In attempting to eradicate his son's memory, he had failed. My grandmother said that her husband told her just before he died that there was not a moment when he did not think about his son, alive, nearby, but severed from his father and mother. Hovering around the simple utility of my cutting board, I can see Grandpa's attempt to perform an act of penance. He had acted to protect my numb and paralyzed legs from the world, something he could never bring himself to do for his son.

As I sat down to write the experiences of one life the fuzzy details of these other lives began drifting onto the page. To understand my own lifetime in two bodies I would need to learn more about the struggles of my grandfather Slagle and the exile of my uncle, and the loss of my grandfather Hockenberry's arm. As Robin Crusoe discovered the footprint on the beach of a soul not his own, I found many such footprints indicating that I was not alone.

For years as a journalist I have chased the story. This story was chasing me. Its influence pulls like a tide collecting waves on a beach one at a time. After nearly twenty years in my life, enough waves have lapped on to the shore. The tables have finally turned. The tide begins to ebb. The journey I never imagined could be taken, a journey into a family, could now begin. Unlike in Kurdistan, no one would demand to know why I had come.

Tying Knots

*M*y grandfather Hockenberry had no left arm from the age of twenty. From the moment in my life when I was aware of his existence, I always tried to imagine the place where his arm ended, but there was no such place down below my elbow. Only by losing an arm could someone acquire the knowledge of what it feels like not to have one.

Grandfather Tom Hockenberry had worked on the utility poles that crisscrossed the nation following World War One. When we would visit Grandfather and my grandmother Beatrice in Ohio, I used to curl up on the backseat of our old Chevy so that I could see only the sky and the utility poles out the rear window. As we drove, the sky would move above slowly, while in the foreground the trees and signs and old barns rushed by in a blur. During the early sixties, the folksy commerce along the two-lane highways still came right up to the pavement. You could see into motel windows and into people's kitchens, where they were sitting at the table. Little produce stands, piled with fresh apples and tomatoes, edged almost into the path of traffic.

In the middle of the foreground rush, between the roadside and the sky, were the utility poles and the wires carrying telephone calls and electricity. The wooden, creosote-stained denuded former trees flashed past while the wire strung between them moved parallel and together up and down, racing along the car in a continuous wave. When night fell, the moon raced along with us. I would position my head on the car seat so that the wire's shadow appeared to emerge from the moon itself. I would try to imagine my grandfather climbing the utility poles to do the work I was told he had done before his accident.

In 1920 Tom Hockenberry was a lineman apprentice. It was a good job working for Dayton Power and Light, the utility company in Dayton, Ohio. During the 1920s utilities were riding a construction boom that would continue right on through the depression. Tom was a high-wire man. He climbed the big poles and repaired the most inaccessible equipment on the highest voltage lines that DPL had in those days. He was an apprentice with every indication that he would become a line-man and make a career out of electrical engineering just as the nation was being wired from coast to coast.

The Tom Hockenberry I knew was a quiet man with square, boxy features and thick glasses that made his eyes look larger than they were. He laughed suddenly and was fond of teasing us, which we encouraged at all the wrong times. His stern "not now" was rarely spoken; more often he just looked threateningly from behind his thick glasses if we kids acted up. He liked all of the kids, but he was never, ever, like a kid. My parents would cut up and make faces, run the hose over their heads and cause us all to squeal and run in circles with amazement. My gray, curly-haired grandmother handed out entirely too much candy to be considered an adult. Only Grandfather was serious, unpredictable, and mysterious, and we took this to mean that he was a grown-up. Of all the people in my family, he had grown up at the earliest age. He was the most fascinating by far.

If anything, climbing on utility power lines and repairing high voltage wires represented a boring, practical job for Tom Hockenberry. In 1916 he had run away from home to join World War One. He was an air force mechanic stationed in France. He drove and repaired motorcycles. He had a girlfriend who gave him a gold watch. By all accounts, he raised hell throughout France. Some of those accounts made it back home to Dayton, where his reputation preceded his return from Europe.

"Well, I never liked him," my grandmother recalled. "I thought he was too arrogant. I didn't care for him at all. And so I never went with him, never." Tom tried to get Beatrice Eiche to go out with him, along with every other girl in Dayton who knew he was back from the war. But Bea had a good job at Rikes, a department store, and wasn't about to let some swashbuckling World War One ace turn her head. Bea heard

Tom's stories of motorcycles, war, and high wires and let him find other girls to impress. He did.

There were always a few pictures of Tom around the house from that period. In his military uniform he was tall and thin, but with broad shoulders. His eyes looked softer and smaller because he had no glasses then, or if he did, the lenses were not as thick. The pictures were mysterious not only because they were some of the oldest photos in my parents' albums: they showed a man with two arms, and we knew Grandpa had only one.

On the outskirts of Dayton on a cold November day in 1920, Tom Hockenberry was up on a 40-foot wooden utility pole replacing the insulators on one of Dayton's 60,000-volt main lines. He wore the spiked boots of a lineman and ascended the pole by grabbing the metal bars that stuck out from the wood on either side. There were a lot of poles to finish on that day, and Tom was settling into a quick rhythm of ascend, replace, descend, ascend, replace, descend. On one pole he went to work on the insulators without attaching his leather safety belt to the pole. The dew on the metal bar where his foot was made it slippery. Tom reached with his left arm out to a junction, stretching his body from foot to finger. He slipped.

As he scrambled to regain a foothold his arms flailed. With his left arm holding a large steel wrench he hooked onto the power line and 60,000 volts instantly ripped through his left hand, across his chest, and out his right leg. He was, for a moment, grounded to the tower, and a river of electrons found a path through my grandfather's body. The completed circuit held his body in the air for a moment. It was broken only by his body's own convulsions. Without a safety belt, he fell from the pole. Gravity delivered him the 40 feet back to earth. His body arrived on the ground some time after the electrons blasted through his flesh and bones at the speed of light on their way to the same place.

Electrocution disrupts the body's own electrical system, kicking over the brain's fragile circuitry. But the truly significant effect of 60,000 volts on a human body has more to do with to chemistry than physics. A human body is a conductor of electricity. But it has a very high resistance, much higher than a kitchen appliance like a hot plate or an electric range. Electrical resistance is measured in ohms, and an electric range produces about 300 ohms resistance. The higher the resistance and the higher the voltage and current, the more heat is produced. Depending on the amount of moisture and fat present, a human body has an electrical resistance on the order of 4 or 5 million ohms.

Like the element on a hot plate, a current applied across that resis-

tance produces many times the heat of an electric range. The heat produced by a 60,000-volt current of 100 amperes or more passing through
a resistance of 5 million ohms exceeds 1,000 degrees Fahrenheit in less
than a second. The heat bakes deeply into the tissue, burning bone,
worse than fat, and boiling the blood itself. The very things that would
keep a limb intact, the blood vessels for tissue repair and the bone for
support and movement, are damaged the most. What electricity does to
a body cannot be undone with sutures and gauze pads. From one stumble and a few seconds of contact with the 60,000-volt line, my grandfather suffered severe burns to his left arm, electric shock trauma, and the
kinds of fractures and contusions you would expect from a 40-foot fall.

"He was dead before he hit the ground," my mother would say when
she told the story we grandchildren never tired of hearing in the car on
the way to Dayton. After a moment, she always added her theory on why
Grandpa survived: "It was the force of the fall that started his heart. That
fall must have saved him." The one man who witnessed the accident
said that Tom's body hit the ground, bounced up, and landed a second
time. "He was yelling so loud, the man said," Grandmother Beatrice
recalled clearly seventy-six years later, when she was in her nineties.
"That's something I will never get over, how the man said that Tom's
yell was the most horrible sound he had ever heard come from a human being."

Beatrice Eiche only paid attention to Tom Hockenberry after she
learned of his accident. She went to visit him in the hospital. "I just got
kind of sorry and felt sorry for him. Somebody that was in such bad
shape as he was, and as young as he was, that's what got me. I thought,
my goodness here he is just a young man, and practically ruined."

The doctors amputated Tom Hockenberry's left arm three inches below the elbow. He insisted that the doctors let him keep his elbow joint.
They did, with the warning that if it didn't heal they would have to
amputate again farther up toward the shoulder. At Tom's side now was
Beatrice Eiche, whose feelings about the swashbuckling Mr. Hockenberry had changed dramatically. They were married within a year of
the accident.

If Bea thought the idea of going steady with a two-armed Tom was
out of the question because of his headstrong arrogance, the idea of Bea
marrying Tom after the injury came as a shock to Bea's family and
friends. "They would never say anything to me. They would say it all to
my mother." With her proud ninety-six-year-old eyes she defends the
decision to marry her long-gone husband in a strong voice. "You know,
they couldn't understand me. They'd say something was wrong with me

that I'd want to go with him. They'd ask what was wrong with my mind."
For Grandmother, the argument was still very much alive. "I just didn't
think there was anything wrong with it at all. If I had thought it was
terrible to marry Tom, I wouldn't have done it. But I didn't see anything
wrong about it."

Dayton Power and Light gave Tom Hockenberry $2,500 for the loss
of the arm and a desk job in the records office. The security that came
with the job got the Hockenberry family through the depression. It was
a job Tom Hockenberry held for forty years. As a twenty-year-old, he put
away the memories of World War One and his dashing days in France.
In his pocket was the gold watch from his girlfriend of those days. He
was never without it.

We never tired of staring at Grandpa's stump. It was the first thing we
wanted to see when we piled out of the car in Dayton, even before we
investigated what sweets were available to us from Grandma Bea.
Grandpa could lift you up on his stump, which we would all take turns
riding like a little seat. There was something about the absence of
Grandpa's arm that made the strength of his stump seem magical.

My brothers and I would advertise the "amazing one-armed man" to
the little kids in the neighborhood far in advance of my grandparents'
arrival. Grandma and Grandpa would drive up in their big sedan with
the colored knob on the steering wheel that Grandpa used for driving
with his one good hand. As the adults would begin to relax after an
eight-hour drive from Ohio to southwestern New York, little kids would
begin showing up in the living room, accompanied by myself or one of
my brothers. They would say hello, introduce themselves in quiet
voices, then after a few minutes leave to be replaced by another kid,
another introduction, and another swift retreat.

The price was one nickel per view for my brother David's little
friends. The rest of us were satisfied just to make good on a brag. "My
grandpa has only one arm." "Oh yeah? Prove it." No problem. The stump
was spectacular enough by itself, but if Grandpa could be convinced to
actually tie his shoe with his one hand, something most of us could
barely manage even with two hands, this was real circus material. My
parents insisted that Grandpa would only do a public shoe tying once
per visit, so my brothers and I made sure that a large audience could
be assembled at a moment's notice.

Grandpa would arrange the two ends of his shoelace, and then with
a pinching motion squeeze them into the first knot. Then, with three
fingers and the heel of his hand anchoring his shoe, he arranged the
lace into two sloppy loops, and in another, this time more mysterious

move, he would take the loops in his fingers and in an instant they were squeezed into a confusion of laces and loops. At this point it always seemed as though he had messed it up. I looked to see the doubtful faces of the other kids. But Grandpa never took his eyes off the laces. He reached into the tangled mess and grabbed a loop and pulled. Then he grabbed another. The knot composed itself perfectly. The shoe was tied. The kids were amazed. We won our bet. Grandpa could go back to what he'd been doing before.

It was the very same knot I made with my clumsy hands each morning, but it was done without all of the pulling and yanking. It was a knot tied with the eyes as much as with Grandpa's sole remaining hand. The function of the knot was precise, its structure identical to the knots I made. But while my knots were wrestled from two strands pulled tightly by two balanced hands and wrists, Grandpa reached the same knot by laying a trap for it, and when the trap was sprung, catching the knot with a flick of one hand. There was more than one way to make a knot. I could see that Grandpa looked at knots differently than I did. He was as much a guy who understood some inner truth of knots as he was a left-arm amputee.

Grandpa's stump could grab things and hold them, like the cans of worms when we went fishing. He would put the can in the crook of his stump and pass worms out one at a time to the little boys waiting with their rods and hooks. The limb was strong even though it had no hand. It did things only a stump could do.

"He did lots of things for me that you wouldn't think he could do," my grandmother liked to say. "He didn't want anybody to think he couldn't do anything." Beatrice had never learned to swim, and once at a public pool in Dayton in the early twenties a boy pushed her into the water as a joke. She struggled in the water for a moment until Tom jumped in. Grabbing her with his stump and holding her to him with the three-inch remains of his elbow, he pulled her out of the water, wailing and coughing and sobbing. "He told me not to be afraid. He always told me not to be afraid. I'm so terrible that way."

The force of pulling his wife from the water tore his stump open from the amputation point right up to a place near his shoulder. He began to bleed severely. Tom returned once again to the hospital, where they sewed him up for the last time. He always claimed that the act of rescuing his wife had stretched his amputated arm and made him able to move it more like a real arm. The scar tissue from the burns, he said, was torn away, allowing him considerable freedom.

We grandchildren called Grandpa's left arm his "bad arm," or we called it his stump. But stump was not a word used in Tom's own house. "We used to have fun playing with his little stub." My father might call it a little stub years after his father's death but never to his face. For most of Tom Hockenberry's life there was little if any explicit mention of the missing arm. My father recalled that "It was never a big issue around the house."

Besides a job and money, for compensation Dayton Power and Light gave Tom a flesh-colored artificial arm to wear at the office. There was a picture in our house of him wearing it at work. The symmetry it gave his body was disputed by the lifeless curves of the dull wooden fingers sticking out of the sleeve of his shirt and blazer. I never saw my grandfather wearing this prosthesis. Around our house he openly displayed his stump, uncovered, in his short-sleeved white cotton shirts and his western string ties. If he went out, he would wear a jacket and pin the jacket sleeve to his side.

To wear the artificial arm was not to gain a limb except in a purely cosmetic sense. It was more like losing or burying a limb. "I couldn't do anything with it," Grandpa would say. To put on the arm he would first cover his stump by wrapping it with an elastic cloth bandage, winding it tightly even on the hottest summer days. Then he would strap the wooden arm over and under his shoulder and pull the belts tight. In the mirror he looked symmetrical, but the weight of the prosthesis hung awkwardly off his shoulder. He looked balanced, but with the prosthesis on he felt anything but right. The one part of his arm that could still move and be useful was now buried inside, covered by an inanimate piece of plastic and wood.

The artificial arm had more to do with the people around him than with anything that might make his own life easier. By all accounts he accepted it quietly, without a complaint. "We wanted him to wear something," Beatrice said, "because of the way people think and talk, you know. People are cruel. They can say things that can hurt you clear through." This was a pain that she suffered as a witness to her husband's apparent strangeness. But it was not at all clear if this was something he worried about. It was others who were concerned about how things might look. Their shock needed to be anticipated, as though the voltage of his near electrocution in 1920 was close by, still considered dangerous.

"He didn't like covering it up." Grandma could not bring herself to say the word "stump" even twenty-four years after her husband's death. Grandma spoke with the voice of a pioneer as she talked about the times before her children were born and she and her husband would go places together, encountering the mysterious public with its riddles and expectations. "I thought it was best to keep it covered, maybe so people wouldn't like to see it any other way. He thought so too . . . I think. And so we did cover it up." She paused and looked past her son's face, past her grandson, through the wall and far back into time. "I think every now and then he got hurt about that." By 1949, when his children were in college, Tom Hockenberry had stopped wearing the prosthesis.

The asymmetry of Grandfather was only jarring at first glance. It disappeared as soon as he began working with his stump and the stump began helping his hand. Sometimes the hand would help the stump. They seemed to be friends, and while the hand was the more useful of the two, the stump, with its stocky, muscular bluntness, seemed the stronger. The stump's roundish end looked like an egg and my brothers and I would imagine that there was a hand inside waiting to come out. If a hand did ever come out, we realized, Grandpa would have lost the use of his stump.

We wondered where his old arm had gone. Sometimes I would dream of it in the bushes near the utility pole in Ohio where Grandpa had fallen. In my dreams it would be there, quietly drumming its fingers waiting for Grandpa to come and claim it. Horror movies about disembodied hands and arms weren't scary to my brothers and me. We all wondered, while watching the white fingers on the screen, if it was Grandpa's arm up there. After hitchhiking out west it had made it to Hollywood to co-star in the movies with Peter Lorre. The lost arm and its mysterious stump contained possibilities. Once, after getting scolded, the suggestion was made that I be spanked for bothering Grandpa. With tears in my eyes, and resigned to punishment, I pointed at the stump and indicated my preference. "Could you do it with that arm, Grandpa?"

Tom Hockenberry made one memorable, bitter attempt to join the community at large. He asked to become a member of the Freemason chapter in downtown Dayton. In the old downtown districts of many midwestern cities and towns, the Masonic Temple is still the most prominent of landmarks. In Dayton, Ohio, as elsewhere, the Masonic Temple was the symbol of an ancient fraternal organization that claimed to know the secrets of the stone upon which communities could be built. In the case of Dayton, gray stone etched a skyline and built the levees and dams that would keep the Miami River from flooding once and for all.

In the thirties, the Masons made much of their importance even at a time of electrification, trains, and airplanes. In the thirties, Dayton was slowly beginning to move away from its agricultural and industrial roots.

Dayton's skyline of stone would become the home of Mead, a paper products company. Its corporate colleague, NCR, would become a leader in office automation and would then be swallowed up by AT&T. These modern contributions to the skyline of Dayton would be made of steel and glass towering over the Masonic Temple, pushing its importance into the background.

The Masons were just the kind of upstanding conservative civic group Tom Hockenberry very much wanted to join back in the 1930s. "It was a big thing to be a Mason," my grandmother said. Beatrice Eiche would know such things. The Protestant, conservative Eiche family had always kept a strict accounting of the sins of Catholics and the "coloreds." Beatrice knew their place in her world, which was no place, and she understood that the Masons would have no place for such people either. Tom's name was placed in nomination by some friends. "The Enfields wanted him to join, and they proposed his name."

There was some suspense about Tom's application. Letting a man with one arm into the Masons was hardly a sure bet. Tom was different. It had nothing to do with being physically unable to work with stone or something specific like that. This was understood by all. It was the one time in his life that Tom allowed another person or group to pass judgment on his life. In a secret vote, the Masons would rule on his fitness as the group had ruled on the fitness of countless men before him.

The Masons refused him. The vote was overwhelmingly against allowing him to join. My grandmother, who could not have been more convinced of the need to exclude blacks and Catholics from the Masons, could not have been more shocked by this decision. "That made me sick to my stomach, to think that they always thought that they were so much, that they were so high and mighty, that they couldn't take him in when he was just wanting to do something normal. That was one of their rules." As she spoke, the bitterness of the moment filled her eyes, and a wavering in her voice spoke not of age but of unquenchable, unredeemable anger.

In 1946, when World War Two was over and the effects it had on the limbs and flesh and spines of quite another generation came home from the war, the rules of the Masons changed. The war's amputated and paralyzed sons went into and left the same hospitals Tom Hockenberry had gone to more than two decades before. As a badge of patriotic sacrifice, the loss of a limb became acceptable to the Masons. In 1946, men decorated with purple hearts, in uniforms, crutches, and wheelchairs applied and were accepted into the Masons. The organization remembered that Tom Hockenberry had asked them to consider him normal more than ten years earlier.

"After World War Two, they called and said they would take him." There was no suspense this time. If Tom had expected a call from the Masons in the years that had passed since they had refused him, he gave no hint. His answer to the Masons was clear: he refused them. His request of the Masons had been a one-time thing; they could not have known what they had done to Tom with their simple refusal. Grandma recalled his decision with equal parts triumph and tragedy. "He said, 'I'm not going in. If they wouldn't take me when I was young and I wanted to go. I'm not going now.'"

Tom Hockenberry had been quite a dancer in his early days, and it was his dancing that made Tom seem so dazzling and dangerous to Beatrice when she first met him. After he lost his arm, Tom never liked to dance, a reluctance keenly felt by his wife. That the loss of an arm would affect something associated with the movement of the legs puzzled his family and friends. "He knew I would like to dance so well, so he would do it, because of me, because I wanted to. But he really didn't care about it." Grandma breathed in slowly when she talked about dancing, and her eyes showed a hint of pink behind her glasses.

"Was Grandpa embarrassed?" I asked her.

"I don't know what it was, but it was on account of his arm. He wasn't much to say anything about it. We'd go to dances and everybody would dance with Dad. We wouldn't have any problem, but he never talked about it, and I didn't either." Discussing Grandfather's missing arm was not something forbidden, but it was pointless, like driving down a dead-end street or imagining the fingerprints on a nonexistent arm. What Tom thought about these things no one knows. In this, father and family were in utterly different and nonintersecting worlds.

Tom Hockenberry died in 1969 when I was eleven years old. He went to sleep one night and never woke up. I remember the tablecloth in the kitchen, remember staring at the red squares while my parents told us what had happened. He had been quite ill for the last years of his life, and the effects of diabetes had put a further strain on a body that had taken more than its share of hits. His death was peaceful. My father discovered him lying motionless in his bed the morning he died. They had spoken the night before. Tom had remarked, as he often did, how much a source of pride his son was to him, and that they didn't get to see each other often enough.

Tom Hockenberry's trials and his quiet acceptance of fate was seen as a supreme virtue by his son, my father. The sacrament of that virtue was to never speak of those things. When they knew he was dead, mother and son sat quietly, sobbing. After all the years of dutiful silence, they proceeded to perform the last simple chores of a life lived twice. When my father and grandmother buried Tom Hockenberry, they put away the memories of his life and the mysteries that died with him. Grandpa was buried in Dayton on a small hill under some trees.

Twenty-four years after his death, I sat with Grandma on my right and my father on my left and asked questions that had never been asked before. The mysteries of Tom Hockenberry were all there, intact, preserved with the same dutiful silence that had characterized his life.

"Were there times when people made Grandpa feel embarrassed and as though he was a man without an arm?"

Grandma looked at her son, considering whether to shield him once again from things she believed were true and not for her children to hear.

"Well, you know, I think there were a lot of times like that."

My father had rarely been in this place in his mother's memory. He did not know these things about his father that Grandma was speaking of.

"The only thing I ever worried about was what the children thought. Because I know he was good to them. Land's sake, he was always a good father to them." She spoke in the third person but never took her eyes off her son. "But we had that to put up with. That was my . . . you know, that's what I had to put up with."

"What?" I asked.

"Him being crippled and that sort of thing." She moved her head around and stared at faces and demons that were not in the room with us. Her voice was raised slightly, arguing a point that was still not put to rest. "I married him, and goodness' sakes, he was hurt. I wasn't going to go off and leave him."

My father intervened for his mother, who was evidently speaking about truly difficult things now. He tried to explain. "It was nothing," he insisted to me. "It was never a big issue around the house. We were aware that he was different from other people, but we knew how he had lost his arm, and that was it."

It was as though my grandmother hadn't heard what had just been said. She looked up at the ceiling and spoke in a voice that sounded like both a whisper and a shout. "You know, he hadn't done anything, you know, too terrible. That's what . . . the part that hurt me the most is that he hadn't done anything. Why were people so nasty?" Her son looked like a little boy suddenly, and a tear rolled down his cheek as he said, "I never knew that they were."

Grandma shook her head and dropped her eyes. "Well . . ." She didn't finish.

"I never had a sense that people were nasty," my father said again. No one had an answer for him.

"Do you think Grandpa was all alone?" I asked my grandmother.

"I think Grandpa was very alone. I really do. I've always thought that he had such a sad life, although he never complained much." The awful anguish was that she could not in the end protect her husband, or ease some pain she knew that had poured from his eyes. After a breath she looked at her son and asked him if he knew differently. "You never heard him complain, did you, Jack?"

My father took his mother's hand. "He never complained." He paused and added, "He kept a lot of things to himself." On my father's face was pride. For my grandmother it was confirmation that she would never really know what had gone on in her husband's heart.

"Did you think Grandpa wanted his arm back, Grandma?" I asked.

"Oh, my, yes."

"How do you know?"

"Well, I'm sure of that."

"Why are you sure?"

"Well, wouldn't you think he would?"

"Do you think Grandpa, if he were alive, would have some advice for me about being in a wheelchair?"

For the first time in a while her face brightened. This was not a question she would have to think about. "I'm sure that he'd give you some really good advice, better than I could give you. I know Dad would really have something good to say to you."

"What do you think it might be?"

Her nearly century-old eyes beamed a confidence that showed above all the pain. It was this question that mattered most to her; it retained no mystery, and as she spoke she did not look at me. She looked at her son, across the table.

"He'd want you to, you know, be proud and brave and everything else. Because you have to be. You have to push. If you don't push, you're not going to get anywhere. You just have to keep pushing and getting a little more and a little more and being brave about it."

"Are you a pusher, Grandma?"

"Yes, I'm a pusher."

"Are you brave?"

"No, I'm not brave. I'm a coward. I'm scared." Now she looked right at me. "I've always been scared to live." I looked over at my father. He was no longer watching us. He had taken the gold watch from his father's World War One days out of his pocket. With his thumb he slowly rubbed the back of it and stared into its face.

Sometimes in my wheelchair I achieve a moment of unity between the chair, the arms that push it, and the mind that observes it all, when I feel like a character on horseback in an elaborately constructed Tolstoy or Dickens novel. Riding over a landscape that seems to be endless and always arriving somewhere new and wonderful, I can't help but believe that if I had not insisted on hitchhiking along a road in Pennsylvania back in February 1976, I would have missed the moment of my accident. The thought always produces a harrowing twinge, as though it was a close call, a cliffhanger rather than a fact. I might have missed what my life has become, each subsequent event locked to the preceding one like the sequential rhythm of a horse's hooves.

The world that my grandfather Hockenberry lived in is mostly gone now. If he had lived to know me as an adult, would we ever have talked about some of the things he kept to himself? I could have learned things from him. He could have watched me do things he was never permitted, in his world, to even dare. It is even possible that he would have found openness about disability offensive and frightening. The attitudes and values of a time are buried with it. I roll along Route 88 and wonder if Grandpa would have had a better life if he had lived longer or been born later. I look for the utility polls along the road and find none. Had he been born today, there would not have been a 60,000-volt line on the rural road outside Dayton for him to fall from; Tom Hockenberry would never have lost his arm. He would never have learned how to tie his shoes with one hand. He would have missed his accident. The thought produces the very same harrowing twinge.

'Bye, Bike

*I*n the reality of quantum physics, bodies can act upon each other
even though they have no apparent connection in space and time.
Particles, behaving as though they were once friends, react to the disin-
tegration of another proton, light years away, in a mysterious subatomic
grief, detectable by physicists as thin, curved trails in cloud chambers.
As my body went about the interior task of healing, others encountered
my body's changes as ripples on the surface of their own lives, as though
I were a pebble dropped into a pond.

My mother tells the story of a long-distance phone call answered by
my father and the words ". . . should we come there now?" that caused
her to sit bolt upright and then run to the kitchen, searching his face
for a sign of what and who this news was about. "Is he expected to live?"
my father asked. I was expected to live. "But will he ever walk again?"
My mother began packing. Until my father got off the phone and told
her I was in a hospital in Pennsylvania, she didn't know where she was
going.

My brothers remember learning about my accident at a high school
hockey game and not knowing what to do. My sister recalls staying at
her friend Tanya's house while Mom and Dad went off to Pennsylvania.
A nine-year-old girl thinking about the words "spinal cord." She tried to

imagine what one looked like, and then what one looked like after it was broken.

My grandparents told of their own phone call in the night. "Are you sitting down?" the voice on the phone had asked. Upon being told that I would never walk again, my grandfather Slagle interrupted, "Well, you know, that's not for sure." His first question was about my brain. "Was there a head injury?" he asked my mother. When told there was only a concussion and a mild skull fracture, he was relieved. My grandparents sat alone, looking at each other.

"There was a terrible ice storm that February," Grandmother said. "We were so shocked. I don't think we could realize that this would happen to anyone that we knew, because neither one of us ever knew anyone in a . . . confined to a wheelchair."

In 1976, their son Charles Peter turned forty. He had lived thirty-five of those years in an institution, and for part or all of each one of those days he had been confined to a wheelchair.

I knew none of their grief. The waves from the news of my accident rippled outward on the surface, far from the bottom of the pond where I began my physical journey back. In the first weeks, months, and years after the accident, my body had become a puzzle. Solving it was exhilarating beyond the simple imperatives of survival. Each challenge was interesting in its own way. How would I get up? How would I get dressed? How would I drive? I imagined how each event might go. I would try out each theory and live with the results of each experiment. I searched for some translation algorithm that would allow me to go from what had been to what was now to be. I would calculate the added time of wheelchairs and various compensatory formulae for determining how I would perform this or that task.

I thought of how I might ride the CTA elevated trains when I returned to school in Chicago. Though I was anxious to get a car or van with hand controls so I could drive, I still longed to use my beloved Chicago subway trains to get around. For a boy from suburbs and small towns, the subways represented freedom in a way that could not be duplicated by using Daddy's car or riding a bicycle. I loved the fast-moving subway cars, the electrical sparks of blue light at night surging past the run-down fire escapes of the residential neighborhoods around the el on their way to the steel and glass of downtown. There were no elevators on the el trains back in the seventies. There are only a few even twenty years later. There were stairs, endless, filthy, rickety stairs, and narrow turnstiles leading up and down to tracks and street.

I insisted that all of my physical therapists listen in elaborate detail to how I was going to board the trains. It was easy enough to explain. I would roll up to the stairs leading to the platform. I would get out of my chair and sit on the second step. I would fold up my chair. I would tie a strap around the chair and attach it to my wrist. I would begin to climb the stairs one at a time on my backside. At the first landing I would haul the chair up by the attached strap, then repeat the process until I was at trackside. Then I would unfold the chair and hoist myself back into it.

"The trains themselves are accessible," I told my therapist, Donna. Of all the people in the hospital, she was the least concerned with melodramas of denial and acceptance. She wasn't interested in anyone's mood. She only cared about physical progress. She wanted to know two things in physical therapy each day. Had I been to the bathroom since lunch, and was I ready to work. "If you have to live in a wheelchair, John, crazy and strong is a lot better than sane and weak," she would say.

I was just crazy and weak in the beginning. I insisted that Donna teach me to ride the subway. "I can climb the stairs to the platforms. That's the hard part. I think those turnstiles could be a problem too."

"I see. How many steps are there at a typical station?" she would ask.

In my mind, I counted more than two dozen. "About twenty steps in the downtown loop stations." There were actually more than thirty.

"What about just taking a cab?" Donna asked.

"Isn't your job to encourage me?" She wanted the details of my plan even if her job was definitely not to encourage me to climb up long, filthy stairways to ride the subway.

"Do you think that this is something you will be doing more than once a day?"

"I'll do it as much as I need to."

"Is this how you will travel to job interviews?"

"I have lots of time to pick a career."

She listened each day without much comment until the morning before I was discharged. When I finished my push-ups and weight lifting, Donna went over to the equipment closet and pulled out a wooden step unit consisting of three small steps. She placed it on the floor mat next to me and suggested that I try to push myself up the three steps to the top. "You'll need to be able to climb up bigger steps than these to get on the trains. You might as well get started with these," she said.

The wooden steps looked like a toy from a church Sunday school room. I placed my hands on the bottom step and started to hoist my hips up the three- or four-inch height of the first step. I pushed with my arms, and my lower body stretched. It did not move. I pushed my arms and shoulders into the effort and still my lower body was just hanging there. The experience was like trying to escape from quicksand. I could thrash about above, but my lower body just hung there, its connection to me muddy and liquid. The power of my arms was soaked up and lost.

I pushed with all my might, and still nothing. Donna's expression did not change. With an effort so extreme that I can still recall the dizziness and the red burst of blood rushing into my straining face, I attacked the three inches. I was spitting and grunting as I breathed. Out of the corner of my eyes I could see that everyone in the therapy room had stopped to watch. I would not fail. I flattened myself against a thick psychic wall with no handholds. My mind was focused on a single act of will erupting like a torch from my fingers, wrists, and neck.

I raised my hips enough to catch the edge of my tailbone on the lip of the step and slid the rest of the way onto it. I smiled triumphantly. I could feel my face red from the effort. Donna looked at me and nodded. "How many steps are there at a typical station?" Her question was a cannon shot to a wall of glass. I understood in that instant that I would not be riding the trains again. If I did, it would only be after the construction of many elevators, or after a physical effort that I was far from being able to imagine. My mind's theories about the future were erased. My smile went away. I looked at Donna and her image was blurred through tears. For the first time since my accident, and probably for years before that, I sobbed.

I had learned a little something about denial and acceptance. Donna quietly and tenderly helped me back into the wheelchair and took me over to a set of parallel bars where she strapped a pair of braces on my legs and placed my arms up on the bars. "Conquering an experience is different than having the experience," Donna said. "If you have to climb Mount Everest to ride a train, it's not the train ride you will remember. Are you sure you want to ride those trains that much?" she asked. My lungs and arms were sore from pushing up those three inches. I wanted to ride them that much, exactly that much. It wasn't enough to get me even halfway up the stairs to the tracks.

"Lift," she said. The tears still ran down my face, and as I lifted myself into a standing position, droplets of tears and sweat landed on the floor below me. The last time I had been at that height was on the gravel piles behind the gas station at the roadside stop in Pennsylvania an hour and a half before our car went over the edge of the embankment. The feeling of being six feet, one inch tall was visceral and unfamiliar. I was a torso balancing on a stick. It had only been a few weeks since I had last walked, yet standing was no longer ordinary. It was a different world. The heights of cupboards and windows were made for this position. To stand was to punch through clouds and stare at the sun.

My arms held me there. My body hung below. The leg braces made solid what I could no longer command my muscles to stiffen. Like dime-operated binoculars at a tourist attraction, I stared out of my own eyes. I greedily looked at everything on tiptoes of the spirit. In a moment, my arm muscles would tire, the dime would run out. I would have to sit down. Standing was a place to visit. I did not live there anymore.

As time went on, my physical changes and the emotional changes for the people close to me who were also dealing with the shock of my accident came together. Gradually that first summer, friends came to visit. Some people from school drove the three hours from Chicago to Michigan to see how I was doing. Friends from high school smuggled a rotisserie grill into my room one day, and in half an hour barbecued chicken, passed out beer for the whole floor, and packed away the grill, all before the nurses discovered what we had done.

Some of the people who visited were even glad to assist me in addressing some of the more subtle physical puzzles of being a paraplegic. Stephanie, a girl who had lived down the hall at school, hitchhiked to Michigan along the same route Rick and I had taken eastward. She showed up at Mary Free Bed without warning one evening. She had long blond hair and wore wire-rimmed John Lennon glasses. She wore a thick, drab, army surplus jacket.

Something about my accident motivated her to visit. I never knew what it was. Perhaps I was suddenly vulnerable in a way I had never appeared to be before. Back at school Stephanie and I would have long talks about the philosophies of John Locke and Thomas Hobbes. While she might break spontaneously into a joyous interpretive dance in front of the stereo, I would sneer and deride what I considered to be the pathetic cluelessness of hippies. Stephanie was idealistic and spiritual while I was intimidating and argumentative. We were distant, cautious friends.

In my hospital room, with a wheelchair sitting next to my bed, I was certainly not intimidating anymore. Stephanie and I talked in my room for a while and then decided to go outside. She had no car, and I was still too nervous to be seen in public in the neighborhood around the hospital, where anyone in a wheelchair was stared at like an escaped convict, so we decided to just go out behind the hospital where there were some trees and a small garage that sheltered a patch of grass.

The security guard saw us leave. I mentioned that we were going to sit out back and talk for a while. He looked at me and Stephanie and smiled. Then he walked over to the linen closet and handed us four hospital blankets. "You might want these," he said. "It's getting dark and it's a little cold out there still."

Sex was one detail of life as a paraplegic that was rarely discussed in the hospital. I had no sensation "down there," so what I would do "down there" now, besides jam catheter tubes into my penis, I didn't know. Stephanie was very interested in this subject. She wanted to know all about everything, and we did discuss it for a while. Then I removed my aluminum back brace, she removed her pants, and on a crisp spring night out behind a hospital garage I laid on my back and she gave my limp, much abused, and completely numb penis a workover that I had never in my wildest adolescent moments even dreamed of. I could listen and watch, but I could feel nothing.

Perched above my own shoulders, I was watching a pornographic movie in which I was the co-star. My head was in a torpid haze of teen-age arousal. My body felt nothing. I rammed and poked and licked her, while she sucked and squirmed and groaned. Nothing much happened. When we had been outside for more than an hour, I heard the voice of the security guard calling from behind the wall. I could not tell how long he had been trying to get our attention. "Are you all right?" He sounded very nervous. Stephanie groped for her army jacket and covered herself. I didn't know exactly how to answer this question. On the one hand, I had just had the blow job of the decade and had felt nothing. Stephanie was still at it, like a surgeon losing a patient on the operating table who can't stop shouting at God and giving CPR. On the other hand, sensation or not, it was also just another awkward silly teen-age moment; kids fumbling with their bodies in the backseat of an old Buick, or in this case, the back of an old hospital with an empty wheelchair nearby. In a deep, confident voice, Stephanie told the security guard, "We're fine, sir. I'll bring him back." The security guard offered a warning before going back inside. "They are looking for you, so John, you should put your, umm, brace back on. I'll leave the back door open."

With much difficulty, Stephanie and I put my brace back on, hoisted me back into my chair and rolled me back to the hospital door, which had been propped open with a brick by the guard. In the dark, under the incandescent parking lot light behind the hospital, Stephanie kissed me good-bye. "I think it will work," she said as she brushed the blades of grass off my hospital-issue T-shirt. She sounded like Jane Goodall talking about one of her chimps in a *National Geographic* special. I was embarrassed to have been busted getting my rocks off. But this was medical science. I was carried away by the idea that we were on the frontiers of knowledge, discovering what the human body could do when pushed to the limit. Or at least how red and sore it could look.

The idea that paraplegia could turn sex into a medical research project, and that people might hitchhike across state lines to visit my bedroom, was some significant compensation for the fact that I might not be able to feel what was going on. I had never been good at getting dates when I could walk. I was suddenly way ahead of my time. Back in the mid-seventies I discovered something that would be the credo of the decade to follow: numb, mindless sex with people who act like therapists. I said good-bye to Stephanie. She went off to Ann Arbor to visit some friends. I never saw her again.

One person who never visited during the time I was in the hospital was Rick. My friends at school said that they had tried to get Rick to come along with them to visit me, but he would always make an excuse. I missed him and the adventures we'd had back in Chicago, but I knew in my heart that he would not come. My friends didn't tell me that Rick had taken up residence in the narrow corridor/crawl space in "the ranch," my bedroom, at school. He would lie on the old, rumpled twin mattress I had placed on the floor and call me on the phone. I never knew until years later that he was there in my space, surrounded by my pictures and other things. He spoke often with me over the phone. As long as he didn't have to look at me, the accident had become an emblem of our intensified bonding. We were the two daring boys who had swung out over a chasm and had scrambled back over the crumbling edge in the nick of time. What I didn't know was how much Ricky thought that only he had made it, that in his mind I had fallen into the chasm.

We spoke continually of our plans for when I got back to school. Yet neither Rick nor I would speak of the accident and what it meant. Gradually it became clear that I was being swept away in an experience that he had no part in. His world changed too. He spent days in the corridor on my bed, speaking to no one. We talked like boys. I was going to buy a big stereo. He was playing guitar a lot, making bigger drug deals and writing more poetry. Over the phone I could tell that life back at school was going on without me. He could tell that I was changed even though he would not look at my body in those first months.

I wanted to get back to school and catch up. Rick said he wanted me to come back, but both of us were afraid, and we never spoke of what was really going on. In this we were children. We could not speak of the accident. Instead, in two different voices the accident shouted at each of us. The voice I heard was angry and defiant, challenging me to reinvent my life; the voice Ricky heard was full of guilt and remorse over the event that had nearly killed his best friend and had changed him. Like tough boys, we pretended not to notice. It was just another thing we winked knowingly about, another thing that made us cool.

My parents could not avoid watching the changes taking place for their oldest son. But while they would visit me in the hospital regularly, much of the change they observed involved their friends and acquaintances, who treated them as though they too had experienced a trauma. My parents noticed how people stared when I went on outings with them. Friends and neighbors, as well as the therapists, freely offered advice. Some of it was pretty bizarre stuff, discussions of amputation and special schools, miracle operations, experimental brain implants and nerve research.

There was also a lot of talk of suicide. Long before Kevorkian made a cottage industry out of physician-assisted suicide, some people would talk openly about suicide with me. They would ask if I had thought of killing myself, imagining that if I had considered it, the experience of being in a wheelchair would be more comprehensible to them. "I don't think that I could deal with it," they would say. Many people would make this macabre suggestion to my parents, saying openly that if I found it too difficult to continue my life, they should be ready to accept my wanting to die. This suggestion was offered as a precaution, like making sure there was plenty of iodine or aspirin in the medicine cabinet in case of headaches or knee scrapes. Although the suggestion was offered in the spirit of liberal freethinking, it was chilling to think that going on with my life made less sense to some people than a self-inflicted death.

I could flex my arms, laugh it off, and roll away. But what about somebody like my friend Roger, who constantly needed others to take care of his basic needs. How might Roger laugh off the nagging suspicion that the person dressing him believed that suicide would be a more elegant solution to his predicament than going on with his life? Was it the experience of quadriplegia that engendered thoughts of suicide, or did hopelessness come from the experience of being surrounded by people who considered that struggling to live with a disability was, in the end, not worth the effort?

There is a line from the Woody Allen movie, *Annie Hall,* where Allen's character, Alvie Singer, tells Diane Keaton that he can't imagine why or how people who are disfigured, crippled, or paralyzed can go on with their lives. The line got a laugh. Alone in the theater I wanted to cry out, "Woody, it's all right, you would know what to do." I said nothing. The fact that he wrote the line into his movie meant that I was the last person he would ever believe could explain something like that.

I wished sometimes that I could tell people that I had contemplated suicide and decided after many theoretical proofs and much soul-searching that it was wrong for me. They wanted their view of the simple awfulness of disability to be confirmed by my experience. The truth is, I never once contemplated suicide. Suicide is something you argue yourself out of, not into. It had nothing to do with my new life, though many people had a hard time believing this. Thoughts of suicide arose from an experience that presented no solutions and offered no hope.

Far from being a blank wall of misery, my body now presented an intriguing puzzle of great depth and texture. To rediscover my changed body was to explore the idea of the body and its relationship to the mind in a way no night class, self-help book, or therapist could. My body may have been capable of less, but virtually all of what it could do was suddenly charged with meaning. This feeling was the hardest to translate to the outside, where people wanted to believe that I must have to paint things in this way to keep from killing myself. The common, tiresome sentiment, "You are dealing with things so well," offered by nearly everyone carried this implication.

I was "dealing" with nothing. I was inside an experience that felt universally human. There was nothing odd about what I was doing . . . there was nothing worth staring at. I was just reacting to each physical, human problem and solving it with the materials at hand. It was this that looked odd to other people. To me, it was the one thing that wasn't odd, the very thing that kept my sanity in place. What was different was that the path was not so well-worn. The future seemed like an adventure on some frontier of physical possibilities. Each problem—getting up, rolling over, balancing in a chair, getting from here to there—needed a new solution. I was physically an infant endowed with the mind of an adult. I stared at my own numb feet with the wonder of a baby staring at the clasping and unclasping of its own hand. Solving each problem offered a personal authorship to experience that had never before seemed possible.

To people on the outside it was all a mechanism, a trick for avoiding the cruelty that had caused my accident, an unfairness that was horrible and hopeless and might reach out suddenly and grab others like them. To the outside, life in a wheelchair was life minus legs, minus dignity, minus dreams. It began to have meaning by adopting the code of denial, plus depression, plus anger, which equals acceptance. The dignity of human existence was restored according to this code only after one denied what was happening, got angry, got depressed, and then saw the light.

But from the inside, trauma did not appear to need any additional meaning, it made sense on its own, and trauma did not seem quite so unusual or unexpected. Far from a digression in the stream of existence, trauma intensified existence, bringing forth elements of experience too easily clouded over by the seductive predictability of day-to-day, so-called "normal" life.

From the beginning, disability taught that life could be reinvented. In fact, such an outlook was required. The physical dimensions of life could be created, like poetry; they were not imposed by some celestial landlord. Life was more than renting some protoplasm to walk around in. It was more than being a winner or a loser. To have invented a way to move about without legs was to invent walking. This was a task reserved for gods, and to perform it was deeply satisfying. None of that was apparent to the people who stared. To them, I was just in a wheelchair. To me, I was inventing a new life. To them, I was getting by in dealing with my predicament. To them, I was standing on a ledge and not jumping off. To me, I was climbing up to get a better view. There was no place to jump off. Whenever I look down, I can see my feet. They're along for the ride. There's no reason to be afraid.

Some stops on the road back to this mythical "normal" life were better left off the itinerary. There were experiences, I discovered, that did not really need to be reinvented. The addition of a wheelchair only made them worse or pointless, like trying to water-ski on wheels, only to drown, or rolling across a bed of hot coals with the idea of attaining some Buddhist state of self-awareness and getting four flat tires instead. There were others.

When I left the hospital with my red wheelchair and my blue van, Claudette was finishing her last year in high school. She came from a big family. Claudette and two of her nine sisters had gone to the public high school, and all of us were friends. Her parents had a huge house near the school and a cottage on Lake Michigan. They spent much of the summer at the cottage with the little kids, leaving the large three-story house unoccupied for weeks at a time.

I drove over for a visit late one afternoon. There were three or four steps into the house. I parked my blue van in the driveway and let the lift down. "You can just leave it down like that if you want," Claudette suggested. Parking the van with the side lift down completely blocked the driveway. "Don't worry," she said, "My parents won't be back from the cottage until tomorrow."

Before the accident, if I had been sneaking over to Claudette's house the neighbors would have shook their heads and raised their eyes at the unsupervised girl in the house with the older guy hanging around. But with the wheelchair and the fancy looking high-tech lift, the neighborhood began to view my visit as something of a humanitarian mission. Now they shook their heads and raised their eyes at the boy struck down in his prime. When Claudette had trouble lifting my chair up the four steps leading into the kitchen, the man next door stopped mowing his lawn and came over to help. "I read about you in the paper," he said sadly. "It looks like you're doing just fine, though. Think you'll ever walk again?"

"No," I said, and then added: "Thank you for helping. It's okay, really." This only made him shake his head more. I had never had such a humbling effect on adults before. I thought of asking him if he could spare twenty bucks. I didn't know how Claudette and I were fixed for cash. I looked at her and concluded that this would be a long evening. "I think it's great how you're just going on with your life like this," he said. I wondered if Claudette's parents would approve of how I planned to get on with their daughter's life that evening.

It was as much her idea as mine to have the house to ourselves, but there had never been a wheelchair in Claudette's house before. To get me in and out of the rooms, we moved all of the furniture. We produced a floor plan that was accessible by moving the couches, lamps, and chairs in all of the rooms. Before long, the house looked as though it had been attacked by a small plow. There was a problem with the TV. There was one in the basement, and one in Claudette's room upstairs. The only television on the main floor was in Claudette's parents' master bedroom.

In a Catholic family of thirteen kids, Mom and Dad's room was something of an inner sanctum that under normal conditions teenagers would not even want to visit. But these were not normal circumstances. Claudette and I were remaking the world to accommodate a new reality. We barged in. We moved the bed. We moved the TV. We moved the stereo from the living room into the bedroom. We moved a dresser. Her dad's tobacco pipes were on a table next to the bed; there was no couch. "We can use the bed as a couch," she said. Before the end of the evening we would use the bed, the TV, the liquor cabinet, and for smoking marijuana, Dad's tobacco pipes.

Well into a second tall vodka and grapefruit juice I needed to visit the bathroom. No amount of rearranging would make the door wide enough. But when we decided that I might just use the now-empty vodka bottle next to the bed, I realized that I had no catheter with me. Before the accident it was always a challenge for me to hold on to my car keys; now, having to remember to bring a catheter with me at all times pushed my mind to the limit. Even though being able to take a whiz was far more physiologically crucial than remembering my car keys, the fact that there was no more sensation in my car keys than there was in my bladder meant that the catheter was just as easy to forget.

Soon it was an emergency. Two teenagers stuck in an abandoned house with no catheter and one teenager filling up fast. I called the nearby hospital and explained that I was at a friend's house and had forgotten a catheter and could I send my friend to pick one up? "Do you have a prescription?" the voice on the other end of the line asked. Were there young people out there who recklessly used catheters without a doctor's supervision? "Can't you just sell me a catheter? I promise I won't overdose. If you have it ready soon, perhaps I won't explode. This is an emergency, and could you throw in a tube of KY jelly?"

Claudette had to take my driver's license and fill out a number of forms to prove that she wasn't just taking catheters for some nonmedical reason. It required an act of Congress for me to take a whiz. She returned after about an hour. I filled the vodka bottle. We instantly forgot about any emergency. Since I couldn't move, we brought everything we needed into the room. We removed our clothes, and climbed into her parents' bed with an assortment of snacks and musical instruments. In no time the room looked as though we had been living there for weeks. Before we fell off to sleep she told me to remind her to get up early. "My mom is supposed to come home at about nine A.M." I watched her set the alarm for six.

When I opened my eyes, the sun was shining through the yellow contents of the vodka bottle. I heard voices in the background. I blinked and looked around me. The place where Claudette's parents had conceived her twelve siblings looked like a room in a transient hotel where a Mafia hit had gone down. I looked for my clothes. Claudette came into the room in a robe. Her face was stricken with terror. "My mother is out there. The alarm was set. I didn't want this. I don't know what to do. I think that I'm not . . ." Her voice trailed off.

The next-door neighbor had helped me into the house the day before. I wasn't going to get his help now. I put on my pants and thought of all the furniture Claudette and I had moved the night before. I knew there was a path for me to get out of the house, but there were still the stairs at the door. Claudette had been sent upstairs to her room. I had no idea how I was going to get out of that house. The only person I was sure was in the house besides Claudette was her mother who, aside from being the absolute monarch in her house of thirteen kids, ran the largest antiabortion group in the whole state. She was a public figure, and there was a blue van with a wheelchair lift blocking her driveway and a red wheelchair in her bedroom. I wondered what her position on mercy killing was. The only help she was going to give me in getting out of her house was to supply a pine box after murdering me.

In the end, Claudette's oldest brother, Jimmy, a junior high school student, helped me out of the house. As I rolled through the kitchen with my shoes in my lap, Claudette's mom could be seen in the shadows, clutching her seven-year-old daughter who I later learned had discovered Claudette and me in her parents' bedroom. A little voice said, "Maybe Claudette was just trying to help him, Mommy." The voice was answered with a severe "We'll talk later, honey."

The agonizing pace of my departure made the whole event a thousand times worse than it would otherwise have been. One of the tables in the kitchen that had been moved the night before had been put back, and it now blocked me on the way out. I didn't dare try to push it and risk scratching it, so I stopped in front of it, completely helpless. I felt like drooling in order to complete the picture. "Move the table, James," his mother commanded. "I'll put it back. Just get him out of here."

I started to open my mouth and say that I was sorry when Jimmy leaned down close to my ear and whispered, "Don't say anything. She's about to blow." I kept quiet. I also resisted the urge to suggest how Jimmy might easily lower me down the steps. I felt so worthless that I would have been happy if he'd just thrown me into the driveway. He bounced me down, and the shoes in my lap flew off into the bushes. There were a few more agonizing moments while he retrieved them from the shrubbery. I rolled over to my van and on to the lift. The operation of the lift, as usual, drew a crowd of neighborhood kids who stood and gawked. From inside the house the voice of Claudette's younger sister said, "Mommy, can I watch him work the van?" Even the guy next door came out and commented, "You ought to put one of those on the house." Right. The little kids all clapped as the sliding door of the van closed like the automatic hatch on a spaceship. I was a guy in a van, but it felt more like the trench coat of the dirty old man on the corner who led the little youngsters astray.

I drove home to my parents' house. There were just a few more weeks before I would return to school and the world outside my family and the town where I had gone to high school. My mother watched me emerge from the van and detected some slight unease on her son's face. "Where have you been?" she asked. "I stayed over at a friend's house." I rolled up to the house. "You left your catheters here, you know. Didn't you have some problems?" I had completely forgotten about that little overnight crisis. "I got some from the hospital," I remarked, hazily recalling the nonprescription midnight catheter run. "You know, honey," my mother began, "if you had just called, I would have brought you a catheter." She was trying to be helpful. Having Mom show up with a catheter and a tube of KY jelly would, no doubt, have given me some of the same psychological scars that Claudette was now dealing with.

"That's okay, everything turned out all right."

My mother's reaction to the accident had been perfectly natural. She wanted to do everything before I did it. As a mother, the idea that I was having an experience that she could not conceive of was the most troubling part of all. For the first time, it made her question the quality of her advice, which only encouraged her to offer more advice on subjects that she would never have spoken openly about before the accident. She would go to the library and check out every book she could find on the subject of wheelchairs and the people who had used them. She was cramming for an exam to become an instant amateur neurologist, disability activist, and paramedic.

She looked for biographies of FDR. There wasn't much to read on the subject. The books about FDR rarely mentioned the fact that he couldn't walk. Most of the other wheelchair-related stories she could find were schmaltzy heroic fables short on detail, while the more clinical papers were technical discussions of lobster nerve tissue and the spinal cords of rats.

My mother did send away for a paperback book of crip sex, published by a crip-sex project at the University of Minnesota. It showed explicit pictures of couples in varying positions. It looked like something the security guard at my hospital could have published if he had thought to carry a Polaroid with a flash around with him. At least his book might have had the naughty feel of normalcy rather than the wooden wit of a medical textbook. These pictures were accompanied by steamy captions that described how "the presence of catheters need not impede the act of copulation; here the catheter is clamped off and folded back out of the way." This book could have been called "The Joy of Clamps": two totally paralyzed people lie side by side unable to do much of anything to each other, so they explain to therapists all of the lurid things they wanted to do to each other. This was a precursor to phone sex.

If I resisted the psychological profiles and jargon of therapy, my mother, if anything, embraced them. If the hospital had printed up little bar graphs to measure how she was doing, she would have hung one on the door of our house for all to see. My parents got lots of unsolicited advice. One of the therapists mentioned to my parents that I would lose all of my friends now that I was paralyzed. I could always tell when some neighbor or hospital staff person had nailed my mother with one of these comments or theories about the dubiousness of my future life because she would arrive with flowers and begin scouring the room with a broom and toothbrush. "Mom . . . what's up?" "Oh, nothing . . ." She would begin, and then allude to what she had been told with an oblique question, "Honey, how good are your friends? Maybe you should think about getting some new ones."

"Mom, who have you been talking to?" And it would all come out in a tearful rush. It would generally take a day of discussion to repair the damage from one mention of suicide or amputation. Some things will never go away. There was the time I sold my ten-speed bicycle. If I could see few things clearly looking into the future, one of them was that I would have limited need for a state-of-the-art ten-speed bicycle. There are all kinds of temptations to modify or adapt things from a walking life so as not to let go of them in a world of wheelchairs. Bicycles are not one of the things that translate from one world to the other. Adapting my ten-speed Fuji seemed to miss the point of both bicycling and wheelchairing. I did not need another wheelchair.

For a boy in a wheelchair to try to sell a ten-speed bicycle, even if it was in perfect condition, to someone not in a chair was a sales challenge I hadn't anticipated. People immediately assumed that I was in the wheelchair because of the bicycle. "No," I would say, "I am selling the bicycle because I am in the wheelchair." This would strike people as far too poignant a circumstance to simply proceed with a sale. They would look at me, look at the bike and get this faraway look in their eyes, and say they would call later. Either they couldn't bring themselves to buy a bicycle from a cripple, or they thought the Fuji must be jinxed. It was like buying a parachute from a blind person who said, "Packed it myself. Never ever had a problem before."

My mother took most of the calls from people who answered the ad. She was relieved each time a prospective buyer declined, or failed to call back after inspecting the bike. She hated the walking people who came to look at her paraplegic son's formerly prized possession. She secretly wanted to chase them all away with a broom.

I finally sold the bike to a high school friend who knew me well enough not to be maudlin about the whole thing, and who knew that the bike was in perfect shape. My mother sat quietly on the front steps of our house as I explained the features and suggested a test ride. The buyer took a couple of tight turns and raced up the hill and around the block. He arrived back smiling and anxious to close the deal. I took the money, wished him well, and watched him ride away without a thought. I counted the money and imagined what new stereo component I was going to add to the gluttony of audio equipment already in my room. I looked up to see my mother sobbing on the front steps.

"What's wrong?"

"I just was remembering how much fun you used to have riding your bicycle and I was watching just now . . ."

Her voice trailed off into a face that was equal parts hurt and anger. It was as though the boy who had purchased the bicycle was stealing it in broad daylight. His ability to ride was the consequence of some monstrous crime that had deprived her son of the same ability. She watched him ride away, and wanted to stop him as though he had snatched a purse.

"Hey, Mom. It's okay. I can't ride it. Someone should."

I gazed at my mother from the other side of an irrevocable experience. The gulf was wide and unexpected. It had only been a few weeks since I had been riding my bicycle. Now I was selling it as a useless artifact from a previous life, as outmoded as a second-grade lunch box was to a college student. I had become a different person. Below the surface, my most basic physical expectations had shifted as an earthquake shuffles plates of stone. Clearly, I had loved riding my bicycle. Somewhere inside I missed it. But where? I now responded to a profoundly different set of physical rules. They were rules that even I did not yet know.

My mother missed seeing me walk. Did I really not miss walking? Perhaps I was in shock. Some kind of mental defense mechanism was at work, keeping me from physically missing what I no longer had, a kind of clearing-out process to make space for the new. My mother's feelings were far deeper. She had been introduced to the idea of a loved one never walking far earlier than I had. I didn't understand it at the time, but she had been robbed of her younger brother. He was the playmate she never had, the younger sibling she could never talk to as a child. Her brother Peter had never really walked by himself, never talked.

When the young man rode away on my bike, in my mother's eyes he was an accomplice to a very old crime. To this day, in my mother's eyes, that crime is unsolved.

I could neither explain why I did not cry when I sold my bike, nor comfort my mother's tears at seeing me sell it. In her eyes, she saw someone else when she looked at me. Her son was not the person in the wheelchair. Where was he? What had I done with him? It was much easier for me to discard the image of me walking because I had an image to replace it with. But she could not give up the old picture so readily. She did not reject me, but rather the idea that the world is subject to such change. I could no longer doubt it. I looked up the street, waved my hand, and in a soft voice half-jokingly said, "'Bye, bike. 'Bye, bike." Laughing through tears, she finally said, "Being a mother is worse than being in a wheelchair."

To this day my mother still gets the teary lost-bicycle look. She still has moments when she claims to wonder if I will just stand up and walk over to her again. The thought is as absurd to me as it is real to her. The waves from the original splash of the pebble continue to move slowly outward from the moment of my accident like faint aftershocks from the big bang that started time. Physicists claim that those aftershocks are still detectable on the very edge of our capacity to measure our world. From below the surface I see those waves only dimly, as a fish might theorize about a cloud passing briefly in front of the sun in a sky it has never seen.

Formulae for change and grief and trauma efface the possibility that we each might discover our own way through difficulty, and by doing so reclaim our own lives from the oppressive forces that tell us who we are and what we should be from the moment we are aware. Change arrives for each soul in its own way, devoid of pattern. Each person confronts trauma as though it has never before happened. It is this which allows the mind and body to fashion a solution unique and appropriate to the identity of a person. If the shock of that change, like the death of a loved one or the loss of one's legs, is a fork in the road, it is a monogrammed fork.

When my mother gets that sad look, I take my hand, wave up an imaginary street, and whisper to her, "'Bye, bike. 'Bye, bike." It always gets a laugh. This is the quiet memorial to an idea of normal that my mother was raised with and forced to believe in. I, too, was raised with this idea. It was what I left behind in a burning car on a road in Pennsylvania.

Fear of Bees

*P*eople often ask me what I would prefer to be called. Do they think I have an answer?

I'm a crip for life. I cannot walk. I have "lost the use of my legs." I am paralyzed from the waist down. I use a wheelchair. I am wheelchair-bound. I am confined to a wheelchair. I am a paraplegic. I require "special assistance for boarding." I am a gimp, crip, physically challenged, differently abled, paralyzed. I am a T-5 para. I am sick. I am well. I have a T4–6 incomplete dural lesion, a spinal cord injury, a broken back, "broken legs" to Indian cabbies in New York who always ask, "What happened to your legs, Mister?"

I have a spastic bladder, pneumatic tires, air in all four of my tires. Solid wheelchair tires are for hospitals and weenies. No self-respecting crip would be caught dead in one. I use a catheter to take a whiz. I require no leg bag. That's for the really disabled. I have no van with a wheelchair lift anymore. Those are for the really disabled, and thank God I'm not one of them. I need no motor on my wheelchair. Those are for the really disabled, and I am definitely not one of those. From mid-chest down I have no sensation. I am numb all the way to my toes.

I know what they're all thinking. My dick doesn't work. The truth? My dick works sometimes. My dick works without fail. I have two dicks. I have totally accepted my sexuality. I have massive problems with my sexuality. Actually, there is no problem with sexuality. It's just not a problem. I think we can just drop this subject of sexuality because it's not an issue. Not at all. The truth? I had a little problem there in the beginning, then I learned how to compensate. Now everything is fine. It's actually better than fine. To be perfectly honest, I am the sexual version of crack. There are whole clinics set up for people who became addicted to sleeping with me. All right, the truth? Not so fast.

You do not have to feel guilty for causing my situation even though your great-great-grandparents may have been slave owners. You do have to feel guilty and fawning and contrite if I ever catch you using a wheel-chair stall in an airport men's room or parking in a disabled space. I feel as though I caused my situation and deserve to be cast from society, on which I am a burden. I am a poster boy demanding a handout. I am the 800 number you didn't call to donate money. I am the drum major in Sally Struther's parade of wretches. I watch the muscular dystrophy telethon every year without fail. I would like to have Jerry Lewis sliced thinly and packed away in Jeffrey Dahmer's freezer. I am not responsible for my situation and roll around with a chip on my shoulder ready to lash out at and assault any person making my life difficult, preferably with a deadly weapon.

I have unlimited amounts of "courage," which is evident to everyone but myself and other crips. I get around in a wheelchair. I am a wheel-chair "racer." I am just rolling to work. I am in denial. I have accepted my disability and have discovered within myself a sublime reservoir of truth. I can't accept my disability, and the only truth I am aware of is that my life is shit and that everyone is making it worse. I am a former food stamp recipient. I am in the 35 percent tax bracket. I am part of the disability rights movement. I am a sell-out wannabe TV star media scumbag who has turned his broken back on other crips.

I am grateful for the Americans with Disabilities Act, which has her-alded a new era of civil rights in this country. I think the Americans with Disabilities Act is the most useless, empty, unenforceable law of the last quarter-century. It ranks up there as one of the most pansy-assed ex-cuses for a White House news conference in U.S. history. I think that the disabled community is a tough, uncompromising coalition of activists. I think the disabled community is a back-biting assembly of noisy, mutu-ally suspicious clowns who would eagerly sell out any revolution just to appear on a telethon, or in the White House Rose Garden, or in a Levis' commercial.

I cannot reach the cornflakes in my cupboard. I cannot do a handstand. I cannot use most revolving doors. I cannot rollerblade. Bowling is more of a waste of time than it used to be. (One of the chief advantages of being in a wheelchair is always having an excuse not to go bowling, even though I do miss the shoes.) I'm telling you these things because I want us to share, and for you to understand my experiences and then, together, bridge the gulf between us. I want you all to leave me alone.

I'm a guy in a chair, crip for life. Everything you think about me is right. Everything you think is wrong.

What is "normal" but another stereotype, no different than "angry black man," "Asian math genius," "welfare mother," or "gay man with a lisp"? Each stereotype thrives in direct proportion to the distance from each class of persons it claims to describe. Get close to the real people and these pretend images begin to break up, but they don't go easily. As each stereotype breaks down, it reveals a pattern of wrongs. Losing a stereotype is about being wrong retroactively. For a person to confront such assumptions they must admit an open-ended wrong for as long as those assumptions have lived inside them. There is the temptation to hold on to why you believed in stereotypes. "I was told gays were like that as a child." "I never knew many blacks, and that's what my parents believed about them." "I was once frightened and disgusted by a person in a wheelchair." To relinquish a stereotype is to lose face by giving up a mask.

We trade in masks in America. Especially in politics. Politicians love to talk about the "American people" and what they allegedly want or don't want. But who are they, really? The America evoked most often today by politicians and pundits is a closet full of masks denoting race, nationality, and a host of other characteristics. America's definitive social unit of measurement is no longer the family, nor is it the extended family. On the other end of the scale, it is not the village or hamlet, neighborhood or block, city, state, or region. I grew up in America at a time when its logo was the racially balanced commercial image of four or five children, one black, white, Asian, female, and disabled (optional) romping in an idyllic, utopian, and quite nonexistent playground.

You can still occasionally see this image in the children's fashion supplement to *The New York Times Magazine*. These are happy measuring sticks of a demographic formula, perfect faces of social equilibrium to distract from the fact that each child is usually clad in the designer fabric hard currency equivalent of the GNP of Guyana or Cameroon. In the eighties the fashion chain Benetton crossed the old American emblem with the UN General Assembly and produced its own utopian logo of a meticulously integrated, multiracial youth army, no disabled (not optional).

We once portrayed these idealized young people as seeds of a racially harmonious society we dreamed would come. Now those children shout down the long narrow lenses of music video cameras, or gun each other down on the streets. Our communities have become multiracial, just as the dream foretold. But they are not utopias. Integration is no guarantee of harmony. It is what most of the world has known since the end of World War Two. It is this nation's last, cruel lesson of the twentieth century.

Today, if one measures America at all, it is in audience units. America is the union of all the multiracial groups of ostensibly "normal" people, ranging from submissive and polite to angry and aggressive, who can be seated in a television studio in front of a talk-show host. There they stare at, and react to, the famous hosts, the famous guests, or anyone else on stage. Mad people, older people, teenagers, victims, predators, all of the species in America's great political aviary pass in front of the audience. America turns its thumbs up or down, then goes to a commercial break. There is no verdict. There is just the din of many verdicts. As the camera scans the audience, the people who can be anticipated to have a distinct opinion, or more likely, an outrage, are handed the microphone. "Why don't you just leave him if he beats you?" "It's people like you skinheads who spread hate in this country." America punctuates each of these outraged questions and challenges with applause, jeers, and shouts.

I caught the delivery of verdicts from one such clump of Americana between commercial breaks on the "Oprah Winfrey" show some time after my accident. I had always thought of myself as a face in the audience. On this show I saw myself on the stage with a group of four married couples, each with a disabled partner. Three of the couples contained a partner in a wheelchair; the other was a blind woman and her sighted husband. The theme of the show that day was something like "One of them is fine and the other one is defective. How do they manage?" The audience applauded with an enthusiasm they reserved for First Ladies, and Oprah herself had that deep, breathy voice that television talk-show hosts reserve for the inspirational subjects—the serious themes that justify all of those celebrity interviews and fluff. Here, "Crips and Their Spouses" was gripping television.

The couples represented an odd composite of the crip population. This was Oprah's idea of the crips next door, and that next door, in this case, was not necessarily the state institution. Just your average run-of-the-mill crip and spouse combo package. There were no Vietnam vets on this panel, no wheelchair jocks, no quadriplegics, no gunshot ghetto homies with their stripped-down Quickie ultra-lights, and, of course, they had neglected to call me.

Three of the couples might as well have had lamp shades on their heads. They were nonthreatening, overweight, jolly, well-adjusted types with a hint of acne, all wearing loud, baggy shirts. These are the people the audience was used to giving a wide berth on the bus and then ignoring. One of the women was in a dented, ill-fitting wheelchair with gray hospital wheels. They said things like, "Hey, Oprah, it just takes more planning. It's no big deal." They laughed a lot. The audience imagined working near one of these people; it did not have to imagine being one.

One of the couples was different; a thin guy in a wheelchair and his pretty, young, unparalyzed wife. They had dated in college before his "accident." They were neatly dressed and clearly held the most fascination for the audience members. "How difficult was it for you after his accident?" Oprah addressed herself to the young woman when she wanted to know some detail. No, she had never thought of breaking up with him after the accident. "It's no different than anything else that might make a relationship difficult." The audience began to applaud while Oprah nodded. On their faces was a kind of sentimental approval. The audience wanted her to know that she could have left him . . . she would have had the perfect excuse . . . no jury would have convicted, certainly not in that audience. She seemed slightly sensitive about this point because she insisted again that she had not thought of breaking up the relationship, and that it really was just another thing, like a joint checking account, for a couple to deal with.

The joint checking account line really got them. "I just want to say that I think you are such an inspiration to us all," an audience member addressed the panel. It didn't really matter what the panelists said, especially the young couple. It only mattered what the audience thought about the young man's plight and his courageous girlfriend. It was far more important to assume that he was broken, that she was tied to him now selflessly, and that they would make the best of things. "Yes, Oprah; we manage just fine," she said in her small voice with her husband's nodding assent. Oprah addressed the young man once. "You must be so happy to have someone like Amy," or whatever her name was.

I was rooting for these folks to hold their own. Though I was just a little older, I could tell that I had logged lots more wheelchair time than the young guy on TV. I could feel what was coming. I saw the audience greedily looking them up and down. I saw what we were supposed to think about them. He: strong, brave, and struck down in his youth. She:

stronger and braver for spending her youth with him. On their faces you could see that the conditions of this public execution were just beginning to dawn on them.

But it was just Oprah. It was all in good fun. I was making too much of a television talk show. They weren't forced to go out onto that stage. A voice inside said, "If you weren't so angry and dysfunctional, John, maybe you would be invited to go on 'Oprah' too."

It didn't take long for Oprah to deliver. "So there's one thing I want to know." She looks directly at the young girl as the hungry crowd buzzes with anticipation. Oh, my god, she's going to ask. Like a car accident in the movies, the world slows down at this point. I can see the smile freeze on the face of the young woman. The crowd goes wild. The camera cuts away to Oprah.

"What I want to know is . . ."

She pauses for sincerity. The crowd is totally with her. The woman must know what's about to happen. She must have been asked a million times. I wondered if the guy knew. The guy probably had no idea. Or maybe it was a condition for going on the show. I'm screaming at the TV now: "Tell her it's none of her damn business. We're counting on you out here. Tell Oprah to stuff it!"

Oprah delivers.

"Amy, can he do it?"

Loud gasp from the crowd. I imagine that it must have sounded this way when Sydney Carton's head was lopped off in *A Tale of Two Cities*. The camera immediately cuts to the woman's face, which has blushed a deep red. She tries something of a laugh, glances at her husband, who is out of the shot. Eventually, when the noise dies down, she says, "Yes, he can, Oprah." She giggles.

The camera pulls wide, and the two onstage seem very small. He takes her hand for comfort. The crowd bursts into applause. Even the other crips on stage are applauding. He withdraws his hand, as though it had been placed in hot oil. The camera cuts back to Oprah, who is nodding to the crowd half-heartedly, trying to get them to stop clapping. She looks somewhere between a very satisfied Perry Mason and a champion mud wrestler. Now we know what the show was really about. It wasn't just Oprah; the whole crowd seemed to care only about this. The oddest thing was that after the question and the embarrassed answer the audience seemed to think they now knew how "it" was done. What did they know? They knew that they had the guts to ask this question; they didn't really care about the answer.

Oprah, here's something I have always wanted to know. Do black guys really have giant dicks? The angry voice yelled at the television and then turned it off. Is that what people think when they stare? What constitutes "doing it"? There was no answer for them. There was no answer for me. Questions like these were the weapon. They need no real answer and apparently are always loaded in the chambers of people's curiosity. Stereotypes bring forth righteous anger and deep humiliation. At the same time, they are completely understandable, like an old piece of furniture you have walked by every day of your life.

Once on a very hot day on the Washington, D.C., subway a woman sat looking at me for a long time. She was smiling. I suspected that she knew about me from the radio, that she had seen some picture of me somewhere. I am rarely recognized in public, but it was the only plausible explanation for why she kept watching me with a look of some recognition. Eventually she walked up to me when the train stopped, said hello, then proceeded in a very serious voice.

"Your legs seem to be normal."

"They are normal, I just can't move them."

"Right, I know that. I mean, I can see that you are paralyzed." I was beginning to wonder where she was going with this. "Why aren't you shriveled up more?" she asked, as though she was inquiring about the time of day. "I notice that your legs aren't shrunken and all shriveled up. Why is that?" I was wearing shorts. She looked at my legs as though she was pricing kebab at the market. "I mean, I thought paralyzed legs got all shriveled up after a while. Were you just injured recently?"

"Uh . . . twelve years ago."

This was a line of questioning I was unprepared for. I continued to smile and listen. I wondered under what circumstances I would ever roll up to a perfect stranger and ask the question, "Why aren't you shriveled up more?" I really didn't have an answer for her. I said something like I try to stay active, eat plenty of salads, vitamins.

She said she knew people in wheelchairs who were much more shriveled up. I can only assume that the expression on my face was one of extreme annoyance and skepticism. Her reaction was to redouble her efforts to convince me that she had some degree of expertise in these matters. She started to click off her credentials. She had worked for the outpatient clinic at a local hospital. She had been responsible for wheelchair access at some community women's health film festival, and she was once roommates with a woman who signed for the hearing impaired. I should accept her as a progressive, hip, knowledgeable person where disability was concerned, and acknowledge her theories on shriveled muscles.

I wondered if these disabled people she claimed to know were close friends and if that's what she called them, her "shriveled-up" friends. This was a whole constituency I had failed to encounter. I looked around the train and wondered if everyone who saw me in shorts was thinking, What's this guy trying to prove by not being more shriveled up?

In quite another context, I was once on the other end of this transaction. I was interviewing African musician Hugh Masekele and critic Greg Tate on the radio around the time Nelson Mandela was released from a South African prison. It was a moment of dramatic change, and I wanted to know if American blacks and black South Africans would become closer now, even to the point of some musicians feeling free to visit South Africa to perform. I can recall that Tate smiled and told me something to the effect that black Africans and black Americans are as close as they need to be and, in any case, were not interested in performing some sentimental act of reunion for the benefit of whites in the media. In my follow-up I tried to reassure him that this was NPR and that I wasn't one of those insensitive journalists who was ignorant about the black struggle. He was aggressively unmoved. "We don't need white people to tell us when it's time to go home to Africa." No amount of cajoling him into accepting that I was progressive and hip was going to change that point. It was just as true that events in South Africa would bring great changes in political outlook and identity for blacks on both continents, but we didn't get into any of that on the radio that night in 1990. Was there a correct answer or a correct question? Whatever lessons might been drawn from the encounter, it was a minor milestone in nationally broadcast awkwardness.

All stereotypes have some, albeit distorted, basis in fact. With the lady on the Washington, D.C., subway, I had to admit that I knew what she was talking about even if I had no shriveled-up friends, or if I was not prepared to admit that she was anything more than an ignorant boob. People in wheelchairs do lose muscle tone, and legs can become quite thin, especially in neuromuscular disease. My legs are intact even though they cannot be controlled by me. Their own muscles move around spastically. Because this movement happens fairly regularly, the muscles are exercised and therefore they retain their tone and shape. Discussing the clinical details of muscle-tone retention was one thing. I was just wondering how anyone could ask such questions of a perfect stranger.

"Hi. I notice that you have been out jogging, and I'm wondering if you are developing a red chafing rash along your groin right about now? I have a lot of chafed friends with groin rashes, and it looks to me as though your legs are not stiff. You are not holding them wide apart as though you're in pain, and I'm noticing that you are not grabbing at your underwear discreetly to ease your discomfort. Am I right in concluding that you are not experiencing a burning, itching sensation in your groin area at this moment?" Not everyone would want to call the police immediately if I rolled up and inquired about their groin discomfort, but I bet I wouldn't have any long conversations on this subject.

If I were not so haunted by these experiences I could simply dismiss each intrusive questioner as just another dangerous psychopath or ignorant clown. More often than not, the intrusions are humorous, and they usually contain nuggets of some elusive truth. Each encounter is a parable about the increasing distance we humans all hail from even as we are more closely packed together on this planet. Perhaps the correct answer to the woman on the train was to take a deep breath and calmly explain the details of my legs and muscles as I understood them. Yet to do so I would have had to admit that there was a category of shriveled-up people, and that I was not one of them. I would also have had to concede that it was perfectly permissible for her to walk up to me and say something outrageous when that was the last thing I believed.

In her question she was demanding that I acknowledge a relationship with her that I wasn't prepared to admit I had. At the very least, I did not realize that I was a part of her own confrontation with the experience of disability. I was a part of this woman's experience of disabled people. That experience was so powerful that she suspected I might be having it along with her. But I was not. "No, I am John! I am a person, not a wheelchair. You must deal with me as I think of myself." This was how I responded. I could dismiss her even though I completely understood what she was talking about.

Encounters with strangers who claimed the right to ask bizarre detailed questions about disability had long ago become common for me when, in 1993, a man boarded a commuter train in New York bound for Long Island. He opened fire on the passengers and killed seven people. The event was a headline for the people of New York City and part of the footnoted background noise of crime for much of the rest of the country. His murderous rampage was psychotic and horrific to be sure, yet trapped within the bloody savagery was a plaintive cry that someone acknowledge his relationship with the rest of the world. He surely had no cause to express that relationship in lead and gunpowder, but what was not reported about the LIRR killings, and which was reflected in extensive conversations with people of every race and occupation for weeks later, is that no one in 1993 was in the least surprised by the fact that a black man in America would be that angry, that he might be carrying a gun on a train, that he might look at the faces of the people around him with unreasoning hatred even though he did not know them.

We accept our masks so completely that we scarcely recognize the faces of the real people behind them, including our own. Getting beyond them requires a leap that people are rarely prepared to take. For me to accept why someone might have had their own preconceived notion about shriveled-up people in wheelchairs is to accept that it was somehow natural for crips to be considered diseased. For an African-American to enthusiastically accept a white person's celebration over seeing black Africans and black Americans coming together is for them to concede that slavery and apartheid were some brief natural mistakes of history and that all some white guys need to do is adjust the political control panel and everyone will be free to kiss and make up . . . preferably on "Oprah," "Donahue," or "Nightline."

Often these meetings of the mask end in anger or bitterness. It is much harder to use such encounters to inform. In order to convince you that another view is possible, I have to accept your degrading stereotype about wheelchairs for a moment. That is the one thing I have declared at the outset that I will not do. I can explain myself to the drivers on the road who honk or presume that I am lost, to the woman inspecting me to see if my legs are shriveled up, or I can dismiss them angrily. It is their choice to be curious or dogmatic. It is my choice to inform or punish.

It is the rare encounter in which both parties leave feeling that they know more about the other. Usually, the stereotype remains real along with the accumulated bits of anger from each face-off. In America in this half-century, we can claim to have made the effort to integrate our communities and to learn more about the diversity within them. But along with these changes it has also become clear that we, in America, are all experiencing this slow accumulation of anger. The tide rises, droplets at a time. Each failed encounter is a capillary tied off, raising the pressure to the heart and denying oxygen to the brain. It has been this way for a long time. It gets harder to laugh at all of this, but it is still possible.

Once a flight attendant noted how adept I seemed to be in getting on planes. She had seen me move from my wheelchair to a small movable seat, to be rolled down the narrow aisle of the airliner; then she saw me move with quick, confident arm motions into the passenger seat.

"You really don't let anything stop you, do you? I saw you get on that plane and you just didn't stop at all. I just think that is great."

"I travel a lot."

"I guess you are the first handicapped person I have ever seen up close. Have you ever thought of killing yourself?"

I wondered if this question appeared in this flight attendant's official training manual under the heading of "Handicapped Patrons: Suggested Conversation Starters."

"Do you ask lots of people on your airline if they think of suicide?"

"Oh, goodness no, that would be crazy. I was just wondering about you because you get around so well that you must have really done a lot of praying to get this great attitude."

My great attitude was eroding fast. There was nothing to do but say something like, "Well, you know, I just think that if you take the energy to do things instead of just staring into space, life can be pretty interesting." Brilliant, John. No wonder you can't get on "Oprah." I was hoping that she would just take my word about not committing suicide during the flight and leave the pilot, standing nearby, out of this conversation when she came out with her other big question.

"Can you, I mean, can your body, I mean are you able to do it with a woman?"

This line did not sound like one from the manual. Some business-class passengers had gotten up from their seats and were slowly walking up toward the lavatory. She continued to look at me, expecting an answer. I could say yes and giggle like on "Oprah"; I could take some time and clinically explain the situation and perhaps gain the attention of the business-class passengers, or we could exchange phone numbers. But what is the real correct answer?

"Paralyzed from the waist down" describes so little of the experience of a spinal-cord injury that most crips use it as a kind of shorthand joke. In my case I am paralyzed from the nipples down. When people learn of this they are shocked to realize that there is no international checkpoint at the waist. It is an arbitrary demarcation. In actual fact, relatively few people are paralyzed from the waist down. Everyone has their particular line separating sensation from numbness. Each line of separation is invisible to the eye. In some people the aspects of temperature and pressure and muscle control are separate. Some spinal-cord-injured people can feel pressure but not temperature in some parts of their body, and vice versa. There are people with almost total sensation but with no motor control . . . a partially damaged fiber-optic cable . . .

picture but no sound . . . bad reception. All of these metaphors aid understanding, but none is precise. The trace of each paraplegic and quadriplegic's sensory border zone is as unique as a fingerprint. Each person has a different answer to the question: What does paralysis feel like?

Not being able to sense the rhythms of your body is to be cast off from the familiar. But the shock is in learning that nothing physical has really changed beneath the skin. Your body is your body whether you can feel it or not. There is actually no reason to believe that loss of feeling makes you any different from the same old bag of water and flesh that you have always known. The bag fills. The bag empties. Life goes on.

In sensation there is the illusion that we are complicit in the body's biology. It is sensation that lures humans into endowing their bodily processes with intent and intelligence. Sensation makes a heart "burn," puts butterflies in the stomach, and a frog in the throat. Sensation creates the little gatekeeper in the brain working the body's control panels. Sensation is the neural confirmation that the brain needs the body more than the other way around. In feelings, the brain is permitted to believe that it gets to vote on processes it has no part of. The body requires no brain to get most of its work done. The infuriating truth about a brain-dead person is that they are perfectly alive. The fact that they cannot have a conversation is a requirement only another brain would demand; the same brain would make no such demand of a pet fish and yet continue to feed and take care of it. When people no longer want their fish, they flush them down the toilet with no attendant scandal, or simply eat them with some nice steamed vegetables on the side. But there is no endless Kevorkianesque discussion of the "brain dead fish" and the necessity of removing its life support. You kill the fish, you kill the person. It's your call. The brain is capable of making such decisions. People make life and death decisions all the time. The brain wants more, though. It wants the world to act as though what has no brain is not alive. This is folly, and just a trifle arrogant.

The brain can neither explain life, nor explain it away. While consciousness is something of a mystery, it is not permitted to intervene in the mechanics of the body. The identity of limbs and organs is mechanical, and in the case of the large intestine and bladder, fluid mechanics. Loss of sensation reveals these mechanics.

A friend visited me in the hospital shortly after my accident, and as she sat on the bed next to me and we talked, I placed my hand on her leg, which was next to mine. I had assumed that it was my leg I was touching, but when I looked down and saw hers I realized that without sensation I could not tell the difference between my leg and someone else's. Her leg is not the same as mine. But because of an injury to my spinal cord, her leg and my leg felt the same to my hand, that is to say, numb. I recall with a hearty Protestant blush the times, and there have been many, when I have placed my hand on a leg under the bedsheets and while caressing its skin realized that it was my own leg, not that of a companion sleeping beside me. Guiltily, I withdrew my hand from my own leg which, truth be told, gets relatively little attention. To have been tricked by one's own body is unsettling. On the other hand, part of the attraction of touching someone else's leg, assuming they were not also paralyzed, is that it would respond to my touch. My own will not. It is the strangest sensation of all.

The spine is a knotted code of some evolutionary ladder. There, in a mysterious order, the functions of the body are laid out on a schematic. At the bottom is sensation for the feet, move upward and you encounter nerves for the muscles of the leg, the buttocks, hips, abdomen, chest, arms, and neck. In the fine print is another message. One of the lowest set of nerves just above the tailbone controls sensation of the bladder and genitals. Just above are the nerves of sensation for the muscles of the large intestines. The abdominal muscles fall silent one by one as you proceed up the vertebrae until about the fifth vertebra in the thorax.

At this point, there is an additional nerve connected to the genitals. It controls some involuntary functions. The toggle switches that open the bladder sphincter, that open the rectum, and that control orgasm are on this 220-volt nerve. The strictly voluntary nerves at the bottom can control things until certain physical limits are met. But when the limit is reached there is no more discussion. The higher nerve fires.

The childhood battle between release and anal retention takes place between the sacral vertebrae and the thoracic. The higher nerve always wins. Orgasm works in this way. Foreplay happens in the lower nerves, then at a perfect moment the higher nerve takes over and in men, at least, one decisive little sphincter opens like clockwork. An orgasm arrives with the rush of a train and the control of a free fall. It has nothing to do with sensation. Sensation is only the illusion of control. What we think of as advanced—our sensation—is on the bottom of the ladder.

The crucial functioning of these systems has to do with the loop between the voluntary nerves on the bottom of the spine and the involuntary nerves in the middle. If the loop is unbroken, then sphincters remain closed. If the loop is broken, then neither voluntary nor involuntary systems are available. Lower injuries between the base and the middle of the spine generally mean that while the body retains more muscle control, more use of legs and abdominals, it is incontinent, impotent, and incapable of having an orgasm. Injuries above the middle mean more severe paralysis in terms of pure muscle loss, but because the voluntary and involuntary nerves can talk to each other on what's left of the spinal cord, bladders stay closed and an orgasm is possible if difficult.

The effect of this curious neural ordering is to divide the wheelchair crips (males particularly) into jocks and sex gods. The lower injuries make all of the layups on the basketball courts . . . the higher injuries, the quadriplegics, get all of the dates. In my case the injury was in the middle. My bladder is spastic, which means it is closed until opened by a catheter. Sexual function is erratic, unpredictable, but orgasm and ejaculation are reliably achieved through some aggressive manual stimulation. Without sensation, though, making this happen can be frustrating. It is hard to know what I did right, or if it doesn't happen, what I did wrong.

There is a kind of harrowing ambiguity about a body without the familiar warning sensations associated with the control of bodily functions. The body is suddenly a saboteur. To be in public becomes a trip behind enemy lines with a time bomb taped quite literally to one's abdomen. To go out and have a large meal and a few drinks in public is a kind of intestinal roulette until one becomes fluent in decoding far subtler and more direct messages and warnings about what is going on in the body.

Much of the independence seen among spinal-cord-injured people today stems not from any newfound magnanimity on the part of society or a breakthrough in wheelchair technology, but from the development of plastic. During World War One the souls whose chest and spinal fractures could be stabilized could look forward to a short life of gradual kidney failure. After just a few weeks, the kidneys would back up or become infected from uncontrolled draining. Death would come within a year in most cases.

Plastic was a material that could be fashioned into tubes and inserted up into the bladder to empty it. It revolutionized the prognosis for the spinal-cord injuries in World War Two, and the victims of polio. More details buried inside the cold phrase, "paralyzed from the waist down." What inkling was there that an injury to the spine even involved the bladder? Bladder stuck shut . . . wait a minute. The nurse told me that I should be grateful that it was stuck shut and not stuck open. She was right.

It makes all the difference in the world if paralysis results in an uncontrolled bladder that is stuck in the open position versus an uncontrolled bladder stuck in the closed position. Mine is closed. It means that I will fill until emptied. But I must insert a tube inside just as the nurse did, every four hours or so for the rest of my life. Why some bladders are stuck open and others are stuck closed reveals some crucial details about the spinal cord, to say nothing of the laundromat.

Loss of control is a dark fear, particularly in America. Why we should so fear losing control in a world that we have no control over anymore is one of the central questions of American culture. The notions of control and power are themes of American policy. Going with the flow and becoming attentive to the subtleties of one's economy or politics are not themes of American policy anywhere in the world. The frustrations in our superpower identity, the frustrations of homelessness, bankruptcy, and incontinence are all facets of the same fear. People who lose control are deviants or failures. People who have control are heroes, role models, victors over adversity, people "with their shit together."

It is the keenest insight gained from a loss of sensation to discover that the icons of control over the body are illusions. For all its urgent tangibility, sensation is the illusion of control over the body rather than the mechanism for that control. Sensation in the body is more a curtain than a window. It hides more about the body than it purports to reveal. The nerves in the skin and muscles give you the "sense" that your limbs are extensions of the brain, which they most assuredly are not. Phantoms of pain and pleasure determine our actions, while the body's processes inexorably continue. Sensation is life's ultimate mask, at life's ultimate costume party: consciousness.

In demanding simple names for complex experiences, our society loses the precious details. A person asked to define the word paraplegic will undoubtedly remark that it is someone who has lost the use of his or her legs. The handicapped, the disabled, the confined to a wheelchair, the mobile in a wheelchair, the physically challenged, the mobility-impaired, the broken in half, the chronically stared at, the person with disability, the about to wet his pants, the intestinally challenged, the numb from the nipples down, the shrapnelly challenged, the amputee, the confined to a car wreck: all of these names could also accurately describe someone in a wheelchair, on a wheelchair, or with a wheelchair. The obsession with finding the right name leads us away from the unique. The whole is diminished by ignoring its parts.

My seven-year-old niece, Sarah, was once sitting on my lap, having long ago gotten used to Uncle John never walking. As a child whose notions of normal had not solidified in concrete, she was free to think far and wide about the implications of my physical condition. Much farther and wider than even I. She grabbed my thigh and looked into my eyes with a questioning, probing gaze that only a child can give. "Can you feel that, Uncle John?" she asked.

"No," I told her incredulous, shaking head. She moved her hands up on my legs and pounded with a force that she was convinced would have caused her own leg pain. The look in her eyes was exhilarating, as though she were on the edge of some experimental breakthrough. "Can you feel that, Uncle John?" She tried a fist out on her own thigh and winced. "Wow." She thought for a moment and then pinched a loose bit of skin above my left knee. "You feel nothing, Uncle John?" "Nothing, Sarah."

She was deep in thought, examining the implications of such a truth. She was satisfied that I had no sensation, but she still needed further elaboration. She suddenly burst out with a last question: "So if a bee stung you right here, Uncle John . . ." She pointed to a place on my thigh where one summer she had been stung. It was her ultimate test, her ultimate definition of pain. I shook my head. "Nothing, Sarah. Ten bees could sting me there."

She turned around on my lap. "Mommy, Uncle John can't even feel a bee stinging him on his leg." Her mom was occupied with making sandwiches or having a rare conversation with an adult. She had noted with some alarm Sarah's blows to my legs, wondering if her persistent daughter might continue the investigation with a fork or other sharp object. "That's right, Sarah. Uncle John can't feel anything on his legs, but it's not all right to hit him." Sarah was lost in thought until she said triumphantly, "Then you aren't afraid of bees."

In a future world where the thoughts of little girls can matter as much as those of presidents and generals, the fear of bees as a metaphor for spinal-cord injury might even be an appropriate topic for "Oprah." It would truly be an indication of the millennium if in supermarket parking lots in the twenty-first century the signs on the parking spaces in the front said: RESERVED FOR PEOPLE UNAFRAID OF BEES. If you need a name for me, call me John. If you want to know if I can "do it," perhaps that can be discreetly arranged. If you want to say one thing more about me, you may comfortably note that I am a person not afraid of bees.

Loose Screws

With a body no longer able to squish, squat, or slink into tight places, fitting into the physical world presented unexpected challenges. Round wheels tracked the earth's bumps and inclines with a thud and a lurch. The width and shape of a wheelchair is fixed, so it was no longer possible to squeeze past the rough edges and unpredictable dimensions of space. The world, so easily traveled on legs that could float over all the little chasms, catwalks, and scaffolds of physical existence, was suddenly strewn with boulders. My eyes could no longer judge security and stability in this new place. On wheels, what looked possible and safe quite often wasn't. I was a square peg in a black hole.

Miscalculations in a wheelchair meant collisions with people and things around me. These were as visible and disruptive as a tall semi wedged under a freeway overpass at rush hour. Every doorway, every restaurant entrance, every check-out line, every street corner was another physical cliffhanger. Was I rolling straight? Would I hit the magazine rack? Would I be able to get the person's attention in front of me without shouting? Would they just move out of the way, or would they insist on pushing me? Everywhere there was something or someone to crash into, an opportunity for someone to stare and conclude that I was lost, confused, escaped from the hospital, or in need of help.

The eyes might theorize about physical movement, but a newly paralyzed body learned a harsher truth and imparted it to a frightened and newly insecure mind. A wheelchair's pause at the edge of a tranquil riverbank could quickly crumble into unforgiving danger. Improperly judge the steep angle on a gravel incline, and suddenly the river's edge threatened to swallow a sliding wheelchair. A puddle too muddy, and wheels were rendered immovable by muck. I often played out these scenes a stone's throw from my parked and waiting van, which might as well have been in Anarctica for all the good it was to me in these situations.

In the fall of 1976 I returned to school, where I discovered this new topography on Chicago's sidewalks. Leg bones no longer dampened the vibrations of walking. It was my ribs and spine that vibrated like a loose deck of cards as each bump and pile of streetcorner gravel was absorbed into the metal of the chair and up through my back. These were not the smooth linoleum surfaces of malls and hospitals back home. Returning to roll on the very same South-Side Chicago streets and sidewalks that I had walked on just a few months before was as jarring as trading in sneakers for metal roller skates. Rolling made noise; it had no rhythm at first, and it took up the whole sidewalk. I could only stroll with my friends in single file. I was either behind them or in front of them. I could hear them talking but from my position I could rarely make out what they were saying.

I was paying more attention to the roadway, anyway. It was crucial to be aware of the curbs at each intersection. It was on the concrete lip of each of these curbs that the most gripping of my early physical dramas were played out. Sometimes there were ramps but more often there were the familiar old-style concrete slabs lining the sidewalk. If the curb was too high, I would go out into traffic and meet up with my friends at the next intersection. Lower curbs could be jumped, and when I insisted on doing this, all conversation stopped.

I would get a running start, tip my front wheels up just as I had learned to do in the hospital, and hurl myself over the curb. Usually this worked even if it wasn't the most graceful way to take a stroll. Many times there was not a happy ending. The crumbling curb surface, a slightly inclined sidewalk, or a poorly executed approach could all cause the chair to topple backward, or bounce and fall over sideways. Falling was a major trauma to the people who watched it happen and no amount of saying "I'm all right" would convince them otherwise. To me, falling was just embarrassing. To others, it looked like a medical emergency.

Once, I failed to get my front wheels high enough and ran full force into a curb. The sudden impact caused me to pitch forward and land in a crumpled paralyzed heap with my chair upside down and on top of me. As I struggled to assure the alarmed pedestrians that I was all right, a nearby construction crew began placing orange traffic cones all around me. I was inside the cones, smiling and hoping that my pants wouldn't slide down as I lifted myself back into the chair. The crowd stood outside the cones; no one was smiling. I was an unusual sight. I couldn't blame them for staring but I also couldn't reassure them that this little tumble was no more serious for me than a scraped knee. "Should we take you to the hospital?" one of the construction workers asked? "Why?" I asked. "Why?" He looked as though I had taken leave of my senses. "Because you can't walk, son," was the answer.

Jumping real curbs was far more difficult than the sample barriers back in rehab. It required a precise combination of balance and brute strength to aim the chair properly, lift the front wheels at just the right moment, and with the rock-solid muscles of wrists and forearms, propel the rear wheels up any surface they contacted. In the beginning I did not have enough strength, and so my strategy was to hurtle the chair at the curb and hope it just sailed up onto the sidewalk from its own headlong momentum.

Each intersection required a strategy, a calculation of the best approach, and the potential downsides. If the able-bodied hiked casually through the world's physical terrain, I approached it as a golfer playing sudden death on the back nine at Augusta. Where the world was simply concerned with reaching a destination, I was playing each hole for keeps in front of a staring, open-mouthed audience.

My friends would offer to help. "We'll just lift you," or "I'll push you up the ramp," or "Why doesn't someone go into the store and get what you need and you can wait here in the van?" It was always simpler to utilize the combined effort of the group in getting where I was going, but I would have none of it. What they saw as working together and saving time by pushing me and scouting ahead for obstacles, was to me demeaning, impossible, and in my imagined golf tournament, ruining my score. In those first months, I insisted on doing everything solo, playing all eighteen holes without a handicap. Unfortunately I was a pretty lousy at it, and because I insisted that my friends let me learn, they could do nothing but watch.

I found myself in a waist-level, ramped universe that few people visited who were not in chairs. The business of the world was conducted above my head, just out of earshot. Even making eye contact was difficult from my position. Like phantom particles of the atom on their way to an outer orbit around the nucleus, children would appear at eye level on their way up to adult civilization. It required the energy of a cyclotron to move me into that world and even more to move it into mine.

The noisy college parties I was invited to were always upstairs. To get to the party, I would be carried up one or two flights and set in the living room. It was something of an event that I had even made it. People holding paper plates of canned chili would stumble over me and say how glad they were that I had come. "How are you doing?" people would ask. "Fine," I would shout back. This was usually the end of the conversation. I wanted to make small talk. There seemed to be no small talk to make. It was here, among friends, in the former haunts of my recently walking self, that the changes began to sink in. It was the details in this new, unexpected world that came to mind when people asked, as they often did, how I was doing. They wanted to know the gruesome headlines about how many people died in my accident, was it my fault, was I in any pain. But no one wanted to talk about the subtle shifts in my world, so I didn't, either. If I was in denial, so were the people around me. Ignoring all of the changes seemed to be the cool thing to do. At parties the loud music made it almost impossible to hear the conversations taking place above my head anyway. I sat quietly while people brought me plates of carrot sticks and beer. "How are you doing?" It was hazardous for me to drink anything at these parties. A full bladder meant finding somewhere to use a catheter in a strange apartment full of people. Once, while taking a whiz in a dark corner of some living room, a very stoned person sat down next to me and watched as I filled an empty beer bottle. "Intense," he said after a moment. Apparently he thought I had found a novel new way of injecting heroin.

Up two flights of stairs, I was captive in a world I did not belong in, and where I was not free. Was it wrong to feel this way? Was it a sign of mental health to pretend the stairs didn't matter? Was it a sign of defeat to avoid them? Was it bad to feel different? Was is all right for everyone else to pretend that I wasn't? I was Lancelot on wheels doing battle against an incongruous and inhospitable physical world, where each detail contained its own lessons, and even the simplest event might be seen as a metaphor for the larger struggle of humanity against the elements.

In Dickens's "A Christmas Carol," Tiny Tim tells his father Bob Cratchit that he hoped people who saw him with his crutch during the holiday were convinced that his suffering would warm their souls and teach them a lesson about the meaning of Christmas. It was another celebrated illusion created by Dickens, along with his Christmas ghosts. Tiny Tim, the original poster boy, thought he could harness the power of people staring. But people stare at anything unusual. Their interest began and ended with the one fact I thought the least about, and had nothing to do with what it took to operate in the world. People weren't interested in playing extras in my melodrama. They wanted a key supporting role in a near-death experience. The more I sought meaning in the little details of my new life, the more the people around me thought I was nuts. "Move on with your life," they said. But my life wouldn't budge, and there were steps everywhere.

The University of Chicago had a lot of steps and almost no ramps. I went back there knowing full well what I was in for. The University tried to help out and gave me my own parking space, but the only way to keep someone else from parking in it was to keep my blue van there all of the time. The choice was between giving up the parking space and giving up driving. In October 1976, I also had my choice of the only two buildings on campus a wheelchair could enter. All of my classes had to be moved to one of these two buildings: the biology hall, which smelled like formaldehyde from the fetal pig dissections going on there all day long, or Pick Hall, a sixties concrete modernistic atrocity observed with contempt or avoided with relish by the tenured legends I wanted to study with in the anthropology, math, history, or Russian literature departments. They much preferred the lead-trimmed windowpanes, stone steps, vaulted ceilings and archways of the old quadrangle buildings.

At first the professors would all try to avoid moving their classes. The administration would then ask if I wanted to file a formal request that they do so. Requesting the classes at all, I thought, ought to be formal enough. "Formal request" sounded like someone named Vito was going to visit one of their seminars with a lead pipe. That actually might have helped. One professor suggested that I be queried as to whether I was "absolutely sure I wanted to put the Department of the Humanities to all that trouble," which was an unexpected spin on the meaning of the word "humanities."

I insisted that all of the classes be moved. The least cooperative professors were the ones I was drawn to. The less a professor wanted to move, the more I wanted to be in the class. If a class was closed, I suspected that the professor had filled it to keep me out. If a professor did move willingly, I presumed that some deal had been made. The substandard professor was being forced on me as a favor to the senior member of the department, whom I really wanted to study with. A professor who moved to accommodate a crip must have something wrong with him. A professor who wouldn't move to accommodate a crip must possess some special academic expertise that was being denied me. Attending such a class was just the battle I was looking for.

It was not surprising that I ended up with the least flexible, stodgiest, academic dust heads at the university who, from the very first day and at my insistence, were thoroughly miffed that I was in their classes. It was an illuminating crash course in psychology, and in the end the fall term had very little to do with the Russian literature, anthropology, mathematics, or particle physics I had signed up to study.

It was all about guilt. Fighting to get every professor to move forced me to like them. I had insisted on dragging everyone over to the biology building to discuss the fine points of Dostoevsky while breathing the smell of formaldehyde. I had put the department and the other students to a lot of trouble. If I overheard them complaining about the dead pigs next door, I felt terrible. The whole situation was an inescapable emotional trap. They could complain, I couldn't. If I missed a class I felt much worse. How was it that I did not anticipate all this? The hardest thing was sorting out what was worth getting angry about and what was better ignored.

By late November, when the winter came, plows pushed piles of snow up around the sidewalks, blocked the two reliable ramps on campus, and surrounded my van with a mountain of snow that was about as assailable as the Great Wall of China. For much of the winter of 1976–77, there was no building a wheelchair could reliably enter at the University of Chicago, and the wheels of my van were encased in three feet of solid ice.

I decided to leave school. The magical place that college had been in the few months before my accident had vanished. In the months I had been away our close-knit family on 55th Street at the lakeshore had drifted apart. Each of my friends had been drawn into the tensions and struggles of school. I had my own struggle, and much as I thought my friends were a part of it, in the end the ghosts I chased on wheelchair battlefields were seen only by me.

Those battles stayed long after I left the university and began to think about how I might eventually find a job. I had previously worked in a car wash, as an orderly in a nursing home, a dishwasher in a restaurant, a scene designer in a theater, an actor, a photographer for the school newspaper, a union welder for a steel fabricator, a worker in an office-furniture factory, a bartender, a truck driver and a forklift operator for a lumber yard, and I also gave guitar lessons to people who were worse players than myself.

My hardwon AFL-CIO welder's card would not get me a factory job now that I was a paraplegic. I hardly thought anyone at the steel company expected me to return. I hadn't ever really wanted to be a welder; it was the union wage that had brought me to the dusty steel factory as a teenager. But after the accident, the absurdity of being a paraplegic welder only made me think about how I could be one anyway to prove a point. Lazy Pasito and Lecherous Ray, whose crew I used to work on, would have advised me to stay home and collect disability. They spent hours on the job talking about how they would spend the ten thousand dollars they could collect if one of the heavy cranes ever came down on one of their hands. Having another hand and retaining the ability to jack off and "squeeze tits," as Ray would say, made it worthwhile. "Ten grand would set me up for life," Pasito would say back in 1974.

At the office-furniture factory where I had worked there was another equally morbid work ethic. I was assigned to the tool and die shop, keeping inventory of the thousands of machined-steel stamping dies used to form the parts for the desks and chairs that the factory produced. The dies would be loaded and clamped between the jaws of the giant steel presses. Raw sheet metal would be fed into the die, and with the push of a big brightly colored button the press would come down on the metal. With each stroke of the press, the metal would be punched, bent, shaped, and cut into pieces that eventually became chairs, desks, and file cabinets.

The presses produced hundreds of tons of force per square inch. They were powered by heavy electric motors which turned even larger and heavier flywheels that spun above the press operator. When the operator engaged the press, the flywheel's gears moved it like a clutch on a car. As a safety feature, each press operator had to wear chains on his wrist. The chains were connected to cables that automatically pulled the operator's hands away from the metal jaws each time the press came down.

The men in the tool and die room made the stamping dies from heavy, precisely cut blocks of tool steel to the specifications on blueprints dense with lines and tiny numbers, many with two and three decimal places. When it was time to install the stamping dies on the assembly line where the press operators ran hundreds of parts per day, the die maker would supervise the installation and stamp out the first parts to see if they met the exacting demands of the blueprints. Because they were simply checking the new dies and not mindlessly running parts through them when the line was operating at full bore, the die makers were permitted to use the presses without wearing the wrist safety chains.

One young die maker asked me to accompany him out into the stamping plant on such an installation job. He was an apprentice, a few years older than I was and held me in some contempt. For me, the tool and die shop was only a summer job; for him it was a career. Though I was fascinated by the machines and held the work of the die makers in high regard, he could not see me as anything but a college boy, an over-tall, uncoordinated, daydreaming teenager. Dorrie, the foreman, was convinced that I would lose a finger before the summer was over. He observed my natural clumsiness as another idiotic edict from management that he would have to live with.

The apprentice told me to put on my goggles. He engaged the press. It stamped the 16-gauge steel with a powerful crash heavy with bass notes. He let a half dozen or so parts fall into the bin, then shut off the press. He picked up each part, and using his measuring tools checked each bend, curve, and punched hole for precise dimensions. This was his first die. He was excited to see that what he had read from the blueprints he had actually produced in a 120-ton press to an accuracy of 1/100th of an inch. Though the press motor was turned off, the fly-wheel retained its momentum and continued to turn. The apprentice took his flashlight and a paintbrush and inspected one cutting and bend-ing surface on the die that could be expected to take a lot of punish-ment. He looked for signs of fatigue and leaned his body closer to the press.

As he did so, his hip hit a button that engaged the gears to the fly-wheel. Hanging next to me were the safety chains. I noticed them jerk backward as they did when they were on the line. But there were no hands in them and so they just dangled out of reach. I glanced up at the flywheel. It was pushing the press down. I looked at the die. The press had closed. The apprentice was still standing there. I looked at his hands. They were still inside the press. A red liquid was clouding the reservoir of oils and coolants that bathed the cutting surfaces with each cycle of the press. The press had severed three of the apprentice's fin-gers, two on one hand and one on the other. He stepped back, looking at the blood shooting out of his hands. I peered inside the press ex-pecting to see his cut-off fingers. There was nothing. The 120-ton press had obliterated any trace save a pink stain on the still-sharp, glistening metal.

The accident caused an uproar on the shop floor. The apprentice was rushed to the hospital. The foreman rushed out and supervised his departure in an ambulance. In the heat of the moment Dorrie yelled at me, "If I ever see you not using the safety chains, college boy, I'll send you home." In his eyes it seemed as though he thought it unfair that the apprentice, who would need his fingers for his livelihood, should lose three of them, while a college boy on a summer job earning gas and movie money should get to keep all ten of his. I felt that I had to prove to Dorrie that I, too, needed my fingers—"I play the guitar, you know." But I said nothing.

Witnessing the loss of someone's fingers in a stamping press was shocking enough, but it was the next day that made an even stronger impression on me. I was waiting for the whistle to blow to start the day shift. The usual noise and conversation suddenly stopped. I looked up and the apprentice was walking toward the time clock, his hands buried in reams of tightly wrapped white gauze. He pulled his time card from the rack with his teeth and punched it into the time slot. As the clock stamped his card, the die shop broke into spontaneous applause. The apprentice was a minute early. The die makers went up and congratu- lated him. For the first time, I noticed that most of them had their own stumps of fingers and smashed bones to show him. He smiled broadly. He was not an apprentice anymore. He was now one of the guys. I was horrified. Dorrie said to me, again with the frustration I had noted the day before, "He's more of a man than you'll ever be with all of your fingers." I put my hands in my pockets.

The apprentice's injury seemed less like an accident than an episode in a deeply felt ritual of human sacrifice. The job had taken his fingers. Because he was injured in the line of duty, he was a hero. In that tool and die shop, trading fingers for a lifelong career was a fair transaction. In the welding shop, Pasito and Ray would each gladly trade a hand for ten thousand insurance dollars and the chance to kiss their jobs good- bye forever. In the job market, one could be a wounded hero-worker with a purple heart, or a maimed welfare case on disability, set up for life in front of the TV. These were the comfortable, familiar images that required no explanation.

There was no explanation for the loss of much of my body. It was something that just happened. Was society prepared for people who simply got disabled, and then simply applied for a job so they could buy milk and do the things everyone else does? Simply getting a job seemed much harder than learning all the fancy crowd-pleasing wheelchair tricks for hopping up curbs and getting over other obstacles. It meant convincing someone to become part of the aftermath of a car wreck they had not been a part of. I had neither broken my back in some war zone and vowed to charge back up the hill nor had I parlayed some insurance money into a small fortune. I was disabled as the result of a random occurrence. This randomness was what frightened people. My arrival in some employer's office out of the blue to apply for a job was a small aftershock that echoed the original moment of the accident. At first they all wanted to look. Then they only wanted to look away.

Workers could trade in their fingers in the line of duty for lifetime employment, or sell their hands for cash.

The State of Michigan required all disabled people to be evaluated and certified as employable, and therefore eligible for job placement or college financial aid. This involved spending a few days being interviewed and taking tests at a local psychiatric hospital. I gave my job history to a soft-spoken pale-skinned man looking at a file with my name on it. I indicated that my primary interests were mathematics and music.

"Mathematics." He paused and then looked at a big book with a list of careers deemed acceptable for the people who were sent to him for evaluation. "Have you ever used an adding machine?"

"No," I said. "But I'm sure I could figure it out." He handed me a ten-page booklet and led me over to a table with an old ten-key adding machine on it. "Let's see how long it takes you to finish these," he said, and walked away. The book was filled with column after column of four- and five-digit numbers that I was instructed in big black letters to add, subtract, multiply, and divide. The machine churned out the sums on its white cash-register tape. After the first few pages, the trainer returned to my table. "You call this mathematics, working a cash register?" I confronted him with my college background in calculus and advanced topology. He wasn't interested in my knowledge of the subject at all. "This is the only test we have involving numbers," he said, as though my question was predicted on the clipboard he was holding. "Don't you like these numbers, John?"

The only thing challenging about the number problems was that there were pages and pages of them. This test was more about enduring hour after hour of mind-numbing repetition than using mathematics. As I proceeded through the problems, the trainer set two bowls on the table next to me. One contained some half-inch metal bolts, the other about an equal number of matching nuts. "What are those for?" I asked. He said nothing, but I could see what they were for by looking at one of the mentally retarded boys at the next table. He was slowly screwing the nuts onto the bolts and placing them in a dish. There were more than a hundred of each, and the assignment was to first screw the bolts on, call the trainer, then after the trainer gave his permission, unscrew all the nuts and place the nuts and bolts back in their own bowls. The idea that I was going to have to take this test made me quietly fume as

I punched the keys of the adding machine. I was not going to screw nuts onto bolts. That was where I was going to draw the line.

The same trainer who was observing my irritation at the adding machine was inspecting the joyful nut-screwing progress across the table. He acknowledged the retarded boy's work with effusive praise. "Great," he said in the overloud voice the health care industry reserves for its most degrading compliments. My outrage turned to jealousy for the favoritism shown to the mentally retarded man. I couldn't help it that I was not retarded. Why couldn't the trainer just agree that the tests I was taking had nothing to do with my training and aptitudes? I told him that I had already taken the SAT's to get into college, so why did I have to take the nut-screwing test? He looked at me silently. After a moment he said, "Are you refusing to take the eye-hand coordination test?"

"I'm just saying that the test seems to me like a waste of time since it is clear that my paralysis doesn't affect my arms." He pointed to the retarded man at the table, who looked up and smiled. "Frank isn't paralyzed at all, and he agreed to take the test. Do you want me to put down that you refused?"

It was hard to accept that the state of Michigan's decision on whether I was eligible for financial aid was based on whether I agreed to screw a bucket of nuts onto a bucket of screws, but this appeared to be the situation. It was also quite clear as I looked at Frank across the table that the "eye-hand coordination test" had as little to do with his future life's work as it did mine. It was no less degrading for him to take the test than for me to take it. The test wasn't about aptitude at all. It was all about the clipboard and the trainer and whether Frank and I refused to do what he told us to do. Retarded Frank was delighted to try anything. I expected the tests to have something to do with my future work, whatever that might be. That I would assert such a claim of self-determination into the trainer's domain only ensured that I would fail his tests.

To act like Frank was the answer. He would still be happily screwing his nuts and bolts long after I had been sent to prison for murdering the trainer and kidnapping his wife and kids. Frank looked at me with the same smile he gave the trainer. I couldn't tell if it was the look of a teacher's pet, or the light by which he made his way through the institutions where he had already spent most of his life. He had seen this trainer before in a thousand different incarnations in scores of other institutions. Frank knew how to win. I was simply not in Frank's league.

The letter eventually placed in my state file indicated that I was a deeply disturbed individual with the inability to follow instructions. I suppose there are people I have worked with since that time who might strongly concur with that assessment, and would be happy to hand me another bucket of screws. According to the trainer's report, I did not exhibit behaviors appropriate to the workplace. I had been recommended as a doubtful prospect for vocational rehabilitation. "John has great difficulty accepting his situation. He did not consider that our tests were appropriate for him. We expect that this will be a serious problem for him on the job." The letter is still in my file in the state of Michigan and the Social Security Administration in Washington. I was asked by caseworkers to explain its conclusions years later. Each time, remembering the trainer with the clipboard and Frank's smile, brought back the same fear and frustration of those moments. I am still trying to prove that letter wrong.

Crip Job

I moved to the West Coast in the late seventies to get away from family, snow, and the places I had known as a walking person. I had heard that Berkeley, California, was a mecca for the disabled, and that there I would not find the architectural problems I had encountered at the University of Chicago. In my view, any school that would go out of its way to attract crips must have something wrong with it, so I immediately ruled out Berkeley along with all of the other schools that came recommended by people in the Department of Vocational Rehabilitation. Wheelchair access was not going to be my consideration in selecting a school, just as cooperation had not been my guide in selecting professors at the University of Chicago.

I settled on the University of Oregon in Eugene because it was rainy there and because no one had suggested it to me. The last thing I wanted was for people to think I had run away from the snowy Midwest to a sunny California sanitarium. The constant rain of the Pacific Northwest was an acceptable compromise for a paraplegic who was simply too much of a WASP to actually embrace an easy way of doing things.

I lived by myself in a little one-bedroom apartment in Springfield, across the MacKenzie River from Eugene. I had my camera, an enlarger, my guitars, a Fender Rhodes 77-key electric piano, and some books. I lived on $420.80 per month, the check I received from the insurance policy of Margaret Zinn. I spent my days and nights practicing the piano with my headphones on. Loggers and their families lived in the apartments around me, and there was lots of screaming from arguing spouses and roomies and their sobbing children.

There was a single window in the apartment looking out on the parking lot and a large fir tree. I put the piano in front of this window. Here I spent my hours alone, practicing for an audition at the University of Oregon music school. This was the apartment where I set the hot dish on my thigh while cooking Thanksgiving dinner. This was the place where my grandfather sent the cutting board to protect my legs.

My apartment had a single high step at the entrance. A metal folding ramp placed in front of the door allowed me to roll in and out. I had very little furniture. I slept on a mattress placed on the floor. My kitchen table was a flimsy chest full of clothes that I set plates on at dinnertime. My electric piano was the only shelf in the apartment. It held piles of sheet music and anything else I could put there. I often placed my camera there, on top of some music books next to the window, so that I could easily grab it on the way out the door.

I practiced Bach and Beethoven on the piano during the daylight hours. At night I would read or watch television until after midnight, then venture out into the parking lot of the shopping center next door to practice wheelchair skills that were too embarrassing to fail at during daylight. Physical skills were best acquired at night when no one was around. I would practice jumping curbs and fancy transfers in the dark. Even here, at three in the morning, police and security guards would be tempted to call an ambulance, or want to know what I was doing. But that was better than having to work a crowd of staring, tragedy-faced pedestrians.

In my solitude I would go for days without talking. People in the apartment watched me come and go. I didn't know them. They didn't ask about me. I didn't ask about them. I was alone. I fell in love with the Kentucky Fried Chicken lady on the local KFC television commercials. "Share a bucket of extra crispy with your friends," she would say. The other person I would speak to was the bank teller at the drive-up window where I would cash my monthly check. I would linger at the window talking about the weather until someone in the line of cars behind me would honk their horn and I had to move on.

As I had been advised back in Michigan, I reported to the local welfare office to register with the people who would monitor my financial aid at school the following year. There was a vocational rehabilitation agency in each of the fifty states. The caseworker in Springfield who was assigned to me was nice enough until she read my file from Michigan and wondered why someone with my attitudinal problems was living unsupervised. "We think it would be better for you in a structured setting," she said, looking at my file as though the trainer from Michigan had advised her that I should be placed in solitary. I imagined my face on wanted posters in the post office.

"I was just told to come here and register," I said. "My setting is fine. I'm planning to go to school next year. I'm looking for some financial aid." She thumbed through my file and nodded a bit. She asked at one point if I had thought of what job I might get in the future. I told her that I hadn't thought of it too much except that I was interested in mathematics and music. She explained her agency's recent success training people in wheelchairs to be dispatchers for taxi companies and the police. "Would that interest you?" she asked. I thought of the bucket of nuts and screws again, and decided not to sneer and insult her in any way. With a stack of papers in her arms, she stood up and came around to the front of her desk. Holding the papers was difficult for her. I could see that she had rheumatoid arthritis and that her hands were bent and deformed and looked quite painful. "Because you are in a wheelchair you are totally disabled according to the state of Oregon definition, and therefore eligible for the full range of services we offer here." Her tone suggested that I had just won the Publisher's Clearing House Giveaway. "What does 'totally disabled' mean?" I asked.

"It means that things will be much simpler for you than they are for me. I'm only partially disabled." She held up her bent and crumpled hands. She pushed some papers toward me on which she had circled numbers. "You can get this much money in addition to your regular monthly check. You will have to report here every month and allow one of our field workers to visit your house to make sure that your kitchen is appropriate for the federally mandated diet. And here is the maximum number of food stamps you can purchase." It all added up to more than twice the $420.80 I was getting. It also meant that I could go visit my beloved bank teller at the drive-up window many more times per month.

All I really wanted was financial aid for school. The food stamps seemed like a good deal too. But the rest of it seemed like planning a life around people with clipboards paid by the state to grade me on my attitude. After insisting that I didn't think I needed to be on welfare, I compromised and agreed to accept only the food stamps.

Taking food stamps to the grocery store enhanced the general performance anxiety of life in a wheelchair. In 1977, pulling out food stamps in a check-out line was like offering to trade one of your kidneys for a bag of groceries. Cashiers stared at them, the shoppers behind me sighed and looked uneasily at their watches, and everyone, it seemed, stared at my groceries to make sure I was buying the approved products. I felt guilty if I was purchasing anything besides ten-pound bags of grain and powdered milk. I could never bring myself to buy crunchy peanut butter with food stamps, only the smooth stuff. Once, when I realized that I had only food stamps to pay for the marshmallow fluff I had placed in my basket, I put the jar back on the shelf and slinked out of the store.

I knew that people stared; I could only imagine what they really thought. But someone in Springfield was apparently paying close enough attention to figure out how to burglarize my crowded apartment. My camera was clearly visible on the top of my piano by the window where I would watch people as I practiced. One night I was lying on my mattress on the floor of the bedroom when I heard a noise in the front room and the sound of the window being forced open from the outside. I called out, "Who's there?" Only the sound of breaking glass answered me. I tried to imagine what was being taken. I wanted to run into the other room. But I couldn't, so I tried to use my voice as a stand-in for my body. "Hey, I'm in here and I'm coming out there right now." I stumbled to raise myself into my chair but in my haste it tipped forward and fell over sideways with a thud and a crash.

"I'm coming out there." I shouted again. Normally a burglar would expect that you would either come in the room or you wouldn't. A burglar would not expect to hear lots of grunts and thrashing around in the next room and a long discussion of how someone was coming in "in a minute. Don't think I'm not."

When I finally got into the chair, I was red and flustered, and I burst into the now empty room still shouting. The window was broken. The glass was on top of the piano and some jagged pieces had fallen onto the keys. I rolled over to the door to try and chase after anyone still in the parking lot. As I opened the door, there was a loud crash. The metal folding ramp in front of my apartment had been removed from its position on the ground and set up against the door. When I opened the door it fell into the apartment, blocking my exit. Across the parking lot a pick-up truck started up and roared out of the driveway with its lights off.

The parking lot was quiet. I pushed the ramp out through the door; it crashed uselessly, half-folded up on the pavement in front of the parking lot. I looked around the apartment and for a moment it appeared as though my screaming might have prevented the burglar from taking something after all. Then I saw that my camera was no longer on top of the piano. The burglar had reached through the glass and grabbed it from the window sill as plain as day. Whoever it was had not even needed to enter the apartment, but apparently they had been sufficiently impressed with my rolling skills to barricade my door with my wheelchair ramp to ensure their getaway.

That someone would calculate a theft based on a study of my physical limitations made me angry. I felt violated and invaded by everyone who looked at me. After only three months in Oregon, the Kentucky Fried Chicken lady still didn't know me; the bank teller lady still had to look at my deposit slip to remember my name. The person who knew me the best had just used that knowledge to rip off my camera. Why had I stupidly placed the camera in the window in the first place? I would never have done such a thing if I were still walking, I thought.

An immunity and a separateness was implied by the wheelchair. Having separate parking spaces and bathrooms and ramps and doorways and governmental departments made me feel like a footnote. Rules didn't seem to apply to me. My world was constructed of obstacles and barriers that other people could not see, even though they stared at me all the time. Some time after my camera was stolen, I was using the men's room at the University of Oregon when I encountered one of my favorite professors. I had been in his class for several months. We had been talking about cultural relativism, listening to fugues, comparing Beethoven's quest for the light with Mahler's end-of-the-world bleakness. There in the men's room, he looked at me, and with the same voice he might use to underscore a flash of inspired scholarly insight he said, "Why, John, I never thought about you having to go to the bathroom. Isn't that interesting?"

If he didn't think of me as a biological creature, what did he think, that I went to the hardware store instead of the bathroom? What did anybody think? What did they learn from staring? As much as I hated being robbed while I sat helpless in the next room, at least the burglar had been paying attention to the right details.

The first job I applied for was something I could do at home. I wrote letters to the two local newspapers, the *Eugene Register Guard* and the *Springfield News*, proposing to write a weekly column on the humorous adventures of life in a wheelchair. I had been writing letters to friends and relatives telling them of my misadventures and it seemed as though a weekly column might make the most of some of these stories, and give me a paycheck. "I would also provide an information service to people in the community who have disabilities," or so I told the editors in my pitch letter. One of the papers responded by saying that they already had a medical reporter who wrote all that they needed on such matters. The larger of the two papers didn't respond until I called and talked to an editor. His first question pretty much told the story. "You want to tell jokes about crippled people, in our newspaper?" "That's right," I told him, and the conversation ended soon after that. It was 1977.

In the crip world, there are jock jobs, crip jobs, and then there are the real jobs. Jocks get a lot of attention in their sporty wheelchair basketball chairs or their tennis outfits. There are the crip skiers, and most impressive of all are the runners in their three-wheel track chairs. Endorsing products, conducting workshops, and participating in wheelchair sport competitions around the world, crip jocks spend a lot of their time giving motivational speeches, usually to business sales groups. "Triumph Over Adversity, Inc." employs lots of crips.

Crip jobs are "for crips." Like the little blind midget who sells magazines at the State Capitol building, or the taxi dispatcher in a wheelchair, these jobs are crip-designated. They are the "Oh, it's so nice that he has a job" jobs. Crip jobs are also all of the positions in the disability industry, which spans the government aid and advocacy agencies: the lesbian quadriplegic on the city human rights commission who makes sure that no one calls the magazine salesman at City Hall a little midget, the blind head of the council on employment for the handicapped, the veterans who nabbed government jobs and show up at the paralyzed veterans conventions. Rehab hospitals always have a crip "counselor" who is a nice-enough person trying to set an example of a working disabled person but who, for a new crip, is the patient who never checked out of the hospital. To new crips, these role-model types seem to have gotten lost in the telethon. The paraplegic counselor in my rehab hospital in Michigan was such a crip worker. He was the one who used to horrify my parents with stories of how I would lose all my friends. After his accident he decided to become a social worker. We patients all understood. He wasn't fooling us. Being a social worker only meant he must have been too much of a chicken to apply for a job pumping gas. At the hospital, that would have impressed us. But of course no one would have given him a job pumping gas.

Real jobs are ones that are not crip-designated, that take on humanity at large. Quadriplegic lead dancer for the New York City Ballet. The armless pitcher. Deaf Beethoven, blind Stevie Wonder. If Helen Keller had been a waitress instead of a professional role model she could have qualified. If senators Kerrey and Inouye had been power forwards for the Lakers instead of cashing in their combat veteran amputee sympathy gigs for a government job they would qualify. Simply being a senator does not push the envelope. After blind brain surgeon and paraplegic figure skater, the ultimate real job is president of the United States. FDR was a crip in the White House, although you would never know it from the history books. Crips all understand that Franklin Roosevelt had to hide his disability or he would have been told to sell magazines at 1600 Pennsylvania Avenue rather than be the President. An added "real job" bonus for Roosevelt is that as the victorious Commander-in-Chief in World War Two he was probably responsible for making more people disabled than any other crip in history, if you don't count Hitler's reputed epilepsy, or Pol Pot's male-pattern baldness. Crips are impressed by such things. It breaks the mold.

The first and only job interview I ever had was for a crip job, as a trainer at a nursing home for developmentally disabled adults on the Oregon coast. "Developmentally disabled adults" is a polite way of describing people who might have had a chance at employment if their personalities hadn't been obliterated through years of psychoactive drugs like Thorazine and Seconal and institutionalization. I talked to the medical director of the facility, who said that she was very excited about having a "real disabled person" to work with the "clients." I had worked as an orderly emptying bedpans and urinals at a geriatric nursing home years before my accident, and she took this to be evidence that I was experienced in the health care field. She hired me immediately. If I had told her how good I was at screwing nuts onto bolts I might have gotten a raise.

The trainers were supposed to run programs to train the clients in various skills. Suddenly, I was the one handing out the buckets of screws and the coloring books and marking things down on my own clipboard. I was also supposed to look after the bedpans and the urinals. I was assigned to the night shift to work with the other trainers, who seemed to be just like the nurse's aides I had worked with at my old nursing-home job in high school. My co-workers actually had been nurse's aides until just a few weeks before, when they were brought over to the futuristic training wing to be paid twenty-five cents more per hour. The promotion to trainer meant that all of the geriatric staff hated them and us and acted as though we thought we were too good simply to be orderlies and aides anymore.

The evening shift supervisor was a thin, attractive young woman who never smiled and who took her job extremely seriously. She was from the rehab world and represented the philosophy of "No More Mr. Nice Guy," the then-current rage for those dealing with mental retardation. We were to hold the clients to task and punish them by putting them in "time out" if they weren't compliant. Indulging the clients in any way was to play into, and therefore exacerbate, their personality defects, which was another way of saying that with all of their time in institutions, they were much more experienced in manipulating people like us than we were in training people like them. We were under express orders not to give any of the clients attention that they hadn't earned through screwing screws and writing in workbooks. It was strict behavior modification in this wing. All infractions were to be recorded and all progress charted.

Alice was the supervisor's name. She made it clear that she hated the idea of having someone in a wheelchair working on the floor. "This role-model business is Maureen's idea," she said, referring to her supervisor, the woman who had hired me. "It's a stupid idea and I don't support it. We have a lot of work to do each night on the floor and if you can't pull your weight I will fire you tomorrow. If you think you are going to roll up and down the halls delivering the message to our clients that disabled people don't have to work as hard as anyone else you can just pack up and leave right now."

This orientation speech was delivered in front of everyone I was going to have to work with. For my first day on the job, it was a little chilly. Alice sounded a lot like Dorrie back at the tool and die factory. Ginny, a gray-haired trainer who used to work in the north wing, came up to me afterward and told me that Alice could be a little tough at first. She told me that it wasn't my wheelchair that was the problem. "We don't have many men working here," Ginny explained. "She's not used to having men around. Alice fixes her own Plymouth, you know." To Ginny, this was decisive. "We think she's a lesbian."

I had gone into this job intrigued with the simple idea of getting a paycheck. But this ultimatum delivered from out of the blue by my boss was a chilly return to the nether world of social services, where your preassigned category arrived before you did. I was back to screwing a bucket of nuts onto a bucket of bolts while a grumpy, skeptical health care professional with a clipboard watched me and took notes. To her, I was closer to the care center's clients than its workers.

I resolved to work like a maniac to prove that I was as good as any of the other employees. I trained clients. I hauled clients in and out of bathtubs. I chased masturbating clients out of the dining room.

I settled disputes over the Portland Trailblazers and over who would watch what on television, emptied urinals, and cleaned up laundry problems that a mother of quintuplets would find challenging. If I was assigned the work of a single trainer, I would perform the work of two or three.

It was my first experience in responding to a skeptical non-crip world with the obsessive energy of a combat general. Like General MacArthur in Asia, knowing when to quit was always the most challenging part of the puzzle. Before I was hired at the care center, the second shift had been far behind in its programs and paperwork. A week after I was on the job, we were far ahead of schedule. Proving Alice wrong about me on the job was just the beginning of my planetary-scale vision of ultimate triumph. After a month we were living together. After three months we were married.

In hindsight, and with so much to prove to each other, it was probably inevitable that Alice and I would end up married. Once the chill in the workplace thawed we actually found we had a lot in common and were quite compatible. I had been on the job a month, commuting between Florence, on the coast where the Care Center was, and Eugene, sixty miles inland, when I started looking for an apartment in Florence. I told people at work that while I looked, I needed a place to stay a night or two each week. Most of the people on the evening shift lived in cramped trailer houses, but Alice offered to let me use the living-room couch in her two-bedroom house in the woods.

On our first real date, we sat in her living room and talked and played the guitar and drank beer. I got out of my chair and we rolled around on her new carpet. She sang what was then her favorite song, "Giant Step" by Taj Mahal. Her sound was straight-ahead folk music. Her voice was deep and full. I played along, fingerpicking the strange dissonant chords that Rick and I used to play. The blend of the two sounds was magical. She said that she fell in love during the refrain.

I told her the story of my accident and why I came to Oregon. She told me about her Jesus-freak mother named Hallie, and her stepfather and the real father she never knew. For hours I lay on my stomach talking and listening. I rolled over and noticed that there was a dark wet stain on Alice's new living-room carpeting. It was my first authentic social contact with someone besides my drive-in bank teller or the chicken lady on TV. On our first date I wet my pants. At the care center, Alice's job was to put people like me in "time out" and start them immediately on a toilet-training program.

Instead, she just laughed. I fell in love when she handed me the dry pair of jeans from her bedroom. "I think these will fit you." They did. I drove home to get dry clothes. I had come between Alice and Heidi. Alice had come between the two women in my life and me. During an emotional weekend, Alice broke the news to her boyfriend Steven. It would be easier for me to break it off with the bank teller and the Kentucky Fried Chicken lady. I had passed through their lives without a word.

We got married in the office of a judge in Newport, Oregon, on a rainy Memorial Day weekend. The witness who co-signed the marriage license was a complete stranger I had grabbed off the street. I got my future mother-in-law's approval a few weeks before the wedding while Alice paced the floor. Hallie spent all of her time looking for signs from God. Alice's mom was a full-fledged evangelical. If I was nervous about being the son-in-law in the wheelchair, Alice was nervous that her mom, the born-again Christian mother-in-law, was going to loudly and publicly ask Jesus to make me walk again right there. Hallie prayed about everything. She especially prayed for God to make her daughters accept their mother's constant praying. There was no point in encouraging her to stop.

Hallie and I hit it off immediately. We had something in common. Hallie was used to having people stare at her, as anyone would who had done as much hollering through a megaphone as she had, on busy street corners, while holding graphic antiabortion posters of torn-apart fetuses. But Hallie was completely free of worry over what anyone else thought. People stared when I jumped curbs. They stared more when Hallie spoke in tongues. I had something in common with my mother-in-law. "Let them look," she would say. "We're all blessed." Which would set Alice right off. "We're not blessed, Mom." "Okay, honey, whatever you say."

The judge's chambers were wheelchair-accessible, which felt like a real sign from God. The marriage ceremony took about three minutes while rain beat down on the window in the county courthouse. When it was all over, the sun came out and we went to a little café and had cups of clam chowder. My stomach growled with nuptial butterflies. I watched the ocean. There was no honeymoon. We spent the weekend at the home of some friends who were renting a farmhouse. There we played music and sang "Giant Step" for everyone. My new world in Oregon was so different from the one I had left back at school in Chicago. It felt like home, even if I had allowed the snow to chase me and my wheelchair out of the Midwest. Alice and I were two misfits resigned, until we met, to go though life without a match. It was a far-from-perfect match, but it was closer to perfect than anything we could have imagined back then. When the weekend was over, we went to work and told no one that we were married. For months it was our little secret.

10

The Staring

When Alice and I finally told the people at the care center we were married the employees were shocked, while the clients were thrilled and not surprised at all. The other male trainer, Delbert, had been hitting on Alice for weeks; she had been ignoring him. "It's not fair," he said. "You're in a wheelchair." The elderly women trainers had to admit they were relieved to find out that Alice wasn't a lesbian, and they told me so. "We never believed she was . . . you know." But it was the clients who claimed to have predicted that Alice and I would end up living together from my first weeks on the job. David, a young man with profound cerebral palsy, howled and drooled when he found out. On his signing board he frantically pointed out a question, "Do Al drive truc now?"

Shortly after coming to the care center I had traded in my big, bulky, blue van for a little orange Toyota pickup. With only a bench seat in the cab, there was no place to store the wheelchair except the pickup bed, well beyond my reach. My solution was to bolt a bike rack on the side of the truck bed and hang the chair off the two hooks, strapping it in place with a bungee cord. I liked the solution. The chair was out there making a statement; I had a pickup instead of a hospital "Ironsides" lift van. It was a form of liberation. I loved the orange truck.

The clients did too. What I saw as radical and liberating in the truck they grasped and celebrated along with me. They fought, taking turns to wash it, sit in it, or if they were able to, go for long rides along the nearby Pacific Coast. It was hard for most of the clients to accumulate enough good behavior tokens from Alice to be able to go on outings. Three in particular, Jeff, Jeanie, and David, saved up all their tokens and spent them each weekend on pickup rides.

David loved all kinds of trucks. I would stuff his flailing spastic legs into the front seat, strap him in, and off we would go. He shouted and drooled out the window as we drove down the coast. I had to be careful. If he saw an eighteen-wheel Kenworth or Peterbilt he liked, or if I simply made a joke, David would flail so violently that he could knock the car into reverse or slam on the brakes. An afternoon outing of driving around and joyous convulsions would send David exhausted to his room as though he'd had a grueling workout, which of course he'd had.

Jeff and Jeanie both used wheelchairs. Jeff pushed with the only arm he could use. His chair was heavy, with a bulky drive that allowed him to move both wheels with his single good arm. Jeanie could move both of her arms, but she was weak and had grown so fat in the hospital that even a crack in the sidewalk brought her wheelchair to an abrupt halt. Jeff was the more profoundly retarded of the two, while Jeanie was capable of thinking through a variety of simple problems. The two were inseparable, having been in the same institutions since they were very young children. Together they were a well-rehearsed comedy sketch, as well as concrete evidence of how men could get by in the world with far less upstairs than women. Jeff couldn't tell you whether the sun was up or down, but because he could act cool and talk sports scores with the guys, he was one of the care center's model citizens. Jeanie was considered more of a behavior problem. She was shy and terrified, always apologizing for being stupid, but she could calculate basketball shooting percentages and tell you the exact birthdates of every U.S. president.

They both shrieked with joy the first time I drove up in the orange truck. Jeff said that it was the "coolest" truck he had ever seen. Jeanie looked at my wheelchair hanging on the bike rack and after a moment's thought noted that it was going to get covered with mud when it rained. "Oh, Jeanie, don't be stupid," Jeff yelled. "People with trucks like the mud." I had to admit it was the first time I had thought about my chair being out in the mud. I would think of Jeanie every time I had to hose the chair down after a long trip. "You're pretty smart, Jeanie. I wonder what you are doing at the care center anyway?" "No John," she would always reply, laughing. "I'm stupid. I'm too stupid." "She's even stupider than me, John," Jeff would say.

One weekend I piled both Jeanie and Jeff into the front seat of the pickup and off we went down Route 101 south toward the city of Coos Bay. Jeff could haul his little body into the truck without a problem, but Jeanie was more of a challenge. "Oh, no, I'm going to fall, I'm going to fall," she squealed with a half-hearted conviction that said she knew one way or another that I was going to get her planted in the seat. "Jeanie, you're so fat you're going to kill John," Jeff teased. Jeanie laughed while I pushed and pulled. Some of the other clients gathered around to watch. The two Down Syndrome adults from the floor came outside and stared at us. They smiled and pointed and shrugged as if they were wondering why we didn't just stand up and climb into the truck like they could. Finally, Jeff, Jeanie, and all of Jeanie's stuff were in the cab. After sweeping the breakfast crumbs out of her chair, I folded first one, then the other wheelchair and threw them both into the bed of the truck. The Down Syndrome clients loved the loud noise of the chairs landing in the back. They seemed puzzled as to why Jeanie and Jeff weren't in them. Startled at first, they jumped back. Then, smiles returning, they clapped and waved.

On the road with the windows down, Jeanie screamed and Jeff turned the radio up loud and I watched everyone who passed by. There were three of us. There were three chairs. Passing motorists caught Jeanie's blotto face and noticed Jeff's undersized head next to her. They could only speculate about me, the driver. I widened my eyes and delivered a searing, semi-crazed expression with the precision of a fisherman casting a trout fly. The cars quickly passed us by while I spied the eyes watching us in the rearview mirrors. Sometimes it was just as much fun to play for pure shock value, like trolling with a bloody fish head. "Jeanie," I said at a stoplight. "I dare you to ask that guy where North America is." Jeanie would lean her head out of the window with her eyes focused on two different points in space, neither of them the face of the person she was speaking to, and ask, "Mister, where is North America?" Windows would roll up and we would be left at the intersection. "Was that all right, John?" Jeanie was always worried. "That dummy didn't even know where North America was," Jeff said with his cool superior voice. "Well, Jeff," I would ask, "Where is North America?" He never knew. Jeanie would answer after a long pause. "It's here, John. It's all around us." If you didn't tell Jeanie she was correct right away she would take back whatever she had said. So I told her she was right.

Jeanie thought some more and said, "Why did we ask that guy where North America was, John?" "Never mind, Jeanie, I was just being silly." She laughed.

Down the Pacific Coast Highway, Jeanie and Jeff watched the ocean in the distance while I watched to see who might be watching us. We drove to a beachfront park. The blustery chill of the Sunday spring morning assured that there would be no tourists or local beachcombers. The parking lot was empty. It was high tide and the distance to the beach was manageable. I was determined to get both Jeanie and Jeff down to the tide line where the sand was wet and hard, and they would be able to roll along the water. "Are we going to go there, John?" Jeanie said. I didn't anticipate how difficult this was going to be.

I could manage the sand only with difficulty, so I expected that Jeanie and Jeff would need help rolling across the dry patch to the tide line. I aimed both of them toward the water and took turns pushing them from behind. A half-turn at a time, we pushed our way toward the water. Jeff pushed and grunted with his one-armed drive and each inch of motion came with a cry of "I'm doing it, John." He would get ahead of Jeanie and each time she shrieked that she was being left behind.

Beneath the gray chiseled marble of Oregon's coastal sky, the three wheelchairs and the orange pickup were alone on the sand. The wind caught Jeanie's shrieks like a kite in a tornado. The infuriating little trinkets she hung from her chair danced and flapped. I alone, among the three of us, was conscious of what we might look like through the windows of the beachfront apartments and boxy little tourist hotels that surrounded the public beach on either side. At close quarters, I pushed Jeanie and Jeff with my own chair, like a switch engine guiding freight cars. Slowly we made progress toward the water.

Across the beach in one of the apartments I noticed two people standing in their wide-open windows, watching and pointing. Jeanie and Jeff were beginning to pick up momentum. Their eyes were focused on the sketchy, moving chalk mark of white foam as each successive wave defined the tide line. The increasingly moist sand was accepting their wheels like crumbly pavement. The wind and surf made it difficult to hear the words, but Jeff and Jeanie were trading their one-liners all the way down the beach. They sat together on the sand as the water streamed underneath their chairs. Jeanie squealed while Jeff rolled his chair around in front like a sentry, the flapping hair on his small head like a Cub Scout's flag. They were oblivious of the skeptical world outside the care center. I was a part of it. It seemed that I was trained to look for, anticipate, or even provoke the very people who would get the wrong idea from what we were doing. I was defending Jeanie and Jeff from a world they weren't afraid of. They were mentally retarded, wards of a state institution, and they seemed more free than I. My arms ached from pushing and so I sat back to rest, staring out at the ocean. It was me who noticed the red twirling lights of the police squad car driving slowly up to my pickup.

A resident of the beachfront property had called in our presence with the suspicion that we were carrying out a suicide pact. The officer approached us with the assumption that we were on an unscheduled, unchaperoned outing. Earlier that summer a group of pilot whales had beached themselves on the sand in an apparent death wish. We were no better at negotiating the sand than beached whales, but I was not prepared for the alarm tripped by our presence. The officer was prepared to pack us all up, and was not expecting to find a health care employee, let alone a licensed driver, with whom to discuss the matter.

"Where do you think you kids are going?" He spoke in a condescending voice that felt to me like a shower of warm, fragrant battery acid. Jeanie saw the officer before I could say anything. "Hi, Officer. We're watching the ocean and the sand dollars." Jeff noticed his holster. "Is that a real gun?" he asked. The officer gestured toward me. "It sure is a real gun and I'll show it to you if you and your little friends here come with me back to the parking lot."

"We won't be needing your assistance this morning, Officer. Don't you have something else to take care of now?" I'm sure I bristled with loathing, for the officer was taken aback, first that there was a sentient being among the three of us, then at the force with which I was attempting to dispatch him on his way to other matters. His tone changed completely. "The residents are worried about what you are doing here. We've received a number of calls."

"Well, Officer, maybe you could call them all back and tell them everything is fine here." On the planet where I dreamed of one day living, the sight of three people in wheelchairs stuck in beach sand rolling toward the ocean at high tide was no big deal.

"Where are you from?" he asked, and pulled out a notebook. It went downhill from there. When I told him we were from the care center up the road in Florence, he had to ask who our doctor was. Jeanie began to howl with laughter. "He thinks you live at the care center with me and Jeff." And, of course, Jeff had to continue looking at the officer's gun. "It's real, isn't it?" The officer had to tell me about how the people living near the beach all thought we were going to throw ourselves into the water.

Of course I had to say, "Why don't you find something important to do with your badge, like arresting some of the drunken rednecks everywhere?" And, of course, the officer got really mad then, and had to tell me that it was his business when three crippled people showed up unexpectedly on one of his beaches. He offered to push us back to the truck. And before I could decline, Jeanie just had to say, "You can push me, Officer."

We rolled back to the truck. I was fuming. He was the enemy. We had made it to the tide line. We had seen the ocean rushing underneath our chairs. To the officer, this was prelude to a mass suicide and I was Jim Jones. He had averted a terrible tragedy. To Jeanie and Jeff it was all an adventure. They had something to talk about for weeks. I alone was humiliated. When we got back to the care center, Jeanie and Jeff eagerly told the other clients about the policeman. For them it was the most exciting part. "He had a real gun," Jeff told Alice. Alice saw the sand all over the wheelchairs and wanted to know where I had taken them. "We went for a stroll on the beach and met a cop," I said. She knew there was more to it. She said she was glad she hadn't been with us.

Alice hated these scenes. There was never a way to reduce the level of gawking. Confounding the expectations of people only increased their staring. Driving around in an orange pickup with a wheelchair hanging defiantly off the side, instead of a conventional blue van with the ambulance lift, made us that much more an object of curiosity. I was getting used to it in the two years that had passed since the accident. But this was all very new to Alice. Her impulse was to blurt out, "What are you staring at?" when people gawked. She hated making a scene, but calling attention to her displeasure only made more of one.

Our best moments were when we were alone. Our worst moments were out among people. The assumptions people appeared to make about me spilled over onto her. Like on "Oprah," she felt people cast her as the nurse, or as the martyr, or as the person who needed to take care of someone else. Upon meeting us, people would ask her how many years we had been married before my accident. This was something I would never get asked; she always did. No one ever assumed that she might have chosen to be with me regardless of the wheelchair. No one considered the possibility that she did not think my accident was a tragedy. The decision I had made to "persevere" and not commit suicide was infinitely more comprehensible to those around us than her decision to choose me as a husband. The question stung her. Each answer, that we had met and gotten married well after my accident, was greeted with a surprise that hurt even more. "Really, well, isn't that interesting. I would have thought you had been married before." It was as though she had joined a leper colony as a way of meeting new people.

We loved to roll downhill together. Sitting on my lap, she escaped from all of the staring. In the waist-level world it was easier to avoid eye contact with the curiosity-seekers above. People did stare more when she sat in my lap; we just didn't notice. We were four arms, four legs, four wheels, one lap, two smiles, connected without rationalization. The wind cleansed our faces. The ride down the hill required no explanation. The wheelchair was a toy in free fall, the derby needed no soapbox. We were doing what anyone would have done with some wheels on a hill. When we came to rest, the toy became a wheelchair again, the staring no longer invisible.

When we went hiking in the mountains of western Oregon, Alice would find the places where no people went. She knew where all the untouched stands of old-growth forest were. The forces which had destroyed the forest on the way to these sanctuaries also allowed me access. We would drive to the end of a denuded logging road and hike a short, crudely hewn, but flat debris-filled trail where the log trucks and machinery had cut their swath. Suddenly we would be deep in a prehistoric cathedral of greenery. Alice was a former tree planter; she had studied forestry. She knew the name of every plant. She spoke of "Douglass Fir" with the familiarity of a relative. To Alice, Doug Fir was not just a species of tree. For me the irony was powerful. A forest had to die to create a path for me to see one.

The first summer Alice and I were together, we went to a country fair just outside Eugene. It was a crowded, hot day in the woods where thousands of people took off their clothes and listened to dulcimer music, smoked pot, had their palms read, and generally scandalized the old-time loggers who lived nearby. For hours I rolled, with some difficulty, over miles of crowded bark-chip trails, past booths of people getting save-the-whale tattoos, selling authentic Indian Tee Pees, plans for building your own dome house, and custom-carved wooden yarrow sticks for throwing the *I Ching*. At one booth, people claimed that the reason I couldn't walk might be untreated food allergies. They offered to bring my body back into balance with an herbal drink that cost fifty dollars for a month's supply and looked like a shovelful of lawn clippings mixed with a quart of poster paint.

In the center of the fair, in a meadow where the dulcimer players performed, the women all took off their shirts and the kids ran around naked. Locals could be seen standing off in the trees staring at hippie breasts like a junior high school gym class left alone with a stack of old

National Geographics. The police lined the entrance to the parking lot with orders to move in if the drug use got too obvious, or if any of the men took their pants off.

Everyone either stumbled over me or offered to push. While this was only mildly irritating to me, it was much more frustrating for Alice, who was glad to get back into the truck and head home. I drove slowly out of the parking lot, through the gauntlet of police directing traffic on the two-lane road adjoining the woods. Just before turning out onto the highway, an officer pointed at the wheelchair hanging from the side of my truck and started to shout, "You can't keep that there." It was hot and everyone was grumpy. He walked over to the truck and started to lift my wheelchair off the rack. I said, "What are you doing? The chair stays right where it is." It wasn't clear if the cop was even aware that he was looking at a wheelchair. "This goes in the truck bed where it belongs."

I started to explain that I couldn't get the wheelchair out of the back of the truck bed on my own. That's why I had the rack. He had not connected me to the chair in any sense other than that I was trying to get away with defying the Oregon state police by brazenly hanging a wheelchair from a bike rack on the side of my orange pickup, instead of putting it in the back. He was pulling the chair off the rack when I hit the accelerator and yelled, "Get your hands off the chair, pal!" The cop started to scream and held onto the back of the truck as I drove forward, carrying him and my wheelchair, which now dangled loosely from the rack. The rest of the police officers sprang into action and ran in front of the truck, blocking my way, drawing their guns and pointing them directly at my face.

I stopped when I noticed that Alice was screaming for me to stop the car, and was trying to get her foot on the brake pedal. The cops surrounded us and demanded that I get out. Trying to explain that I couldn't stand up sounded like more defiance. Two officers opened the door and began to haul me out of the car. Alice was hysterical now. I was screaming expletive-laced vows to kill the entire Oregon state police force. The wheelchair dangled from the bike rack. The locals stopped watching the naked dancing women for a moment and turned to watch this gathering riot. Even the dulcimer music stopped. "I can't walk," I said finally. "That's why I have the chair."

A senior officer stepped forward and told the other cops to put away their guns. "You shouldn't try to run over the state police on a hot day, son," he said calmly. I explained that it was my chair and the officer had started to move it without even letting me explain, and that I couldn't reach the chair if it was in the truck bed. He looked at Alice. "Couldn't she get the chair for you?" "What if I'm by myself," I shot back. "Do I have to have a nurse drive with me so I don't get arrested?" The officer remained calm. He pointed at Alice. "She doesn't look like your nurse."

"I'm his wife, Officer." Alice was apologizing and insisting that it was just a hot day. Tempers had flared without reason. "No hard feelings," she said. The officer had a compromise. "Couldn't we just put the chair in the back this one time, until you get home?" The officer gave me back my driver's license. "Let's not have any trouble. I don't know about wheelchair racks on the sides of pickups, but I know it's against the law to try and run over a police officer in this state. I don't have to check that." We drove away. I scowled at the line of officers. Alice pulled her baseball cap down over her face. We didn't speak the whole ride home.

She hated all of the staring, and especially these violent little scenes pitting me against the world. They were painful, destructive, directed from something deep inside me. I always told Alice that I would never let it happen again, that I would try to be more reasonable, but I knew it wasn't true. Mine was the secret ambivalence of an addict. Each scene delivered an exhilarating high of righteousness, a permission to be angry, something never permitted in day-to-day life. They were wrong, I was right. I could say it without hesitation. But each confrontation also brought with it a surge of poison; each fix tightened an internal knot. A reluctant Sancho Panza to my wheeled Quixote, Alice and I were drawn together and forced apart by our journey. I was fighting for some idea of freedom. She alone could see that I was not free.

Roll Model

*A*rmrests were out.

Crips have few pieces of advice for other folks in chairs; this was one of them. In the mid-seventies the prevailing wheelchair culture for paraplegics involved playing wheelchair basketball, terrorizing drivers who parked illegally in handicapped spaces, and waiting for computer implants to repair spinal cords and make everyone walk again. Armrests made some sense because they were comfortable. Quadriplegics all had armrests, but for them balance was a serious issue because of limited hand and arm function. I showed up to play wheelchair basketball one time and was promptly told by the other crips that I needed to lose my armrests.

There is something utterly intimidating about seeing a person close to your circumstances with a physical command of body and space that you don't possess. These guys were hot dogs. Walter was the captain of the Eugene, Oregon, wheelchair basketball team. He had been a star on Fresno, California's team, a national wheelchair basketball power, and was in Eugene going to school, as I was. Walter was not someone you spotted and immediately said, "There goes a basketball star." He was fat and goofy-looking. But he was a solid three-point shooter, and he was always the fastest downcourt. He had no armrests, and in a one-on-one would play to the bitter end. His defensive moves would often end with him spilled onto the gym floor, holding the ball. Walter told me that using armrests was for pussies, and whenever I came to practice he would point at mine and laugh.

Walter had a way of quickly assessing whether someone he met for the first time was cool or a jerk. Arm strength was a big indicator of character to Walter. He liked to grab one of my wheels from behind just as I started to roll, stopping me cold. His wrists were so strong it felt as though the chair had suddenly broken. Alarmed, I would look at the frame and the axles just to hear Walter say, "When you gonna lose the armrests, pussy?" I was bullied into losing my armrests in the late seventies. People often ask why I don't use armrests. I have only one answer, the one Walter taught me: armrests are for the Tiny Tim, cup-in-hand, poster boy, "Jerry Lewis Telethon" crips.

Once, many years later, I thought of Walter when I was waiting with a colleague for a cab at a hotel in Los Angeles. The doors opened and a man in a wheelchair was rolled by an attendant up to the edge of the roadway to wait for a vehicle. My eyes popped. I leaned over to my non-crip friend and whispered, "There's Larry Flynt."

"Who's Larry Flynt?"

No crip would ever have to ask. It is hard to have role models in a wheelchair. In America you have FDR, of course, but he was the champion self-loather who was never photographed in a chair during his lifetime, and made a deal with the press corps that he was never to be even seen in crutches. If FDR had done wheelies or had worked out advanced transferring techniques on the White House furniture, that information is lost to the crip world, like Mayan dialects or Incan shopping lists. The details of wheelchair history put out with the trash, the FDR legacy is a troubled one.

You had the Vietnam dudes, but they were so involved in the war it was impossible to get them to deal with disability. In the film *Born on the Fourth of July*, director Oliver Stone is obsessed with penises, and writer Ron Kovaks is obsessed with the war and an idea of America he should never have believed if he had had half a brain growing up. Only actor Tom Cruise seems to be interested in the chair itself, but he can walk, so who cares if he can hop stairs in a wheelchair? It's like Patty Duke playing Helen Keller and getting an Academy Award for saying "wa-wa . . . wa-wa." The little crip kid in the movie *Boyz 'n the Hood* had excellent technique but only a couple of lines, and then at the end of the film became a symbol of the horrible end in store for you if you didn't leave the ghetto. Thanks.

So who does that leave? There are endless role-model profiles of famous heroic quadriplegic skiers and football players, and there's James Brady, the former Reagan press secretary. They are the feel-good characters that make it into the mainstream media. In fact, it's mostly athlete crips or former athlete crips who make it into the media. My favorite are the football players. When they act like livestock and run headlong into each other in a semi-comatose testosterone frenzy they are called "team players" following their coach's orders; if these same players break their necks and end up in wheelchairs they are the brave men who took the ultimate risk to win. In the hospital they are like the diving-accident people. "So, like, um, shallow water and you dove into it, fine. And over here men in armored suits butting each other with their heads while running at top speed . . . fine." What's the message here? It's certainly not about whether football or measuring the depth of the water before you go diving are a good idea.

The hero business is targeted chiefly at the nondisabled. It's apparently reassuring to be told over and over again that you can survive a disabling injury and live off the sale of the TV movie. But what about practical details from people who know the ropes, who have hung in there, who have taken the airline flights, gotten a real job, and found the unfindable public bathroom?

In America, for role models, basically, you've got FDR and Helen Keller, you've got George Wallace, Larry Flynt, and few others. Larry Flynt publishes porn, and his idea of disability empowerment is putting pictures of amputees having sex with their stumps in his magazine *Hustler.*

Physicist Stephen Hawking is someone I looked up to even though he is way below eye level in his small body and electric wheelchair. His wisdom is delivered through priestly graduate student acolytes who speak for him. He lectures on stage with an assistant actually decoding Hawking's odd little grunts and moans. It's not as though the decoded version made any more sense than moans and grunts. That's the beauty of Hawking. You have to strain to hear him. You have to strain to read him. He looks like a perfect excuse for the handgun-in-the-mouth exit, but there he is talking about black holes. Hawking does not deliver lectures on self-esteem, or motivation, or the human wellspring of potential. He says things like, "For small cold bodies, self-gravity can be neglected and the degeneracy pressure will be balanced by attractive electrostatic forces between nearest neighbor particles arranged in some sort of lattice."

I suppose that it's possible that this actually does refer to human potential, but if so, only implicitly. Hawking's first book is called *Large Scale Structure of Space-Time,* in which he thinks about, and describes, the fabric of the universe in the densest mathematical language imaginable. Hawking has Lou Gehrig's disease, or ALS, a degenerative disease of the nervous system. He not only sits in a wheelchair but as a professor at Cambridge University he sits in the mathematics Chair that had once belonged to Isaac Newton + chair + wheels + batteries + motor + 325 years = Hawking.

I once attended a lecture by Hawking at the University of Chicago. In the woody depths of Mandel Hall I sat in the front row watching Hawking expound about the arrow of time. Time's arrow, he claimed at the time, may be a function of whether the universe is expanding or contracting, and should the universe ever begin to collapse, then as space would start contracting, so would we also begin to lose the accumulation of time and instead slip into the past.

As usual, Hawking's speech was nearly incomprehensible. This was in 1986, and since then Hawking has stopped speaking through an interpreter, preferring a voice machine instead, and has discarded his notions about the flow of time as untestable. But with all his difficulty in moving around, Hawking is this planet's authority on the behavior of gravity; in Hawking's particular case, gravity is a force he might just as well do without. A weightless world would permit Hawking's body to move autonomously. In his work he does not speak much about weightlessness. Quite the opposite, he studies and theorizes about black holes, places where the most intense gravitational forces would trap all of the rest of the universe like him. Hawking has always maintained that mathematics is a way to ask the truly big questions. He has a particularly riveting grasp of those questions, so interesting that to even begin thinking about them is to hurl oneself off the ledge of physical intuition and to have faith in thought alone. Such questions are worth thinking about to Hawking; what is given and unalterable, like his physical condition, is uninteresting. Hawking is a solid varsity crip, way beyond the Helen Keller league.

Following the lecture, I went outside to find my car and encountered Hawking and a group of university bigwigs heading off to some self-congratulating academic soiree. I rolled up to the group and addressed Professor Hawking. I started to tell him how much I had enjoyed his lecture. His assistant interrupted me before I could finish and said curtly, "Professor Hawking is very busy and must go to his next appointment. Please excuse us!"

I looked into Hawking's eyes to try and appeal the assistant's precipitous judgment and at least get a tiny nod of solidarity. There was none. Hawking's eyes said that rule one to his assistants was to roll him quickly away from any crazy people in wheelchairs who approached him. He clearly didn't want anything whatsoever to do with me, even though I had read his work. My wheelchair disqualified me, just as his qualified him to ignore me.

Why had Hawking confused me with some drooling, fawning fan who cared more about wheelchairs than his Nobel-class physics? I groped in my heart for the badge that would get me through the checkpoint and allow me to talk to him. He thought I was one of those irritating disabled people, one of those telethon crips. But I wasn't. I was a guy who knew mathematics, I had a job, I had a career. I had no armrests. "Hey, wait, there must be some mistake."

I sat there in the cold among the Gothic spires of the gray University of Chicago campus and chuckled at my own thoughts. So I need a badge to speak to Steven Hawking? So what if I was a telethon crip? So what if I admired his physical challenges and integrated them into my own understanding of his work? So what if I was in a wheelchair and not a tenured dust head who's spent too much time in a supercollider? "Hey, Hawking! When you gonna lose those pansy-assed armrests?"

This culture trades in role models. They are useful pointers of hope for people who need to feel that they can escape from various kinds of imprisonment and adversity: the ghetto, poverty, immigrant marginality, physical handicap. If Hawking was sick of wheelchairs and disability, his success made it far more likely that he would be identified as a role model for the very class of people he was trying to escape. Hawking has a real job. He is a physicist specializing in the theory of gravity. Just as matter is sucked inescapably into black holes, so Hawking's triumphs in physics make it impossible for him to escape being known as the man heroically triumphing over Lou Gehrig's disease. Hawking is the little guy with the glasses in the wheelchair. That's how he's known to the world outside physics, trapped like amber in the trophies and footnotes of sentiment.

On the other hand, Larry Flynt is no one's role model. He has escaped being stereotyped as a brave crip. There at the hotel Flynt rolled into view in his gold-plated wheelchair with the maroon velour upholstery. With his moussed blondish hair and gold chair he looked like a big fat trinket: a human paperweight. The person I was with wondered why I knew so much about the publisher of *Hustler* magazine: every paraplegic knows that Larry Flynt has a gold-plated wheelchair. No other crip would be caught dead in one. It is Larry's signature. Even the spokes are gold. To the world, Larry Flynt is the millionaire pornographer. This disqualifies him for heroism. He never gets asked to speak at the Easter Seals convention; he never gets invited to the Special Olympics; he never gets asked to appear with Jerry on the telethon.

Flynt's TV crip movie would truly be interesting to see; you just couldn't show it on TV. Of all the people to lose the use of their penises, Larry Flynt the skin mag mogul really rolled snake eyes when he was injured. "The story of a man who despite his tragic disability continued on with his life. His life was ruined by a gunshot wound, but bravely he would not allow his paralysis to get in the way of publishing pictures of spread-eagled blondes performing fellatio." America likes its heroes all wide-eyed and innocent. Unless Flynt finds Jesus or starts his own telethon, nobody will care about his story. Because he's a pornographer, nobody is going to call Larry a role model. Because he has armrests, he's a wimp.

I looked him up and down in front of the hotel. He did not want to look at me any more than Steven Hawking did. I checked out his arms. They were scrawny. One of his tires was soft. He was being pushed. One of his shoes was untied. He had gold-plated armrests on his chair. If Larry wanted to lose his armrests, he could melt them down and live off the gold.

One place in America where there are always lots of wheelchairs and crip role models is at the Vietnam Veterans Memorial in Washington, D.C. Sunny days make the black granite of "the wall" into a mirror. The slow-ramped descent into the center of the V is particularly powerful in a chair, a slow pan back into history. The names float by above and below. At four feet eleven you are waist level to the slaughter.

I missed going to the Vietnam War by a few years. In junior high school the lottery numbers for the draft were a constant preoccupation. Discussions of student deferments, no student deferments, being brave and stupid and going off to war, or being smart and cowardly and going off to Canada filled cafeterias and playgrounds. It was coming our way. It was a surprise to my friends and me that Nixon actually ended the war when he did. Of all the rites of passage in high school the most vivid was going to the draft board to get the draft card. When the war ended, draft cards were no longer worth burning. The lottery numbers were forgotten. The last year of the lottery was my sophomore year. I know I was obsessed with my number then; I can't remember it anymore.

The war dug a trench through a nation and between two generations. On one side were the veterans, on the other side the nation that had sent them to war. To roll in a wheelchair down the cobblestoned path alongside the monument was to climb into that ditch. It was a different kind of staring as I joined the slow procession of people on their way to the monument. To these people the chair signified veteran, that I must have been wounded in the war.

The Vietnam Veterans Memorial is in a part of Washington with ramps on every corner and wide, smooth pavement promising state-of-the-art access. In purely physical terms, it is one of the easiest places to get around in a chair. As a landmark of the national psyche, it is a closed, frozen space. Rolling through the monument on its first Veterans' Day, I was anointed by a tragedy I never experienced, but the crowds so needed to believe I was a part of it that it felt almost obscene to announce otherwise. I was a fly on a black wall stuck to the names of the dead. The crowds slowed my chair with staring unlike the customary street voyeurs. Offers to help were many, and filled with very personal comments about patriotism and America and pride. "This place is for you, son," a father said within earshot of his wide-eyed kids. It wasn't. It was. People wanted to talk to me about folks they had lost in the war.

The memorial was intended to be a touchstone for those who observed the war as a national scar, as well as those who wore their scars from battle in tattered ill-fitting combat garb pulled from closet retirement for the occasion. I wandered among the crowd of mostly non-veterans. *The Washington Post* described that first Veterans' Day when "the wall" was dedicated as a collective national act of contrition. On the ground it seemed more like an outing where the principal activity was rewriting history. Families exclaimed their patriotism. The protesters came back to apologize to the veterans. The veterans came back to feel like heroes, or anything at all for the first time. Those who ignored the war while it was going on came back to explain to their kids where they were, when. Those who had ignored the protests of the war came back to reclaim lost virtue and revel guiltlessly, and with TV cameras rolling, in "America, right or wrong."

This tournament of emotions sought only the end to a large, undefined pain coined somewhat deliberately as the Vietnam Syndrome, pop-ular then and now. On that day, the curious learned quite a lot about the Vietnam Syndrome and almost nothing about the war, except that 58,000 Americans died there. The monument made that point well. Other points were lost. There were no Vietnamese faces to be seen, even though a short walk across the Memorial Bridge brought you to Little Saigon in the Virginia suburb of Clarendon. Thousands of residents buy fabrics and eat bamboo-steamed rice cakes in one of the largest Vietnamese immigrant communities in the U.S.

Around me, fingers pointed and mothers nodded as something about me was explained to their children. A man asked about my unit and which branch of the service I had been part of in the war. He was not a veteran; he seemed slightly younger than me. He groped for some meaning about the war that I could not truthfully supply. I could have given him a fictitious unit and battle and war wound. His need was great to hear such a story. I thought of thanking him for recognizing the ser-vice of the veterans. His face was tearful and would have filled in any line drawing I supplied. I could not bring myself to either explain that I was hurt in a car accident, or to elaborate some tale of Vietnamismo. In the end I just nodded vaguely without words.

I did not relish this disguise, but I couldn't take it off in that crowd that day. I was an impostor. The actual veterans around me paid me no mind. They weren't confused. In my face, I was disqualified. Youth and the clean pavement around the eyes confirmed that I had not marched the jungles and stared into the pits that haunted these men. I could not blame anyone else who saw me for thinking that I might have been a veteran. I did blame them for needing to think it.

I wanted to see the Memorial for my own reasons and I rolled up to a place on the wall where the writing was thick and tall. I scanned the names. Pictures fanned the mind, connecting one name to another. Where had they died? The names were roughly chronological, and there was a temptation to try and imagine which had died in groups and which were just single names. Some people who viewed the wall saw groupings of buddies. The bad days. The lucky shell that hit the crowded tent. The battle that had gone terribly wrong. The ambush. The pilot who died alone.

The names looked beautiful and sacred and horrible, as the tally of any slaughter would be. I reached out to touch the wall and looked into the granite. Even up close, the reflection in the black polished surface was clear. I saw my face and my fingers and after a moment I saw behind me a small crowd staring and two people with cameras poised to shoot.

I turned around and on everyone's face was a deep sadness. They were watching me. I looked back at the wall. They thought that these names I was touching were my buddies, the men I had left. The men I had tried to save. The men who had saved me. The men who had died because I had gotten the flu that day and stayed at the base avoiding the bloody ambush. I was the bullet to the back, they were the bullets to the brain. I was "pretended to be dead" while they were "fought to the death." I shook my head and tried to jog the racing imaginations of strangers. There was nothing to be done. I backed away.

"It's okay, son. We want you in the picture."

I rolled away quickly. On the way out I rolled past a veteran in a uniform that had long ago ceased to fit. He was sitting with two friends. They were smiling broadly and tearfully at the proceedings. The crowds belonged to them, as did the monument. Their faces were stubbled and unkempt, their eyes drunken with a glow part liquid, part catharsis. Their wheelchairs were old. The treads on their tires were smoothed from long years of slow use, slightly deflated and squished flat at the bottom where they touched the road. On their frames and upholstery were stickers and little knickknacks. A pocket for cigarettes and a little bracket for an ashtray. A holder for a beer can.

We spoke briefly. I shook their hands. One of the men was a paraplegic, the other two had lost their legs. The youngest and thinnest of the three had crutches attached to his chair and the below-the-knee prosthesis was exposed for all to see. Its mechanical ball joint was well oiled and beautiful. It had the serious look of something well used and usefully filthy. There was no question: these men were veterans.

"Car accident, right?" one of them said as he offered me some beer. "I could tell by the chair."

"I wish I could get the VA to buy me one of them chairs."

I was not a veteran: there was no question about that here. We talked a little about hardware and seat cushions. We talked a little about Vietnam. One of the men said that sometimes he was afraid to take off his uniform. He said there were a lot of bodies with no names.

I asked about the memorial and one of the men held up a piece of paper with the names rubbed on in pencil. The impressions were obtained by placing the paper on the wall of the memorial and rapidly shading over the etched granite with a pencil. "It took too long for people to remember us," he said. He asked me if I liked the memorial. I told him that I did very much, but that the civilians kept thinking I was a veteran and asking me questions about the war. All three of them found this quite funny. They all laughed and looked me up and down. "That's the stupidest thing I've heard all day," the paraplegic said.

What I noticed when I looked at his chair was the armrests. They all had armrests except me.

Reaching
the Pedals

*I*n the fall of 1978, two years of practicing the piano would be tested at the University of Oregon music school. Alice and I moved to Eugene. I started school and prepared my audition while Alice got a job at a care center in Eugene. The University of Oregon was accessible: its buildings were laid out in a small wooded valley. The music school occupied the highest point on the campus; the practice rooms overlooked a hilltop of pine trees and lush ferns. Rolling the trail along the edge of the forest, the sound of pianos and bassoons, marimba, and cellos drifted chaotically through the trees. I wanted so badly to be in one of those rooms. I applied to study piano and composition.

I had worked very hard to return to school, but I wanted to do something besides the academic subjects that had been so frustrating at the University of Chicago. It was important now, after the accident, to do something meaningful. Music had been a part of my life since my first piano lessons at age four, but going to music school was all about reclaiming the joy Rick and I had had playing together in Chicago before my accident. It was all I wanted to do. In Oregon, and without Rick, I would find my own way.

My audition took place in the small office of the head of the department with the three members of the piano faculty sitting just two feet behind me. It was a crowded room. They moved furniture to make a path from the door to the keyboard. I told them I would not be needing the piano bench, but there was no place for it in the little room except in front of the piano. One of the professors placed it out in the hall. I sat in my chair with my feet tucked under the wheels. I did not use the pedals. I played a Bach prelude and a short piece by Chopin. Of the three faculty members at the audition, the most intimidating presence was Madame Thal. She was compact and formidable with the body architecture of Catherine the Great. She spoke with a deep voice and rolled her r's in a vaguely European inflection which made it seem to me that she might be personal friends with Rachmaninoff. The other two were a tall man with enormous hands named Victor Steinhardt, who seemed to have the only sense of humor of the trio, and Professor William Woods, the upright, silver-haired chairman of the department.

The Bach piece went well, but after the Chopin, Professor Thal crisply remarked, "It's clever what you are doing there with your hands. I suppose you would have to play it that way." What I was doing was using the reach of my fingers to hold notes that would otherwise have been sustained by depressing the pedal. I would strike and hold keys down to sustain the notes before moving on. It was the only way for me to even come close to the effect of pedaling, but it meant that my hands were stiff and stuck to the keys, crawling back and forth across the keyboard. The training Madame Thal had received called for arched wrists and floating, spidery hands brushing the keyboard from above. My elephant fingers were not much to look at. Professor Steinhardt looked at my enormous wheelchair biceps. "You look as though you could lift the piano with one hand," he said. "You have quite a reach, well over an octave." Everyone seemed impressed by the sound I had managed to coax out from under my clumpy digits. There was still the matter of the pedals. I wasn't going to be using them. Professor Woods remained silent. He had been tenured for eons at the university and had taught child prodigies as well as marching band majors whose first instrument was the tuba. He seemed intrigued by the whole idea of a student who couldn't pedal at all.

"There is too much pedaling in modern performance," he said. "Pedal turns the clear lines of Mozart and Beethoven into mud." His two colleagues nodded in agreement. Professor Woods stood up, placed one hand behind his back, and began to leaf through the book of Chopin pieces I had brought to the audition. He cleared his throat. "Of course, most music for piano requires pedal. You understand that, don't you?" I said that I understood, but still wanted to study piano. I was accepted into the program. Two years of practicing since the accident had paid off. It wasn't Juilliard, but I was in music school.

At my first lesson Professor Woods made it clear that there would be no more stiff compensating fingers simulating the pedal sound. I would begin with the unpedaled literature of Mozart and Bach. It was all written for harpsichord and very early fortepianos where pedal was used sparingly, if at all. "Your arm must be floating in the air, your hands hanging limp and strong off the end of your wrists. You can worry about the pedal later."

Avoiding the pedal meant avoiding virtually all keyboard music written after the 1850s: no Liszt, Schumann, Shubert, or Brahms, and of course no Ravel, Rachmaninoff, or Debussy. I practiced my assigned repertoire, but the lush flowing chords of the modern romantics tantalized me. I dreamed of how I might make the pedals work. Sometimes I would ask Alice to hold down the pedal while I listened to the open strings ring and echo off each other. The harmonics of each string ascended across the sound board like tall crystal ladders in a stately procession of sound, an infinity of tolling bells that vanished when she let go of the pedal. The felt dampers slipped back down on the strings, burying my dream bells in soft wool.

Short of taping the pedal to the floor, there did not seem to be a way to even begin playing keyboard music written after 1800. No device to operate the pedal other than with the feet was available. There were hand controls for operating pedals, but they were for industrial shop tools, drill presses, and band saws. Automotive hand controls worked well, but the chief limitation of any hand control was that you had to take one hand off the keyboard to use it. A trained monkey working the pedals for me was more practical than that. The only solution was to build something completely new.

Professor Woods was intrigued with the idea of a device that might allow me to attempt Chopin or Debussy. He was utterly without any mechanical talent whatsoever. I was the first of his students to haul prototypes into his office and spread blueprints out on the black Steinway next to his desk during a lesson. It was great fun. I planned a recital for the late spring.

The device would need to be portable, silent, quick, and sensitive. It would need to be mouth-operated since head movements would interfere with reading music. In settling on a design I had much to learn about the delicate motion behind the sustain pedal on a piano, and the foot that could operate it properly. My first prototype used an electrical solenoid that ran off wall current. It was fast and powerful, but made a noise like a hammer when it was engaged, and its magnets hummed like a bad refrigerator. It slammed the pedal to the floor with all of the subtlety of one of the presses at the furniture factory. The first time I bit down and threw the switch it knocked one of the pedals clear off my piano at home. There were other problems with a solenoid design: it was disconcerting to have a switch in your mouth that was connected directly to a 120-volt wall socket. I spared Professor Woods inspection of this design.

The device that began to take form, much to the fascination of Professor Woods and the music school faculty, operated by compressed air. A small piston with a rubber pad cut from the sole of a shoe was set directly over the sustain pedal. The piston was connected to an air line that went to a series of valves that could be controlled by biting down on a plastic ball like the old remote shutters for a camera. The air came from a compressor at first, but when even the quietest one proved to be too noisy I found an old scuba tank. I filled the tank with compressed air, where it functioned just like a battery. A regulator doled out air in small, silent bursts. Biting down on the ball opened the regulator, and just enough air to swiftly depress the pedal was released into the air line. Relaxing the ball closed the air line. The pedal went back up, and the air was exhausted with a tiny hiss though a filter under the piano. Depending on how much pedal was required in the music, a full tank of air would last for a few hours of practicing.

The machine was constructed from items available at junk shops and somewhat exotic industrial specialty stores where inventors would go to bring their blueprints to life. There in the steel-caged shelving of these places were other pale-skinned inventors rooting quietly through oily metal bins, examining tubes and coils and gadgets to see if they could be fitted to a task they believed had only been envisioned by them. For the year it took to design and construct the pedal device I was part of this strange brotherhood of inventors.

We were all short on cash, wore torn and wrinkled shirts, and drove old cars filled with the accumulated debris of what might once have worked, might be made to work, and what had never worked at all. "It's for a mouth-operated pedal device. I want to use it on a piano," I would explain. "Yes, of course," my fellow inventors would nod. It was another thing that needed to be figured out. They looked at a wheelchair as an opportunity for applying ingenuity. Disability was not a tragedy, it was an uncharted reservoir of special cases in the vast ocean of unmet needs inventors saw everywhere. When one of my inventor friends stared at my chair it was a binding force. "You could connect a trailer right here and go camping." "There could be a way of adjusting the height of the chair so you could reach cans on the top shelf in the supermarket." "How about solar panels?" "You could put a generator on the wheels and charge your batteries as you rolled." The ideas were mostly impractical, but they were fun to think about. The most useful thing about talking to inventors was that they looked at the chair as I did.

Inventors weren't shy about disability because they saw the physical details as an interesting problem in engineering. As long as the wheelchair said tragedy, everyone was inclined to stare and look away. Problem solving brought people together. None of my inventor friends ever asked about my accident. It didn't occur to them. We talked about all of our inventions: the self-cleaning hubcaps, heated snow shovels, remote baby monitors, automatic programmable pet feeders. In the grand tapestry of form and function, each of these ideas was a single stitch and the inventors were the weavers.

I filled up our house with lumber and compressed air components and eagerly awaited delivery of the custom-made items for the latest design. The man from UPS grew fond of following my progress. With each delivery he would ask, "Is this going to make it faster?" "This will make it quieter, right?" "This will allow you to play longer." He watched the pile of gadgets take form on the brown upright piano in my living room. "You're getting there." He was excited.

The pedal device cost about $525 to build, which was an extraordinary sacrifice for a music student on food stamps. Its debut at the music school in April 1979 consisted of a recital and demonstration which attracted lots of attention but was not a red-letter day in the history of musical performance. The little piano piece "Gymnopedies" by Eric Satie, which cannot be played at all without the pedal, was the music for the demonstration. Aside from one measure where the device got stuck and the notes bled together in an ugly unnatural chord, the thing worked pretty well. At best, my performance was serviceable, but that wasn't the point.

I sat with my fingers floating over the keys. When I bit down, a burst of compressed air would race through the plastic tubing to the cylinder and the piston would silently depress the pedal. The row of felt dampers lifted off the wire strings above the sound board. I had played for years without seeing them move like that. Seeing the dampers lift all at once was thrilling. Unable to walk, I had stepped through a door and back in time. I learned that feet and legs meant more than walking: they gave magic to the notes, sustaining them with the piano's dreamy bell sound, tolling Satie's and Debussy's century of birth to a close. As I unclenched my teeth, the pedal popped up and the dampers lay back down on the strings. In the silence I could just barely hear the sound of the air that had been holding the pedal now hissing as it aspirated out a small opening. It sounded like a tiny breath. To the audience it was a triumph. They gave me a standing ovation.

There was sadness as much as excitement in this small triumph. Just as I could only reach the first step of the wooden stairs back in physical therapy on my way up to board my imagined subways, this device did not begin to solve the problem of the pedals. If anything, it revealed just how difficult the problem actually was, if I wanted to play the piano as it truly should be played. I received an A plus from Professor Wood, who beamed with pride and had tears in his eyes as he listened to me grope my way through "Gymnopedies." We both knew that my device lacked the subtlety necessary for music. It was more spectacle than musical, functional but not suitable for real performances. The idea that the muscles of the legs and foot might be replaced by a few hundred dollars worth of items from the hardware store, even for a task that seemed as simple as the control of a pedal, was more naive than planning to ascend thirty steps to take an eighty-five-cent subway ride in Chicago.

The device was 90 percent workable. To engineer it up to 98 or 99 percent would cost far more than this first prototype and require much more time and sophistication. It would mean supplementing the compressed air mechanism with computer driven, ultraprecise motors. These could not be adapted from other applications or pulled from a bin at a hardware store. They would have to be custom-made at great expense, and there was still no guarantee that using the improved device would be any more musically satisfying.

I could be an inventor or I could be a concert pianist. Both would demand a lifetime of work, and to do one would mean giving up the chance to do the other. I knew as I played the recital that I was not going to take the pedal device to that next step. Conquering the pedal on a piano beyond this rudimentary demonstration stage was only worth doing for the sake of the music. This meant that I had to want to play the music more than I wanted to conquer the problem with the pedal. As I played I knew I didn't want it that much. There would be other things I might want that much someday.

Professor Woods had thought of all this too. He came to me during my next lesson and said how excited and proud he was, but that perhaps I might like to try the harpsichord. "There are no pedals on the harpsichord," he said. Even if I had ever been curious about the harpsichord, this was just the kind of thing that would make me never want to touch one. The no-pedal option, I imagined, was the cowardly one, as though harpsichords were invented in medieval Europe to give disabled war veterans from the Crusades a musical instrument they could play in their Special Education classes.

But harpsichords were not pianos for people with disabilities. There were no pedals on the harpsichord for the same reason that French horns had no pedals. They were not needed. I couldn't credibly construe the harpsichord as a secret weapon built by some conspiracy to keep me from playing the piano. I did try. "They never took me seriously. They were just humoring me all along. I should never have believed them." With very little enthusiasm, I agreed to see the harpsichord professor. I half expected his office to be filled with amputees and people in wheelchairs, like me, steered away from taking piano lessons. It was not the case; I was the only disabled person in the harpsichord program just as I had been in the piano department. "You might find that you will be able to concentrate more on the music now," Professor Hamilton said at our first meeting. He was right that music had been the last thing on my mind.

Without a physical obstacle, I was free simply to play the music. It was a freedom that required no victory or public vindication. I did not have to file a lawsuit, bulldoze a staircase, or become an engineer to play the music of Couperin, Mozart, and Rameau. It was a harpsichord that suggested to me that there was a way through life without all of the confrontations. In the first half of the eighteenth century, during the gloomiest barbaric excesses of the Spanish Inquisition, Dominico Scarlatti had found a way to escape the public executions and courtly debates over how heretics were precisely to be compensated in pain and permanent injury for their imagined insults to God. He played the harpsichord. In the twentieth century I played Scarlatti's harpsichord sonatas.

I made one more pedal device before I put away my tools. About a year and a half after Alice and I were married, I got fed up with driving with an automatic transmission. My orange truck was an automatic, but I wanted to trade it in on a four-wheel-drive vehicle with a four-speed stick shift.

I had heard somewhere that there were hand controls for manual transmissions. I didn't know anything about them. I didn't know if it was practical for me to drive a stick shift, or even safe. I did know that I wasn't about to take anyone's word for it without trying it myself. Determination to try the impossible against all odds may be heroic. It is not the best attitude to have when visiting a used-car dealer. Most people would shy away from vehicles they are unable to drive. I wanted to look at the most difficult, impossible cars for someone in a wheelchair, manual transmission only.

Our salesman showed us a Toyota Land Cruiser. Land Cruisers are very high off the ground. Hopping into the seat from a wheelchair requires the energy of a poll vaulter. Out in the lot with Alice and the salesman watching, and me sweating and grunting, I made it into the driver's seat, although my pants were down around my knees. The salesman didn't even flinch. "Now, with suspenders that will be no problem at all," he said. Alice wasn't quite as convinced. "Are you sure that you want to be doing that every day?"

I didn't feel like discussing my physical capabilities with Alice in front of a total stranger. The salesman was more encouraging. "Think of all the places you'll be able to go in this vehicle." This salesman had already convinced me to buy one car I could barely lift myself into, and so he started to sell me one more car I could not drive out of the lot. "John," she said, "think about this." For just a little more money, the salesman suggested that we could buy a small Toyota coupe along with the Land Cruiser for those days when I didn't want to bother with all the effort that came with getting into the Land Cruiser. "I'll give you an unbelievable price." Both the coupe and the Land Cruiser had manual transmissions.

"We just came here to see if it was possible for you to climb into a Land Cruiser." Alice was a little worried. "Now this guy is going to sell you two cars that you don't even know for sure that you can drive. Are you crazy?" I had driven into the dealership with a pick-up under my own power. I left in a caravan without the pickup. Alice drove one car, the dealer the other. I sat in the backseat and looked at the clutch and brake pedals and thought about the monthly payment we would be making for the next four years.

If I wasn't crazy for buying both cars, I was probably crazy for keeping them later. I called my old driver's training instructor back in rehab to get the name of the manufacturer of the hand controls I'd heard about for manual transmissions, and how I could call them and place a rush order. The company was very cooperative.

"Yes, we make hand controls for manual transmissions." I was elated. I told them about my two new vehicles. "No problem, we have a model that will fit each of those cars." The price was reasonable, and the agent even asked the name of my insurance company so that he could bill them directly and send the two units out that same day. He said they would arrive the next morning, and he gave me a number to call if I had any trouble installing them. "One last question and we're through," he said. "Just tell me which of your legs is amputated."

"Amputated? Right." I hung up. These were not for paraplegics. I had just purchased not one, but two cars that, at the very least, were illegal for me to drive, assuming I could ever modify them enough to get either of them out of the driveway. It took me a few days to tell Alice that the hand controls I had imagined didn't exist for paraplegics. She suggested that if there was ever a reason for a dealer to take cars back, this might be it. Maybe a lawyer could help, she said. But I could not face going back to the dealer, or going public with what had happened. I had nightmares about the story on the local TV station—the poor little crip who was sold two cars he couldn't drive by the crafty, unscrupulous, ablebodied salesman. I could hear Walter and the Eugene basketball crips laughing at me. I decided that I would make another pedal device.

It was back to the hardware store. This pedal device would not need to be quiet or sophisticated, it just needed to work. With a few hundred dollars' worth of aluminum tubing and threaded rods and U clamps and C clamps, I hooked up a linkage that connected the clutch pedal to a lever I clamped onto the steering column. The chief problem with designing hand controls to operate a stick shift and a clutch for someone who had no legs was a shortage of arms. You needed an arm to steer, and an arm to work the accelerator/brake lever that came with the standard hand controls I had been using for years. Working the new clutch lever either required growing a new arm or taking an existing arm off the steering wheel or the accelerator to shift.

I got so I could do the hand shifting quickly, even on hills and curves. The complexity of working the levers combined with the sheer physical force of depressing the brake and clutch pedals of the powerful vehicle made driving a physical and emotional ordeal. Driving the Land Cruiser was more like playing the drums. Passing a driving test in it was more like playing the drums in a nursery and not waking anybody up.

I was certainly more nervous about taking the driving test than I had been about giving my piano recital. If the recital was a public display of what it was possible for a disabled person to do at the piano keyboard, my driving test with the Land Cruiser was about what a crip could get away with behind the wheel of a car. My recital was an A plus in Special Ed. My driving test was the big leagues. Alice correctly pointed out that if I failed the test, the police might want to talk to me about my shop-class solution to the Land Cruiser's transmission problem. They could confiscate the car altogether. It was all or nothing.

My old pre-accident Michigan license was still valid, so technically I was not breaking the law while I practiced for the test. My birthday was the moment of truth. To get an Oregon special license for disability I had to take a written test and a driving test. The written test was fine. When the instructor grabbed his clipboard and came with me out to the parking lot, he wanted me to know that according to Oregon law a paraplegic was required to have hand controls. "You wouldn't believe the people who come out here and want to take a driving test in their old Plymouth using a broom stick to work the pedals." I looked him straight in the eye and said, "Don't worry, I have hand controls."

As insurance against losing my pants while transferring from my chair to the driver's seat of the Land Cruiser I wore white overalls. I didn't want anything to spoil the high-tech effect of the hand controls. The key to passing this test was to perform with such confidence and authority that it wouldn't even occur to the tester to question what I was doing. I just hoped that I wasn't going to have to shift on a hill or downshift into a curve.

It was a bit of a circus act. I leaped into the cab of the Land Cruiser, tossed the wheelchair on the two side hooks where I hung it (just like the bike rack on my old pickup), and closed the door. He was still standing outside watching when I said, "Are you coming?" He climbed in. "Wow, this is great," he said. "So they're making these Land Cruisers for people in wheelchairs now." I didn't want to know who he thought "they" were. "That's right. I used to have one of those vans with the lifts, but I like this better," I said as I started the engine. "You seem to manage just fine. Now, I'll bet the transmission is a little harder to operate." He was looking directly at the tubes and linkages under the steering wheel. "No, it's a piece of cake," I said. "*They* really know how to make these hand controls nowadays."

I engaged the clutch and quickly put the car in first gear. My hands were off the steering wheel for maybe half a second. "Turn left out of the parking lot," he said as he looked at his clipboard, another evaluation by another guy with a clipboard. It was like having a combat flashback; my temples were sweating. I signaled, came to a full stop, put the car in neutral, then when the way was clear put it in first and pulled out. I stayed in first until I completed the turn, quickly put the car in second, then third. It was all straight road. I had it down. Because I never stopped talking, the fleeting instants my hands left the steering wheel went unnoticed. I don't remember anything I said. I just talked, and laughed, and pointed to things out the window to keep his eyes off my steering wheel.

The test was not as much of a cliffhanger as I had expected. In the end I passed because the tester was an overworked bureaucrat with ten road tests to go before he could take his lunch break. As long as I didn't wipe out a family of pedestrians, he wasn't going to create a problem. He handed me the certificate allowing me to get a picture license. "That's the first time I've ever seen hand controls for a stick shift. They really are changing the things you people can do, aren't they?" I had to agree. "Yes *they* are. I don't know what I would do without *them*." On the back of my new license was printed the words HAND CONTROLS ONLY. I was legal. *They* did change things shortly after 1979. Apparently not everybody passed their road test. Today all driver's licenses for paraplegics specify hand controls and automatic transmission only.

The whopping monthly payment for two cars meant that I needed a job and that Alice and I needed to move to a place with a much lower rent. We found a sprawling, forlorn cinder block house on forty acres adjoining a national forest in the little town of Fall Creek. In Oregon such a scenario was the low-rent option back in the late seventies. Across the street a family lived in a broken-down school bus parked next to a tiny cabin used by the adults for playing poker and the kids for going to the bathroom. It was a beautiful setting, even if the houses were pretty bleak. Alice raised garlic and had a garden. We had a rickety greenhouse where she grew tomatoes and peppers. I cultivated marijuana plants and practiced the piano.

Among the trees and away from people, we spent a peaceful year. We would drive the Land Cruiser up to a high meadow and have picnics. Eagles flew overhead. The sound of the creek accompanied the endless stars of the western sky. When the moon rose, Alice and I drove with the headlights off to see the shadows and colors of the night as the birds saw them. When I played the piano or harpsichord the music drifted out my window and mingled with the steady hiss of the Oregon rain. My home was a place far away where anything seemed possible, and what I had was more than enough.

In Fall Creek, Oregon, New Year's Eve 1979 began with a heated argument about Iran. The decade of the seventies was ending with a bang for America. Iran had taken more than just the fifty-two people hostage at the embassy in Tehran. The whole nation was embroiled in the "Hostage Crisis." There was a soft rain out at the house. Some neighbors were over talking about how we should nuke "that fucking Ayatollah." The unemployed loggers of Fall Creek would soon be voting for Ronald

Reagan. They tossed down shots of whiskey. They inhaled full bong hits of harsh marijuana. They pulled no punches. These people were not from Woodstock.

I had brought home a bottle of Wild Turkey for the festivities. After a few shots, and with all of the finesse of a pitchfork in a wasp's nest, I suggested that the Iranians might have had a strategic point in taking the hostages, however horrible the situation was. It was brutal, but there was some logic to it, given the history of Iran's relations with the west. "We put the Shah in power back in the fifties," I said. "Maybe the Iranians are still a little grumpy about that?"

"They're Iran, we're the U.S.A." The fine points of international relations didn't hold great political value here in Fall Creek. "They should be thankful we even allowed them to have a government," one guy named Al said. His live-in girlfriend, Shirley, put down the bong, and when she was finished hacking and turning purple added, "We gave them a government and look what they did to the price of oil." "Nuke 'em." Al concluded the discussion and stood up to leave. "And fuck you. Go live in I-ran," he said. "Happy New Year," I said. They went back across the street to play cards and start getting blasted in earnest.

I was well on my way to being blasted myself. I took another big drink of Wild Turkey and got out of my clothes to take a shower and bring myself back to earth. It was just 9 P.M. The woodstove was burning away. It was a cosy evening. Alice and I rolled outside onto the porch to watch the soft rain. I was naked and full of Wild Turkey. The air felt good. I told Alice I was going to roll down the driveway. "Hurry back," she said, and went back inside. There was no one around. The only activity was the sound of the anti-Iranian poker game going on across the street. It was silent, dark, and the air was equal parts wood fire and prehistoric Oregon mist.

The driveway was full of crushed gravel, bumpy and treacherous. I rolled it easily during the day. It was a little different naked, drunk, and at night. I went all the way down to the highway, where the roadway was flat and newly paved. There, the wheelchair made no sound when it moved. I rolled on the center line, looking up at the stars that could be seen through the clouds. The chill of the air was bracing, but knowing that I was just a quick spin away from the house and a hot bathtub made it tolerable. By this time I was also quite drunk.

Suddenly, I could see my shadow on the blacktop; this meant a car was coming. I had rolled some distance from my driveway, and so I quickly rolled back. I did not want to be spotted buck naked in the rain in a wheelchair on New Year's Eve. But the car was coming on fast, and

I could tell that I was not going to make it to the driveway in time. I quickly rolled to the side of the road to wait for the car to pass. I was right next to the house where the poker game was going on. I rolled onto the shoulder and in the dark did not see the three-inch drop that tipped the chair forward. I spilled out of the seat and landed behind a bush. The car was still too far away to have seen what happened, but the headlights burned away the shelter of the roadside brush like a blowtorch. The car sped by and it was dark again.

I was sure the driver hadn't seen me. I was also sure, until I tried a few times, that I could quickly get back into the chair. I was much too drunk. My idea of a stroll in the night air had become the opening scene of a horror novel. The bathtub I had come from just a few minutes earlier suddenly seemed to be on the other side of the world. I was sitting in the mud. Right next to me was an empty wheelchair, the neighbor's dilapidated school bus, and a house full of equally drunk poker players who wanted to nuke Iran, and me along with it. I couldn't call to Alice for help without attracting attention and bringing them all out of the house. Soon, another car was coming.

I crouched down and pushed the chair behind the bush to conceal it from the headlights. I didn't want to appear like a dead body on the side of the road, or someone who needed help, so as camouflage, all I could do was act crazy or nonchalant, as though I always spent my evenings sitting naked on road litter and broken glass, in the dark, in the rain, in the winter. Three cars went by; the third slowed way down before I saw Alice come out on the porch.

I could hear her calling my name. I could only whisper it back without emptying the poker house. I tried waving and throwing rocks. Finally, our dog found me and barked. Alice could barely lift me into the chair, she was laughing so hard. I was laughing too. "What were you doing down here?" In my most sincere, slurred voice I said, "Trying to look inconspicuous."

After a bath and some drunken retching, I was in bed and on my way to a hangover by 10 P.M. It looked as though Alice would see the New Year in alone, until a police squad car, lights blazing, came down the road and turned into our driveway. In terror Alice ran to the greenhouse and pulled up the fifteen marijuana plants and stuffed them all into the woodstove. The cop knocked at the door. Alice was sure it was about the pot plants, until the officer, with the most serious face she'd ever seen, said, "Ma'am, we have a report of a naked man in a wheelchair, lying by the side of the road. Have you seen anything tonight?" The cop was ready to bring out the dogs and begin dredging Fall Creek.

"He's in bed, officer. Everything's fine." The officer hadn't known whether to believe the story until Alice confirmed it. He was not looking forward to finding a paraplegic corpse on New Year's Eve. "I'm very happy to hear that, ma'am," he said. "I wonder if I might ask you a few questions?" Alice was as relieved as the officer.

"So there was a naked man at the side of the road in a wheelchair?"

"Yes."

"And he's fine now?"

"Yes."

"Well, you need to watch that in the future."

"I will, Officer."

"Happy New Year, ma'am."

She came into the bedroom, laughing, after the cop car roared out of the driveway. "I could have really put you in 'time out' tonight." I started to argue the point by insisting that it was just an accident, and that anyone else taking a stroll in their birthday suit would have been able to hide. "It's the wheelchair that calls out the National Guard," I said. Alice just narrowed her eyes. "No, it's you who call out the National Guard every chance you get." The night breeze blew through the window and with it the scent of something burning. "What's that smell?" I asked. "The pot plants," Alice said. "I wasn't going to take the rap for a naked man in a wheelchair. They're in the woodstove. Now go to sleep. I just saved your career." "What career is that?" I said as I rolled over. "Happy New Year," I said. There was still about an hour to go in the decade.

In 1980 the world changed. American politics turned upside down. Ronald Reagan was elected President. The cold war was in post-Vietnam reruns and the syndication deal was worth much more than the original series. The concept was weak by the eighties, but the special effects were terrific. The superpower arms race had become a laughable way to incinerate more wealth than the world had ever known, produce the most boring and meaningless treaties and summit meetings, and build the most amazing toys the world had ever seen. The winner of this race would be the one who ran out of money first. A volcano erupted in North America in 1980. It was the first leap year since my accident.

A week before the fourth anniversary of my accident, my grandfather Slagle died. I was three thousand miles away. I couldn't make the funeral. I composed a song on the piano as a way of saying good-bye. I played it over and over, sobbing with an intensity I had never before experienced. Nothing that had happened to me, including the accident, was as tangible a loss as his death was. I had been his favorite. He unreservedly endorsed and thrilled over each one of my dreams. What I barely imagined I might once do, he was sure I already had.

John Slagle's son Charles Peter missed the funeral too, but in 1980 I didn't even realize that my grandfather had a son, and I an uncle. The secrets John Slagle kept about why he had tried to erase his son's existence died with him. The wife and two daughters who survived him would spend the rest of their lives sorting out those secrets. I lay on my bed in my room from dawn to dusk on the day of my grandfather's funeral. I felt so far away. Next to me was the little cutting board he had made. I hugged it close. I was his oldest grandson. From now on I would have to take all of my steps without him. In a few months I would be working for NPR, something he would never know. After more than fourteen years in radio and television the thought that he never got to hear one of my stories has never left me. I would have traded every trip, every opportunity, and every triumph for him to have heard me on the air even once. My grandmother once told me that she has always thought the same thing. "When you were on that program 'All Things Considered,' your Grandfather would have planned his day so he could have been with people at five o'clock when you came on, and he could say, 'Hey, listen, that's my grandson.'" In 1979 I would never have believed that I would be able to do the things that I did after my grandfather died. He believed. If he had heard me once it might have been possible one day for him to have spoken of his retarded son with the same glowing voice he reserved for me. "That's my son," he might have been able to say without shame. I'll never know it, but it is something I believe.

Real Job

*T*hose early years after the accident were filled with milestones, bad mistakes, and self-revelation on the way to somewhere. I was walking the edge of a cage, and finding out that the doors leading out were in the center, well away from the bars I was always hitting my head on. I ran from this man-in-a-wheelchair image, even when I didn't understand who he was. I ran straight at the staring people, thinking that I could shatter their assumptions like glass. Their assumptions did not move. Confronting them was an argument with a mirror. I did not like the face that I saw, the fixed image of a man in crisis, sadness, or insanity. I was doing what I was supposed to do. I was confronting the obstacles and making the best of it. That was what I had been told to do all my life, especially after the accident. There was a biblical inevitability to it. The person who confronted a stereotype would end up living it. I became the angry young man, like the black actors compelled to play all the pimps, terrorists, and athletes. If I wanted another part, I would have to write the script.

The script was on the radio; a volcano—Mount Saint Helens—wrote it for me, and I read it over the airwaves of National Public Radio for the next twelve years.

I rolled into the offices of KLCC: Eugene, a local NPR station in the spring of 1980 with no experience and no idea of what to expect. I was wearing my white Toyota Land Cruiser overalls and no shoes. I refused to wear shoes on principle. It was a symbolic thing: I didn't walk, therefore I wasn't going to be forced to conform to the rules of the able-bodied world and wear shoes when I didn't need them. I rolled around with big red and white wool socks on, a Christmas elf from some North Pole telethon.

Our managers at KLCC wore ties, taught students, raised money, served on boards, and spent their weekends color-coding the jazz and classical music records in the library and typing out elaborate rules about how much choral music is appropriate for the breakfast hour, how many fast tunes you can play after ten at night, and why Miles Davis, Coltrane, and Charlie Parker were better played at two in the morning. They left the news volunteers alone. We had a single wire machine. Our foreign news came from shortwave, which we typed up ourselves straight off the radio. It gave our low-budget newscasts the imprint of authority, as though we were decoding messages from our own exotic correspondents rather than just reading the wires, unable to afford many long-distance phone calls.

The news director at KLCC was progressive, to put it mildly. He thought that First Amendment freedom of speech protected virtually all recorded sound. Editing a broadcast to remove pauses, long digressions in interviews, or even coughs and retakes was a dubious exercise in censorship. We didn't have to hit time posts in our newscasts. We ended whenever we ran out of things to read. Something about having a radio station all to ourselves made it seem as though we were at the center of some revolution. But we were in Eugene, Oregon, so we had to find revolutions to get in the center of.

We claimed to have continuing, special, up-to-the-minute coverage of the human rights situation in Chile. We would devote a half hour to a forum of people from the junior college Spanish Club, who said they were the Chilean Human Rights Committee. We were absolutely convinced that they had special access to the late Salvador Allende's closest political allies. We read every leaflet from the Libyan dissidents committee in Eugene, and the Iranian dissidents committee on the air, usually followed by a long phone interview with the head of the committee.

There was a weekly woman's program run by some of the women reporters and the infield members of a lesbian softball team. They produced week-long specials on toxic shock syndrome, and Indian motherhood: Native American techniques of natural childbirth. KLCC was very fond of running special series. There would be weeks when the pesticide series was airing part five while the domestic violence series was airing part eleven and the nuclear contamination series part three. We aired long, uninterrupted debates from the Oregon legislature, which by modern broadcast standards would be considered as sure a way to kill ratings as going house to house and shooting all the people with radios. KLCC News was C-Span meets Radio Free Europe, and it never scored lower than the top five stations in the market.

If you produced it, and it was factually correct, Don, the KLCC news director would broadcast it, which meant you could hear your best and worst ideas played back on the air. It was a shocking experience. One of my first pieces was on fireworks, a fun holiday story for the Fourth of July weekend. It was fifteen minutes long. I had such fun producing and editing it, but listening to it was excruciating. It was a great way to learn. Hearing something awful you produced, on your own car radio, was a strong inducement to learn from your mistakes. That summer I produced my own ten-part series on nuclear power that seemed to run for hours. But to my surprise, people actually listened to KLCC and would mention that they had heard my stories. The general manager of the station never commented on any stories, but he did tell me that I would have to look more presentable when I went out on interviews. He said people in the community were asking him why I didn't wear shoes.

I had never once imagined being a reporter before I became one. It just happened. Being a radio reporter was no crip job; it was a real one. KLCC was a dream radio station, at a unique moment in time, in a very special place. Eugene did not fit anybody's demographic profile, then or now. KLCC had a show, "Songs of Work Struggle and Change," on which labor union music was played exclusively. DJ's at the station had names like Iris and Thistle and Bebe and Cisco. The fact that I was in a wheelchair helped to balance out the unfortunate disadvantage that I was a white male who had never been a tree planter, seen a Holly Near concert, or gone to the counterculture's annual Rainbow Gathering. It would never have occurred to anyone at KLCC to even mention my wheelchair. We were the alternative radio station. Of course we would have people in wheelchairs as reporters. No one would ever have mentioned that I was a disabled reporter any more than they would make an issue of lesbian softball players on the air.

KLCC aired the NPR programs fed each day by satellite from Washington, D.C., but many people at the station viewed them as a necessary evil. NPR was the conservative sell-out network with no principles, on a par with the Pentagon. When Mount Saint Helens erupted in May of 1980 there was an argument at the station over even covering it at all.

The volcano was a "mainstream commercial story" and not sufficiently alternative for KLCC's mission. Besides, the people who produced the Native American show said that it was old news, that medicine men had been predicting an eruption since Washington had become a state in 1889. But NPR paid real money for pieces, and a mountain blowing up and distributing a layer of ash the size of New Jersey over the entire Pacific Northwest was something some of us couldn't ignore. We decided to cover it.

We were the only public radio station with a real news department within two hundred miles of the mountain. Our main reporter, Howard Berkes, was on the air every night. I would sit and listen as the anchors of "All Things Considered" interviewed Howard as he sat in our main studios. When I listened to the interview on my radio, the same interview being heard all over the country, Howard was the geologist, the mountain climber, the reporter who watched a mountain exploding before his eyes and lived to tell the world about it. When I looked through the window of the studio and watched him live on the air, he was just regular old Howard who read the wires, called up the right people, could write a decent sentence, cut audiotape, and wore these strange German pants with suspenders that made him look like Heidi's little brother Wolfgang. In that moment Howard was all of those people. On the radio he could be anything.

When NPR called to talk to Howard I would answer the phone sometimes, and the NPR producer would ask how we were all doing. It was as though she thought we were reading by candlelight and drinking bottled water. We were a good 150 miles from Mount Saint Helens, but as far as NPR was concerned, our antenna was in the volcano's crater. The Pacific Northwest was an exotic frontier to "National Public Radio in Washington, D.C."

The volcano put KLCC on the map at NPR, and network editors began relying on us to produce various regional feature stories. My first NPR story was about independent gasoline dealers who were angry at big oil companies trying to take their business when the price of gasoline began to plummet. I drove to Portland to a meeting of dealers, drove back to Eugene, stayed up all night, and sent a sixty-second story by phone to Carl Cassel, the newscaster at "Morning Edition." They aired the story at 6 A.M. I listened to it. I talked fast to make it fit into a minute. I sounded like I was on drugs. My mother recorded it on a cassette back home in the Midwest. She called that morning. "Your father and I heard you say your name. But what was the story about?" she asked. I told her I was paid thirty dollars for it.

I did stories on the timber industry, the Hanford Nuclear Reservation outside of Richland, Washington, where the plutonium for the first atomic bombs was made, Indian fishing rights, and a group of people on Mount Rainier who were building a space port out of wood to attract extraterrestrial aliens. While Howard covered the volcano, I did everything else. When NPR rewarded Howard's good work by giving him a network contract and moving him to Salt Lake City, the NPR editor asked me to ". . . take over the mountain."

Saint Helens had been the round little sister of mountains Hood and Rainier. Her explosion on May 18 tore a hole in the side of the earth and erased the gentle peak visible from Interstate 5 just before the exit for Castle Rock. Saint Helens traded convex for concave. She looked now like a construction site where the earth moved without the help of workers. In the volcano's crater there was nothing but relentless round-the-clock excavation. Everywhere else, the volcano's ash remade the earth, blotted out the sun and entombed the great trees blown down like blades of grass in the force of the explosion. In the wreckage of a mountain were the bones and vaporized flesh of the more than fifty people who vanished that day. In the moment of the eruption their nerve endings registered the energy of a thousand nuclear detonations, a tiny spark loosed from the uneasy sleep of extinct stars. The sensation passed from their bodies like the image on a strip of film when it is consumed in flames. Charred remains testified that when these trees fell someone heard a cataclysm's unrecordable sounds. Torn open like a pillow, the gray stuffing of the planet drifted through the air and landed thousands of miles from the Cascades.

The ash was smoother than sand and held feet and wheels equally well. Mixed with water, the ash made a cement sludge. The mountain, along the north fork of the Toutle River, had killed all of the fish and removed the river's banks. The migrating walls of soaked ash had dammed, and changed, its course. The river was no longer a life-giving habitat where creatures gathered and thrived. It was like a loose hose gushing water in spasms, a parody of life that once was.

Being a reporter brought back all of the stultifying performance anxiety of my first days out of the hospital. While I was comfortable and confident in the studio, writing, cutting, and mixing pieces, out on the street with my microphone, tape deck, and wheelchair I was terrified. I was terrified of the local television people and the radio old-timers who knew everybody and always seemed to know what they were doing. I was convinced that I had already missed the story the moment I arrived.

Finding and telling stories was easy, getting the nerve to go up and talk to total strangers was not. It was more than bashfulness: I was afraid of irritating people, I was afraid of their ignoring me. I was afraid of wetting my pants. I was afraid of getting a flat tire. I was afraid of running over someone's feet. I was afraid of stairs. I was afraid to succeed. They would think I had escaped from the hospital, that my tape recorder was a toy with no batteries in it. They would think I was panhandling for spare change. I was down here, they were up there. But most of all, I was afraid to come back without the story: the "guy in the wheelchair who tried but couldn't do it." I was trapped between twin stereotypes, theirs and mine.

Obsessing about all of this made no sense at all, but I had about as much control over these feelings as I did over my pancreas. The worst part was knowing that I was not completely wrong. Outside of a meeting of the Lane County Public Utility Commission meeting, a man who had angrily denounced the building of a new nuclear power plant inside the meeting came up to me as I got my microphone ready, and before I could introduce myself, fumbled in his pockets and handed me a dollar. The only solution was to speak loud, be direct, and before anyone could even think of their own explanation for why a guy in a wheelchair wearing white overalls and big socks was rolling up to them with a microphone, say, "Hi, John Hockenberry, NPR, I wonder if I might ask you a few questions."

People almost always said yes. They liked the idea of being on the radio, just as I did, and they really didn't care who the reporter was. I just figured they were doing me a favor. Being a reporter, and acting like one, were two different jobs. I was good at the first and terrible at the second. Deep in my own turmoil it took a while to realize that there were distinct advantages to having a wheelchair. The people I interviewed always remembered me later. "You're the one in the wheelchair, right?" Being remembered as "the one in the wheelchair" went against everything I believed in. Being remembered was the best possible thing for a new reporter.

It also helped if there was some rearranging or logistics required to get me into a house or office for an interview. Together, the interview subject, their staff, or their family, would all pitch in and move the plants, chairs, and desks or pull me up some stairs. Whether they were the mayor, a scientist, a congressman, or just someone on the street, when the interview began the subject was more than ready to talk. It always helped that I was far more nervous than they were. Glad to help me, they usually ended up spilling their guts far more than they intended. It was a form of panhandling.

Once, the mayor of Seattle and I had a long, very friendly, discussion about medical care and spinal cord injuries and he casually mentioned to me that the Reagan administration had just offered to keep the state's federally supported public health hospital, slated for closure, open (a 30-million-dollar proposition) in return for Senate votes supporting sales of AWACS high-tech surveillance jets to Saudi Arabia. We had been talking about wheelchairs, but that detail was news. I was recording, I did the story for NPR. It hit the wires. I got calls from all the wire services and the Seattle newspapers about the story. It was true. The Reagan Administration won their AWACS vote, but I felt embarrassed that I had gotten the story, not the real reporters. It was their beat; I was just panhandling.

New situations were exciting, but they also stirred things up, like bats hanging off some inner cave of my own soul disturbed by a broom. We are imprinted with fears and prejudices—the fear of being too conspicuous, of having the world cut us off and leave us to drift on an ice floe; ancient fears. If we are too much trouble, we imagine the world would be right for doing it. I could struggle to be whatever I wanted to be as long as I understood that the first battle would take place inside. Like using a coffee grinder to make sawdust or a refrigerator to keep fish from freezing in the Arctic, being different meant tearing up the warranty card that came with the product and pressing ahead to see what it could really do.

In the early 1980s Oakridge, Oregon, a town already hard hit by a timber industry mill recession, saw its last big mill close down. I spoke with the mayor, the company president, the teacher at the local school, and an old-timer who had been with the company since the beginning. I needed some general townspeople to comment and the only way to interview them was simply to approach them on the street. Nobody said anything very interesting until I saw two men soon to be jobless in cowboy hats. We went into a bar where it was quiet and I could get to know them.

They didn't really care about who was talking to them. Having grown up thinking that they would always work in the forests, they hadn't any idea what they would do now. My shyness and nerves were nothing compared with what they were facing. As we concluded, one of them said, "Let me ask you a question." "Sure," I told him, fully expecting to be asked about my accident or some detail of why I was in a wheelchair. Instead he said; "Is this your job to just go around and have a beer with people and talk to them?" I told him that I got paid by the piece, and that basically that's what I did. "You get paid to just travel around and ask people questions and have a beer with them?" I nodded. "That's some job. I might just try to do something like that after the plant shuts down. Damn, how could someone like me get into that line of work?"

I had never thought of my job in that way. They were not looking at me in any of the ways I had imagined. It was a revelation. I had to admit that it was some job. I was a guy who got paid to talk to people, not just a bothersome crip on the street. They had said it, not me. I had to believe them. "You should get them to buy you some shoes, though," one of them said. "Those socks make it look like there is something wrong with your feet." I thanked them, told them good luck, and said good-bye.

In the years since, whenever I was worried about what I thought I looked like with my wheelchair and tape recorder, I thought of those two guys. On their advice I bought myself some shoes. The only ones that would not fall off when I climbed in and out of the Land Cruiser were Converse basketball sneakers. I was wearing high-top All Stars back in 1980. They were hard to find then. Later, it was hard to find high-top sneakers that were not purple or pink.

In early 1981 the hostage story, which had so often competed with Mount Saint Helens for the headlines, came home to Eugene. I covered the homecoming of one of the American hostages in Iran, Victor Tomseth, who had been the political officer in the Tehran embassy. He had grown up in nearby Springfield, Oregon, and was coming back to the University of Oregon to deliver a speech. It was to be a ritual of ribbons, as the other homecomings all were. The color yellow and a song by Tony Orlando had become the unlikely emblem of American strength and bravery in the face of an angry, hateful world.

Tomseth was greeted by hundreds of demonstrators in addition to the well-wishers in Eugene. Because Tomseth was the embassy political officer and presumed to be the chief operative of the CIA in Tehran, the demonstrators believed that he had encouraged the Shah to deal harshly with his opposition, and that Tomseth might have been the U.S. point man for the Shah's policy of brutality against student and Islamic militants.

Mr. Tomseth was shouted down during his speech. The whole affair nearly became a riot. It was the one hostage homecoming of the fifty-two that took place that winter that was not reverential. The people in the audience who were anxious to see an authentic national hero were embarrassed and outraged by the protesters, but it was Tomseth himself who candidly noted their concerns and told the crowd that he felt that mistakes had been made in the U.S. policy toward Iran. He was dignified, and not defensive. In his acknowledgment of the protesters he indicated that the hostage crisis in Iran was a far more complicated affair than America had, up till then, been told. He also revealed just how difficult it must have been for him during those 444 days in Tehran, living the consequences of a policy that had gone so completely wrong. It was a view of the hostage affair that was concealed by the adulation the other hostages received. In fielding the questions from the crowd, Tomseth looked relieved to be able to say the things he had thought during the months he was a captive in Tehran. It was clear that he had never thought of himself as a hero and was surprised to learn that anyone in America did.

I had never thought of Eugene, Oregon, as a hotbed of national and international news but within a year of the eruption of Mount Saint Helens, I was making a living working full time as a freelancer for NPR. I quit music school. Being three thousand miles from NPR headquarters meant that I never had to dress up in a suit, roll into an editor's office for a formal interview to convince them I could be a reporter. A job interview would probably have ended my career right there in Eugene.

I was never the reporter in the wheelchair to the people at NPR. They only knew me as a voice over the phone until one day when I missed a deadline and was found out.

Along the Columbia River in the high desert of Washington, the farther you drive from the interstate highway, the more conservative and isolated the towns become. Some of the towns felt as off the beaten track as the outback of Australia. Touch-Tone telephones were unheard of, which is not terribly backward or noteworthy, except to say that where there were old-style telephones, there were old-style telephone booths, with the folding door and a concrete step.

On assignment in eastern Washington, on a slow news day, Mount Saint Helens had one of its smaller eruptions. I knew the newsroom would be very anxious for a small 60-second item. They would be expecting my call. Noon Pacific time was only two hours before NPR went on the air in the East.

I called the geologists' offices near the volcano and got the latest details. "It was a small eruption. Ash had been emitted, and there was a tremor, some movement of a large mass in the volcano's crater." It was something, but nothing to stop the presses over. There were no pay phones anywhere other than old-style phone booths. I tried to get into one and failed. The only way would be to get out of the chair, but then I would be far too low to reach the phone.

At about ten minutes to five Washington, D.C., time, I had run out of hope for a pay phone. I drove up to a small school with a ground-floor entrance in a little town outside Ephrata, Washington. I grabbed my tape recorder, rolled into the school and down to the principal's office. Classes were about to pass. I tried to get the office ladies' attention.

"I wonder if I might use your phone. I am a reporter for National Public Radio. I need to send a story back to Washington. I have to send it in the next few minutes. I won't tie up your phone for long." The ladies were in every way unimpressed with my story, and my request was not something they were going to grant without more discussion. One of them answered me. "Students can only use the phone to call their parents. It's a rule. Are you calling your parents?" "I am not a student. I am a reporter from National Public Radio. May I please use your phone?"

The other lady stood up slowly and walked over to the counter. She looked at my wheelchair. She examined my tape recorder. "Please, I really need to make that call. I couldn't fit into any of the phone booths." It was almost five o'clock Eastern time. "Is this a long-distance call?" "It's an 800 call; it won't cost you anything." In Ephrata, Washington, in 1981, the number 800 represented just one more area code on the other side of the earth.

"Our principal will have to approve this." His name was Mr. Gillespie. "What sort of news report is this?" the lady asked without the slightest hint of urgency. "Mount Saint Helens erupted and I have to file a story to the network in Washington. Please, I need to use your phone right now." She smiled and looked back at her now-smiling colleague. "Young man, that happened almost a year ago."

By the time I convinced Mr. Gillespie that he wasn't going to have to raise the town's property taxes to pay for my call to Washington, D.C., and got through to the newsroom, it was after five-thirty. They had taken the story from another affiliate. I apologized, asking if they were counting on me. They said they had been waiting for me, but it had all worked out. My editor thought differently. When I returned home the next day he telephoned and wanted to know why I hadn't called; why, he asked, had I let him down?

Up until that moment I was just a voice on a phone to him; now he would have a picture. I had been filing stories to NPR for months on Mount Saint Helens and other news events around the region with no problems. "I missed the deadline because I couldn't get my wheelchair into the phone booth to file." I blinked at the ceiling and paused. There was no response, so I continued, "I looked everywhere for a pay phone

I could use. When I found one it was too late. I'm really sorry." My editor said something about not letting it happen again, then rang off.

The cat was out of the bag. My editor never mentioned wheelchairs to me, but he clearly spoke to someone about it. For weeks after that phone conversation other people I knew at NPR called to say they had heard the most unusual story about my missed deadline. "Did you have a skiing accident or something?"

It was the only time I had missed a deadline in twelve years. In those early months at NPR I was operating on a moment by moment assessment of what I could do. It was important not to be second-guessed by anyone else. Because of a phone booth I had come out of the closet, and I no longer knew what to expect. In the little logistical details of countless assignments I was the inventor of what was possible. New truths about what I could do and how I might do it were learned with each new assignment and the challenges associated with each new place I went. Until I missed that deadline, those truths were known by me alone.

Live at Five

*I*n November 1981, I moved to Washington, D.C., to be the newscaster on the program "All Things Considered". I was going to have to write and deliver one five- and one seven-minute newscast each night starting at 5 P.M. Eastern time. Unlike KLCC, I would have to hit the time post exactly. No longer would I be rolling around buying beers and talking to people about the recession. I had a desk job, which meant I couldn't go to work in overalls anymore, and that I always had to wear real shoes.

NPR headquarters occupied five floors in a nondescript office building about six blocks from the White House. For most of its existence, NPR had been some old folding chairs, microphones, and an odd assortment of talented people committed to doing something that had never been done in broadcasting. If Edward R. Murrow, standing under the bombs of the blitz in London during World War Two, was the model for the electronic media at the center of the action, Susan Stamberg reciting the recipe for her Thanksgiving cranberry relish on "All Things Considered" each year was the model for a broadcast network happy to be out of the loop.

It's not as though NPR had any option to be in the loop in those early days. If the television networks were going to scramble over each other just to hear the same grumpy "no comment" from inside the beltway,

NPR was going to do everything else—the documentaries on spray-painted van art, the radio comic operas about the budget deficit, the twenty-minute pieces about a trip to the dentist, the profile of rest stops on Route 66.

When I got to Washington in 1981, NPR was just starting to turn itself into more of a big-time news operation. While public radio was criticized for having a liberal bias, my perspective was skewed by coming from KLCC, where more of a Marxist view was the mainstream. I could expect to find NPR beholden to the establishment, the KLCC diehards insisted. "They censor everything there, you'll find out."

NPR was hardly the establishment, but it was nothing like the information commune I had become accustomed to at KLCC. My first day on the job I was pointed at the typewriter, told where the wire machines were, and asked to pronounce the name of the leader of Poland. "It's not Voy-Check Jaruselski, its Voahhh-tzik," the producer of ATC told me before going off to answer the phone. The crisis in Poland and the declaration of martial law by the government was the lead story throughout December 1981.

It was amazing to see how many of NPR's broadcasts were on tape and how little of it was live. The interviews were all cut for air, and it was not uncommon for a thirty-minute interview to be trimmed to two or three, with every pause and stutter sliced out. At KLCC, a thirty-minute interview might get trimmed to twenty-nine minutes, and pauses were to be left in and not "censored".

I had never worked in an office before, and this one looked as though a few grenades had gone off inside and the fire sprinklers had been left on for a week. On one side of the building, "All Things Considered" had its cubicles laid out around a big semicircular table. On the other side of the building, all of the reporters had their offices. In the middle, the newscasters sat at another semicircular table next to a window where you could watch all of the big shots from CBS going into the CBS Washington Bureau across M street. Right next to the newscast table was the "Morning Edition" area.

With the exception of Nina Totenberg's couch, it was all Formica, foam rubber, and gray felt. The place looked like a warehouse for furniture you might see at a junior college fire sale. Packed into a few thousand square feet, desks, chairs, and floor-to-ceiling piles of old newspapers delivered the unmistakable message that something important was being done here and was not, under any circumstances, to be thrown away.

Listening to NPR out in Oregon, you got the impression that here was a family of committed journalists working to make the news a meaning-ful part of people's lives, to provide an alternative to the lurid sensation-alism of television. In Washington it was not quite like that. The model for consensus at NPR in the early eighties was Bosnia in the early nine-ties. The "Morning Edition" people hated the people from "All Things Considered," and everyone hated the editors in the Washington bureau who behaved like talent agents parceling out three- to twelve-minute doses of their megastar reporters, Nina Totenberg, Cokie Roberts, Linda Wertheimer, Bill Buzenberg, and Neal Conan, to the hungry, suspicious programs. As for the virtues of being different from television, each day when "All Things Considered" ended at 6:28:30 P.M., the producers sit-ting at the U-shaped table would switch on the televisions to see what the networks led with. They would bet to see if ATC's lead matched the big boys. If it did, there were congratulations all around. If it didn't, it meant someone would usually pipe up to say that NPR had a different responsibility for news than the networks. What was not said was that they would all try again tommorrow to get it right.

I was afraid that keeping my KLCC credentials was going to be diffi-cult in this place. For the first few weeks of newscasting I insisted on pronouncing El Salvador with the accent on the last syllable. It was how we had all pronounced it back at KLCC along with the name of the Chilean president, Augusto Pino-CHET. Salva-DOR: we rolled off those final syllables with revolutionary fervor. It was not a popular practice at NPR. I was told that I was hitting the last syllable kind of hard, and would I consider talking normally. I obeyed, but I had bad dreams about my old news director warning me about selling out. In the early eight-ies, NPR wasn't selling out, but it was growing up.

One sign of this maturity was the number of open, screaming fights that took place near the newscaster desk. The producer of "Morning Edition" was fond of throwing aluminum reels of tape across the room when he lost an argument over a story assignment. The "Morning Edi-tion" arguments were always over "what America wants to hear" in the morning, while at "All Things Considered" it was always "Why does *The New York Times* have that story and we don't?" When "America did not want to hear" about some vote in the British House of Commons, the producer of "Morning Edition" was told by the stuffy London Bureau chief, that he should go to work for "Entertainment Tonight". The nearly tearful, screaming producer slammed the phone down and threw it across the room.

Once, just after I started, the executive producer of "Morning Edition" and the assistant editor on the Washington bureau came to blows right next to the newscast area. As they landed punches and wrestled their way across people's desks, knocking over chairs and sending piles of debris flying, I asked Al Smith, my assistant, if we should call anyone, like a nurse, or an ambulance. He said that if we let them alone long enough, maybe there would be another NPR employee in a wheelchair.

This was not likely. There was no room for even one person to turn around in a wheelchair anywhere in the office. I could either roll forward or backward. There had never been another employee in a wheelchair at NPR, and the layout of the bathroom was clear evidence of that. At deadline time I would race to the studio to deliver the newscast. Around each corner was the possibility that I might collide with a producer, one of the anchors, or one of the senators and Congress people who would stop by to be interviewed. Actress Carrie Fisher and I once collided as she stood waiting to be interviewed by Susan Stamberg. I shouted "Excuse me!" without recognizing her. She jumped up and landed in my lap. I couldn't remember her name. All I could remember was that she was Princess Leia from *Star Wars.* "Thanks for saving the universe," I said. She stood up and brushed herself off. "You're welcome," she said. I almost missed the newscast.

A wheelchair stood out in the crowded floor plan of NPR's offices. Some people were very helpful, most were just friendly and curious, others wanted you to know that they were sensitive enough to handle a disability at the office, unlike their insensitive colleagues. These were the people you wanted to avoid. One famous NPR reporter was far too progressive to simply pass me in the hallway. When I rolled by he would dramatically flatten himself against the wall and make a big point of (humorously, he thought) getting out of my way. Another favorite gesture was to pretend he was a matador and wave an imaginary cape at me as though I were a bull. Once he asked if everyone did something like that when I rolled by. On his face was the expression of absolute certainty that this was the way to openly deal with my disability, to bring it out of the closet and make it a part of the workplace. "No," I replied, "you are the only one."

Because NPR was so out of the loop, any hint that we were taken seriously by the giants of the media in Washington was cause for celebration. There were few such hints. Nina Totenberg was, of course, the genuine article. Nina got stories no one else in the business did, and had been doing it from the beginning of her career at NPR. By the time I arrived at NPR, Nina was already a legend, and there was ample evidence of her status for any newscaster. She would file stories for the newscast when she wanted to, at whatever length she desired, and never, *ever* would she be edited by the news desk. If Al and I saw a story we thought Nina might do for us for the lead newscast of "All Things Considered," she would let us know through her editor/agent that we were not permitted to assign any stories to Nina.

Nina always knew what was going to happen everywhere in Washington, not just on her Supreme Court beat. She knew what was going on at the White House, in the Senate, and was the person who would represent NPR at the big events around town. Nina knew everybody. If she didn't know someone, then Cokie Roberts did. Together they were the franchise. Even the NPR White House reporters would have to ask Nina or Cokie to intercede to get an interview with someone in the administration when they couldn't get a callback. Nina and Cokie always got called back.

It was Nina and Cokie who had the friends over at ABC, CBS, and NBC to tell them the results of network exit polls on election nights. At NPR the cut-rate computer system for tracking election results was a half hour behind everyone else. By nine in the evening NPR had a simple formula for declaring a winner. NPR would declare a race if two networks declared. Three editors were assigned to do nothing but watch TV. This was one nightmare my KLCC news director could never have imagined.

Besides Nina and Cokie, the other big name, heavy hitter at NPR was Frank Mankiewicz. He was the president of the whole network. The former campaign manager of Bobby Kennedy is today a senior vice president at the public relations firm of Hill and Knowlton. As a friend of the Kennedys, cohort of the most powerful members of the Democratic party, Mankiewicz was always part of Washington's varsity crowd. Most people at NPR needed Nina and Cokie just to get access to Frank.

The comic strip "Doonesbury" had a character who was the White House correspondent for NPR, but he didn't resemble anyone we worked with. The one other thing during the early eighties that made NPR a potential player in big-time Washington was the rumor that the young woman having an affair with Watergate reporter Carl Bernstein while he was still married to Nora Ephron was an NPR employee. In the newsroom we were too scared to even ask who it might be. She worked on another floor, and unless you were friends with Nina or Cokie you could not expect to find out. The hot-tempered producer of "Morning Edition" knew but would not tell me. All we knew was that one of Ephron's best friends, Barbara Cohen, was the director of the NPR news division, and our boss. In the movie *Heartburn*, based on Ephron's best-selling book, I could brag to my family that my boss was played by

Stockard Channing. In those days it was the kind of thing that passed for fame and glory at NPR.

Newscasting was the most exhausting desk job you could have at NPR. Every night there was my voice right at the top of the program talking about all of the places I had never been, the people I had never met and the stories I only knew about because they were on the wires. It was a struggle to get anyone who was working on a piece for the program to agree to file a spot for the newscast. The producers of "All Things Considered" viewed it as a five-minute grace period before the first piece had to be cut, in the studio, and ready to roll. It was like a commercial break before the real program began.

During my second week on the job, an Air Florida jet crashed into the Potomac River. During the years I was a newscaster, Israel invaded Lebanon, Argentina invaded the Falklands, and the U.S. came close to invading both Nicaragua and El Salvador. Each day I would write like a madman, hoping I had written enough in time to go into the booth where the director would point at me, a light would go on, and my microphone would be live for five minutes from Miami to the Aleutian Islands.

Each day I would be scared of three things: that I would say something wrong, that I would not have enough to read, or, worst of all, that I would wet my pants. The men's room at NPR was narrow and small. The door was difficult to get through, there was no wide stall, and getting back out the door was most challenging of all. After three in the afternoon it was too risky to even go into the men's room. The hysteria of the newscast deadline made it impossible, or simply too frightening, to break away. In a mind-numbing routine everything was written and cut down to the wire. Each day, Monday through Friday, I arrived in the studio with seconds to spare, my yellow sheets of news copy in my lap weighted down with a book so they wouldn't blow away as I sped toward studio 5.

In the old tool and die room I had once seen someone's fingers sliced off by a stamping press. On this job, it felt each day as though a blade was taking a thin slice of my brain. It was hard to make any kind of mark as a newscaster at NPR. The newscast marked you like no factory job I had ever had.

Occasionally I would fill in as a host for "All Things Considered," and things would get more interesting. There was the time I got to ask one of the stupidest questions in the history of radio. It was the day Nina Totenberg broke the story that Supreme Court nominee Douglas H. Ginsberg had smoked marijuana with his students at Harvard. All day long we could tell that Nina had a big story because there were piles of documents spread all over her couch, which only happened when something big was about to break.

She had discovered the marijuana allegation while investigating Ginsberg's background at Harvard, and she was clearly unsure about what to do with it. In the just say no years of the Reagan administration it was politically significant that one of their own nominees smoked pot, but the idea of smoking marijuana disqualifying someone for a job cut a little close to home over at NPR, the Woodstock of news. The Washington bureau sent a message to the Justice Department indicating that we were going to go with the story, and that we wanted their response. Nina was also aware that *The Washington Post* was working on a similar story, possibly for the next morning's edition.

At six o'clock the producer of "All Things Considered," Art Silverman, came into studio 5 and said that Nina was going to lead the six o'clock half hour, and that the story would be told in the form of an interview. I knew nothing of the story except that Nina was flying around the studio on afterburners, and that Chuck Bailey, her editor, was trying to calm her down. "Who's doing the interview?" she asked. Art said it would be me. "Oh, great, the acid head," she said, pointing to me. I smiled and waved. I was remembering all of the times I had asked her to file stories for the newscast and all of the times I had told her that her stories were too long.

The interview was completely written out. Nina always insisted on writing the questions and the answers in such a way that the interviewer appeared to know absolutely nothing while Nina knew everything. I said I wanted to take a look at the questions. "Just leave them as they are," she yelled. It was two minutes until air. The first question was very general: "What did you find out at Harvard about Judge Ginsberg?" The answer was that he hadn't written or published much, and that his judicial philosophy was an unknown. Nina would speculate that this was just what the administration wanted after the very public Robert Bork fiasco. The next question was about Ginsberg's position on abortion, and the answer again was that no one really knew, other than to say that he was a conservative. None of this information justified all of the hysteria I had noted all day long over in Nina's area, so my eyes were drawn to the third question written on the paper: "Did you find anything else, Nina?"

This seemed odd. "Nina, what is this 'anything else, Nina?' question." She shouted back at me. "Never mind. You've got to ask it that way." Art, the producer, looked at me and said that the answer was that Nina had discovered that Ginsberg had smoked pot with his students at Harvard.

"And you're not going to put that first?" I asked. "You're burying the lead. It will make it look like you think there's something wrong with the story if you put it like that at the end." In the last seconds before air time, the Justice Department sent us their response. It came directly from Attorney General Ed Meese. It confirmed the story and said that Ginsberg admitted to "experimenting" with marijuana and that he "regretted" it. With confirmation from the Justice Department there was no reason not to lead with the story, but Nina insisted, "We're going to do it this way." The show began, and we were on the air.

The interview proceeded nicely. Listeners learned about Ginsberg's lack of published opinions and legal theories. They learned that his position on abortion was unknown. I looked at the third question. Never in the history of radio would a question be more disingenuously asked, and I had to ask it. I thought about surprising Nina with something like, "You know, Nina, I heard the guy used to smoke pot with his students. What about that?" or "But, really, Nina how good was he at rolling joints?"

While the microphone was open Nina eyed me with her signature glare, warning me off any deviation from the script. "You'll be ruined in this town and any other if you try to pull a fast one," her eyes said. She was a trembling bundle of nerves. The whole Washington bureau was watching on the other side of the glass. One of the editors held up a piece of paper from the wire machine indicating that the Justice Department had started to move the response on the wires to preempt the story and make it look like they had known about this all along. I asked the stupidest question in the history of radio.

"Did you find out anything else?"

She paused and said, "Yes, John," and began to explain that she knew that Ginsberg smoked pot from a number of sources, but that she didn't know what that meant as far as his fitness for the Supreme Court was concerned. "I doubt there is anyone from Harvard Law School around Judge Ginsberg's age who didn't smoke pot." We had been talking about one professor, now we were off-handedly accusing the Harvard faculty of being potheads. I noted that smoking pot was against the law that Ginsberg would be responsible for interpreting. She responded by talking about permissiveness during a particular era in America, the man's career, and having to think about his future, then saying, "It's hard to say what this means." The interview ended.

The second piece in the program was on tape. The microphone light went off. The studio door opened and the editors rushed in with the news that the story was exploding on the wires. All three networks led with it. We had the correct lead that night, and any of the earlier hesitation about ruining Ginsberg's career vanished. Nina, the producers, and editors decided to lead the next feed of "All Things Considered" with the story and redo the interview to put the marijuana stuff first. The stupidest question in the history of radio was only heard by the East Coast.

The other time I made broadcast history at NPR no one knew about it. It happened on the day John Belushi died. It was a very busy news day, and the reports of Belushi's death came late in the day. I had drunk two large cups of coffee after three o'clock that day without thinking about the consequences. While I was on the air telling America that Belushi had died I looked down and realized that I was wetting my pants live on the air. I never told anyone. I was just the newscaster.

Oddly enough, wetting one's pants on live radio was far from humiliating. There was a certain exhilaration in knowing one crucial fact and withholding it from an audience of hundreds of thousands. Far from embarrassment, it was closer to feeling the way Richard Nixon must have during most of his time as President. I always wondered if Nixon ever wanted to scream out that he was a war criminal and a crook. Only he knew these truths were not self-evident. Later they were self-evident. In the end, Nixon discovered that resigning in disgrace was not humiliating. Upon his death he became a hero for doing the one thing he feared most: self-destructing in office.

After three years of newscasting in Washington, D.C., I was hungry to return to reporting. It had been a long time behind a desk. I had learned a lot about what was possible in radio. I was also coming into contact with other people in wheelchairs out in public. I was not the only paraplegic in the world. It was the first time I had thought about that since I was in the rehab hospital. I had almost a decade of wheelchair rolling behind me. I was ready for something new. I asked NPR to send me back into the field.

My wife, Alice, and I separated in 1984. Seven years had passed between the moment she delivered her tough employee orientation speech to me in Florence, Oregon, and the moment I resolved to leave. When she had been my boss, she told me she wouldn't tolerate an example of disabled people not pulling their own weight. I took her challenge, and during the years we were married I pulled my weight farther than I had ever imagined. We met when I was a hippie music student looking for extra money, dreaming of writing soundtracks for movies and playing French baroque harpsichord. By the time we split I had become a correspondent for National Public Radio; she was a struggling housepainter in Virginia dreaming of living on a fishing boat in Alaska.

Marriage was about more than pulling your own weight. It was about pulling weight that was not your own. Alice realized, long before I did, that this was something I could not, or would not, do. When I left Washington, D.C., for Chicago and the life that would take me to the Middle East and eventually the donkey on the road to Kurdistan, Alice wanted to go along. "Can't I come with you?" she asked as the sun of late autumn streamed in through the window of our Virginia house outside Washington. Off in the distance on the farthest hill, a bonfire was burning. I couldn't look at Alice's tears. I looked at the bonfire. "You can't go with me," I said. "I need to do these things alone." I sounded so sure of what I was saying, but I did not understand why I was so sure, or what it was I was so sure I had to do. For the eight years since my accident I had sought out the places that were ramped and the parking spaces that were reserved and the bathrooms wide enough to use, all in the pursuit of my own personal, physical freedom. What I had discovered was a perfect, personal prison built by freedom's best intentions.

I could feel the creeping dependency on those physical details, and the smallness of that wheelchair-accessible world. It was a tiny fraction of the world at large. The more I traveled this accessible world the smaller it seemed. My prison was made from ramps, bathrooms, doorways, and elevators. My freedom consisted of exactly what America was willing to dole out, on its own schedule.

But real freedom was in not needing the parking spaces, elevators, curb ramps, and bathrooms. It meant going places where there would be none of those, to face what was really possible in life rather than what was permitted. I was drawn to the places where access hadn't even been thought of. Only there could I imagine real freedom. These were the places that I was most afraid to think of going. The first place on that list was Chicago, the snowy, hard city I had been chased away from in my chair eight years earlier. The place where I had left Ricky behind.

Long after Alice and I had split and I had moved back to Chicago, my father became aware of how my life was becoming more and more this solitary crusade into physical frontier outposts of my own making. He once said a curious thing to me. I had been telling him how anxious I was for a foreign assignment at NPR, but felt I was being held back. I was frustrated, and told him so; he paused, and quite innocently remarked, "You know, John, your mother and I think that you use your wheelchair as a crutch."

This was not the kind of remark my father typically made, but apparently he had given this a lot of thought. I was shocked and stung by both his candor and the absurdity of what he had said. It was a key insight, he had struck a nerve, but there was something howlingly funny about the idea of using a wheelchair as a crutch. If anything, being a paraplegic meant that using a crutch was impossible, or perhaps it was a condition devoutly to be wished. I answered slowly, unsure as to whether my father was being completely serious.

"I use my wheelchair as a wheelchair. If I could use a crutch, I would use it as a crutch." My concept of using the wheelchair was a physical one. A better or worse use of the chair had more to do with physical skills, of hopping over curbs or precise slalom moves in traffic on crowded pavements. For my father, the wheelchair was something akin to his father's artificial arm. He answered quickly, "Well, of course, that is true, but I think you know what I mean about using it like a crutch. Your mother and I think that if you weren't in the wheelchair you would never have made it this far."

In one regard this was an endorsement of my ability to integrate the wheelchair into my life, but it was not what my father was saying. He was referring to the very things Alice had noticed in our last years together, how I searched out the places where I was sure to find obstacles. He was talking about pulling my own weight for all the world to see; about going to the front of the line. He was talking about making a scene. He was talking about calling attention to something that in his mind was best kept hidden. The virtue of being different was to behave as though you weren't. He was talking about the very thing he had never once spoke about with his father: his missing arm. That was the rule. It was a rule he never violated, and one that he was proud his father had always followed to the letter.

Since the accident that made me into a paraplegic, my father has struggled to reconcile his father's quiet acceptance of the loss of his left arm with his son's impulse to spray paint the word "wheelchair" all over his life. This struggle was as invisible to me as his father's trials had been to him. Until the moment my father mentioned the crutch, I would never have thought about it. My father has always been very proud of the things his son has accomplished, and never embarrassed by my wheelchair, but its visibility and the manner in which I behaved in it went against something deeply engrained from his childhood, and how he came to accept his father's amputated arm. In my father's mind, the ghost of his father's lost arm remained on earth, haunting all the places where I no longer walked.

The struggles I insisted upon could not be reconciled by Alice and me. In the end, I was not able to distinguish her from all of the physical objects in my life that promised freedom but delivered a sense of confinement. Today she pulls one hundred times her own weight each day in shrimp on a fishing boat in the Gulf of Alaska along with a crew of people who pull their weight and hers. Our years together had been good ones. She would probably be proud and a little sad to know, more than a decade after our divorce, that I am still pulling my own weight.

Lost Causes

*H*eavy snow and inaccessibility had chased me and my wheel-chair away from Chicago right after my accident. They would not this time. The NPR bureau was on Michigan Avenue in an old black Art Deco building. It had no bathroom that I could use. I asked NPR once about the possibility of making a bathroom work in the building. I was told that since they didn't own the building, there was nothing they could do. Every four hours or so it was a big deal to me. It was no big deal to them, so I found a bathroom I could use three blocks away in the downtown junior college building.

The path along Lake Michigan was where I pushed my chair to the limit. The path spanned the entire Chicago waterfront from south to north, nearly twenty miles in all. Just before Thirty-third Street there was a hill where I would push as fast as I could until I felt a tingling in my scalp. I would need to be able to go all out, I thought. I would need the ability to push my arms this fast without stopping. I imagined being chased, or running for shelter somewhere far away. The scene was dim and vague, but I was sure there would be a time when my life would depend on being able to go that fast and far without stopping. When I felt the tingle in my scalp I knew I had made it.

Martha met me at the finish line of the Chicago Marathon in 1985, a year and a half after Alice and I split up and the day after our first date.

I wasn't expecting her to be there. She had invited me over to her house on the second floor of a northside brownstone, where she cooked me a pasta dinner. "You're supposed to have pasta for a marathon." she said proudly. There, neatly folded on her kitchen counter, was the *Chicago Tribune* article on how to prepare for the big race. She had thought this evening through. It was very nice. I didn't even care that I had to haul myself up a flight of steps to sit at her dinner table.

Martha had once picked me out of a crowd with her dark brown eyes. She liked the size of my arms. She said she liked to go camping. She said she knew how to fish and that she had never dated a man who could rig tackle more sophisticated than a marshmallow on a hook. I could tear down a bass rig and bait a hook with a live grasshopper in the time it took to turn a boat around. I had an old brown Mercedes coupe that could go 130 miles per hour without a shake. My tiny apartment had a view of Lake Michigan. Martha was interested in my view and my adventures.

She met me at the finish line with a blanket, a towel, a bottle of apple juice, and a thermos of hot tea. My time was 2:38:46. Good for a runner, bad for wheelchairs, but I was happy. "Did you get hungry during the race?" she asked. "I didn't think about food once." At that moment I was thinking about my sore wrists. "I didn't think that you would after my dinner last night."

This was my second marathon. The only thing worse than running a marathon once is running it twice. The second time you know exactly how painful it will be, and you know exactly how long it will take. Worst of all, having finished a marathon once, it would be impossible to live with yourself if you failed to finish the second time. The first time a marathon is a throw of the dice. The second time it is a slow walk through fire. The first time there was no one at the finish line to meet me, so it was good to see Martha's face there on that cold, rainy November day where the steam from my body mixed with her breath and the gray mist blowing in from Lake Michigan.

From the beginning we seemed to have lots to talk about. We especially talked about how all of our relationships never worked out, so we went on to have a failed relationship of our own. It was my idea that Martha and I move in together. "We'll get a big place," I said. "I'm never home. You'll have your own bedroom and bathroom. I can cook. And we can continue our discussions about how all of our relationships never work out." We did.

Being with Martha taught me a couple of things back in 1986. Chief among them was this proposition: Though you might be willing to die trying, certain battles cannot be won, certain details cannot be overlooked. In the matters of the heart, wooden puppets named Pinocchio cannot, ever, become real boys. There was also the important corollary: Never . . . never keep the keys to an apartment you once lived in, especially if the woman you used to live with still resides there. In 1985, Pinocchio was in love with Martha. Martha may have loved Pinocchio, but she was only going to marry a real boy. I was not a real boy.

During the time Martha and I were together, NASA announced that it was taking applications for something it called the "journalist in space program." There were, no doubt, plenty of people in Washington, D.C., during the Reagan eighties anxious to assign troublesome journalists to cover the asteroid belt, but this was not a secret Pentagon program for suspending freedom of the press. A journalist was to accompany astronauts on a space shuttle mission in the same way a teacher was to be the first civilian non-scientist to get a chance to reach near-earth orbit. The very first civilian candidate, teacher Christa McAuliffe, didn't make it. She died along with the six other crew members on the ill-fated *Challenger* in January 1986.

In the shock of the *Challenger* disaster, the journalist in space program was not shelved right away. For a time NASA proceeded with the selection process. From a pool of about 3,000 applications they selected 100 candidates, and then 40 semifinalists. The project was officially discontinued in 1987, but not before it received considerable media attention on the issue of civilians, and as it turned out, crips in space.

It wasn't long after moving in together that Martha and I began having difficulties. It was a big apartment, but Martha still said that she needed her "space," especially when I was around, which wasn't too often. The weekends would always begin happily and end sadly. The happiness itself would bring on her tears. We would go out and have a wonderful time, and in the middle of dinner, or after the movie, or at home cuddling on the couch she would get this faraway look in her eyes and the tears would begin to roll down her face. "What's wrong?"

"We had such a wonderful time, John. It's just the idea of being with you forever," she would say through her tears.

"Don't think about forever. How about being with me for another week?" I would say. "String enough weeks together and they make a lifetime." Thinking back, it was hopeless, but it was just the kind of challenge that could keep someone like me interested: I felt like Sidney Poitier in the film *Guess Who's Coming to Dinner?* It could work. We could be a part of history. They would make movies about us long after we were gone. Caesar and Cleopatra, Cyrano and Roxanne, John and Martha.

I encouraged Martha to believe that our relationship might work out.

She encouraged me to apply for the space program. She loved adventures. I loved Martha. The fact that she encouraged me to take a ride on a vehicle that had exploded over Florida a few months before perhaps should have tipped me off. Martha needed her space. The space program said it needed journalists. But did the space program need disabled journalists? On this Martha was clear. "Why not?" she would say. "It would be great." I wanted to know why our relationship was looking more and more doubtful. "If we can put a man in a wheelchair into space," I asked, "why can't you and I stay together?" At least Martha was encouraging about the space program.

If you are even the least bit off the mainstream in America, you have got to be able to pick your battles to survive. If Dylan Thomas had been in a wheelchair he might have written about the disability rights movement this way: "If you're not going to go gently into that good night, then fine, you can just sit there raging in the dark for all I care." What constitutes going gently into the night and what constitutes rage unto the dying of the light is a central question in American society, whether you are in a wheelchair, a member of a minority group, or waiting for a cab in the rain at rush hour in midtown Manhattan. More than just picking your battles, you have to learn to choose your lost causes.

Occasionally lost causes choose you. Could I qualify as an astronaut and take a place as a crew member on the space shuttle? Could I find a way to live with Martha? One cause was truly lost, but I discovered to my great astonishment that the other was not lost at all. Lost causes contain considerable truth. What is possible in the world can only be found among the wreckage of the impossible.

We are a society of causes and movements. The powerless are becoming empowered. The powerful are scheming against the rest of us. To be the adherent of a cause is to be categorized politically and socially in America. We are a nation dedicated to the idea of political action. There is no doubt that political movements have catalyzed many of the towering changes we have witnessed in this century. But much of what passes for action turns out simply to be fashionable, more like political play money than hard currency. In America it's hard to tell the real from the symbolic.

In the restaurants of Grand Rapids, Michigan, during the mid-seventies a middle-aged woman, her paraplegic son, and the rest of her family could be seen ordering dinner. The middle-aged woman would always demand to see a menu written in braille. "What! You have no braille menu?" You could be sure to hear her loud voice. You would be sure to notice that there were no blind people in this group. When the demand was made for the braille menu, the people around the table could be seen slinking down in their seats, or holding their ordinary menus up before their faces.

In the town where I went to high school, I was mortified enough by the commotion created when I showed up at a restaurant in a wheelchair. I was grateful to be able to roll into any place and order dinner, but asking for a braille menu seemed to be pushing it. To my mother it was a cause célèbre. It was a mission that brought her great pleasure, but it resulted in few, if any, braille menus. Restaurants were required to have them, my mother insisted. I suggested that all restaurants were also required to have someone on-site who was able to perform the Heimlich maneuver, but I didn't need to have the manager grab the person at the next table and get her to cough up her crab legs to prove it to my satisfaction.

What I failed to immediately understand was that with a recently injured son my mother now considered herself a full-fledged member of the disability rights movement. If she wanted to be the braille menu enforcer, I thought that was fine. But why did I have to be present for these scenes? "It's better when you're here," she said. "I can just see those managers squirming." I would try to point out that in the quest to improve the lot of the disabled, having sighted people in wheelchairs asking for braille menus was a little like teaching guide dogs for the blind to sniff out ramps and bark at entranceways with steps. "I don't care, John," she would say. "Someone has to fight for the braille menus."

During the time my mother was fighting for braille menus in Grand Rapids, Michigan, my parents lived in an inaccessible house. They still do. My brothers and sister all do, as well. The one member of my family who lives in a place that is wheelchair-accessible is also the only other disabled member of our family.

I don't hold this against my family, it is just that for me the political issue of wheelchair accessibility is quite distinct from the actual accessibility of a given structure. Regardless of the legislation and the number of demonstrators willing to surround the U.S. Capitol, I can only get into the building by myself if it has no steps. Period . . . the end. We have all spent much more time, myself included, thinking and talking about general issues of political change rather than making the changes themselves at home.

Lawyers worry about whether the restaurant at the top of the Empire State Building is accessible while people forget about the corner grocery. The former is a news story and a place that a person in a wheelchair might visit once, the latter is not news. But a corner grocery is somewhere a crip might visit again and again. We tacitly accept that things around us cannot or will not change. But we are happy to march for a symbolic cause . . . even a lost one.

In 1990 the Americans with Disabilities act was passed, and a few weeks after the event I went to a bicycle shop in Brooklyn to get a wheelchair wheel straightened and a tire replaced. On the front of the door to this shop was a single large step. I raised my two front casters onto the step, grabbed each side of the doorway, and pulled myself through. One of the workers in the shop saw me approach the door and as I lifted my chair onto the step he rushed over, expecting to catch me in a fall. The young boy stood so quickly that his tools and a bicycle wheel went flying. The noise brought the manager of the shop up from downstairs. He arrived with a look of alarm on his face that suggested that he thought his store was being attacked.

"I thought you were a gang kid," he said. There was plenty of evidence of gang activity around the band of shops and rundown apartments on Smith Street. The street formed a border of gang territory and the residential peace of Brooklyn Heights and Cobble Hill one block west. Gangs were loosely organized, with local names or the more nationally known "Bloods" and "Crips." "I'm not a Blood," I said, attempting to break the ice with some humor. "I'm a crip."

"You, a Crip?" he said in a gruff voice heavy with Brooklyn, accustomed to saying exactly what was on his mind. He looked amazed that I would be a member of a gang, although plenty of young boys injured in drive-by shootings remained members of their gangs even if they used wheelchairs. After thinking for a moment, he said in a voice he might use when correcting a child's catechism, "You mean cripple. You mean that you're a cripple."

"Right." So much for icebreakers. I proceeded to the business at hand. "I need this wheel straightened and the tire replaced. It's for a wheelchair, but the rim and tire are the same as for a bicycle." He looked at the wheel, concluded that it was something he could work with, and handed it to the young worker who was busy picking up the tools he had knocked over a moment before.

"You know," he said after a moment, "you people can go everywhere. I was reading the other day that you people can now really go places."

I was a bit puzzled. "I get around just fine, if that's what you mean."

"No, no, no," he said. "You people. It's a law now. I saw on TV that President Bush says that you people can go everywhere in wheelchairs."

I brightened up. "You mean the Americans with Disabilities Act?"

He jumped in confidently. "Yeah, yeah, that's right, the American disability act." He turned to his young employee. "You know, we watched that on TV the other day. George Bush was signing this law with those people in wheelchairs and there was a midget too." The employee said he remembered the midget. The store owner asked me seriously what the new law meant.

I glanced back at the entranceway step and said in my most accommodating, reasonable voice, "The law means that you are probably going to have to put a ramp up on that step there."

His inquiring expression was gone. With the conviction of someone holding a law degree from Georgetown he said, "No, no, no. That law's for new buildings. This building here is old, it's from before. I don't have to make no ramps here on that step. But all the new buildings are going to be no problem, right?" He went back to working on my wheel. "By the way, is that a racing chair?"

I was glad I knew how to get through his doorway unassisted because the step to the sidewalk wasn't going anywhere any time soon. It did not matter that he was wrong about the law. The Americans With Disabilities Act did not stipulate that old buildings were exempt from its changes. He assumed that he and his business were exempt. There was no KKK-style intolerance in his voice, just the matter-of-fact conviction that he was not a part of any change that was intended to result in the inclusion of 20 million Americans in this nation's public spaces. I understood that more than any staircase or broken elevator or narrow doorway, it was this sentiment that shut down access, and a whole lot more, in America.

We are taught to watch the big picture, to become fluent in the symbols of change, and to celebrate those symbols. At the same time, Americans take as a virtue the routine opting out of any individual act of change. The civil rights movement is a good example: for blacks, the civil rights struggle has been just that, an uphill battle to convince the mainstream of what is right, just, and possible in America. It is a struggle that has swung from one polar extreme to another. From persuasive evocations of truth, justice, and righteousness to the imperative militancy of confrontation "by any means necessary," blacks have had to make the point about inclusion.

But to most people in America, particularly white people, the civil rights movement has never been much more than an arcane debate over constitutional law and the precise semantics of the Declaration of Independence. Were the founders really serious about that "All Men Are Created Equal" business? As if this is something that has to be excavated out of an ancient pyramid and decoded by experts. While blacks argued tactics and embraced politics during the sixties, whites spent lots of time discussing the sociology of prejudice and racism. Liberals and conservatives alike concluded that it was somehow an unfortunate fact of human nature to be prejudiced against people of another race. Racism was a phenomenon better understood as fated rather than as the product of individual human will. This premise avoided the simpler historical fact that whites had acted hatefully toward blacks. Humans are inherently prejudiced, the same impulses toward racism could be found among blacks as existed in whites. According to this view, racism was a matter of science, not morality.

Blacks had no option but to think of the civil rights movement as a struggle against whites. Whites could afford to take a far more detached view. They could see the civil rights movement as a struggle against the primitive impulses of an imperfect prejudiced humanity. The fact that blacks were forced into slavery by other humans, Europeans and Africans looking to make a profit, was beside the point. Were the slavers just acting out their inevitable human nature in imprisoning and slaughtering millions of Africans? Was this also what the Nazis were doing?

Blacks and whites have always clashed over the extent to which the civil rights movement is about pragmatic, down and dirty confrontation and change versus a kind of abstract anthropology to be observed from a slow-moving blimp. Racism as a "social phenomenon" is unquestionably bad, according to this view, but it may always be with us. Like the stubborn mildew on the shower tiles, it is an immutable legacy of social injustice. We just have to keep on scrubbing. But while whites can simply scrub the tiles to see progress, blacks must bring down the whole wall to have any sense of being included in the broader society. One job is performed with a sponge, the other with a sledgehammer. The two jobs are incompatible.

Having spent nearly the last two decades staring at steps, broken elevators, narrow aisles, and legal exemptions, it is clear to me that social change requires more than just some tile scrubbing. Walls have to come down, and the well-meaning people straddling those walls are the last ones to advocate heavy construction. In the end, the civil rights movement has taught whites less about inclusion and much more about how to find exemptions and loopholes in the system. It has taught blacks less about coexistence and partnership and much more about working the system. Blacks and whites face each other uneasily across this institutional fence, each giving the minimum and taking the maximum. When Los Angeles explodes, there is no law to change anymore. So what are we left with—changing our human nature? Or is it sufficient simply to say the right things, to be politically correct?

Today, in theory, freedom of speech protects everything, including racism. At the century's end we use the Bill of Rights more to shield hatred than to protect people from intolerance. Freedom of speech is a pretty moot point if we are just one riot away from martial law. In 1995 it's hard to see how much farther the Supreme Court or the National Guard can go to induce change or prevent civil war if individuals don't begin adjusting their human nature.

A system designed to bring people together has done much to drive them apart. The Supreme Court that heralded a social revolution more than a generation ago has produced a river of political symbols. Its waters race between two ice floes on which the people of a divided nation live. On one, blacks who would have benefited wonder why so little has changed. On the other, whites who claim to have given up so much to achieve equality wonder why so few are grateful. A century after emancipation and thirty years after the Civil Rights Act, it is probably more "human nature" than ever to be racist. With so much emphasis on symbols, relatively few people in the United States have actually had to change their individual ways of doing things.

I point to the step in front of the door of the Brooklyn bike shop. There is no way that this doorway is accessible. I even feel bad about hot-dogging my way up the high step, knowing that most people in wheelchairs couldn't even consider trying to get into this shop. The owner doesn't see any of this. He is sure of one thing about the Americans With Disabilities Act. "It's just for the new buildings." So I have three options. I can sue him over a flat tire, I can look for a new bike shop, or I can go over to his place in Brooklyn and go to work on his front step with a sledgehammer. Which one is a lost cause?

I was working in the NPR newsroom when the announcement about the NASA journalist in space program first crossed the news wires. I had always wanted to be an astronaut. Long ago I had decided that I had missed the launchpad. But this program seemed like a second chance. I was a journalist. I wanted to go into space. I would apply. One of the editors suggested that only science reporters apply, and that I was not part of the science desk. I noted that there was no stipulation from NASA about "science reporters". "Go ahead and apply," she said. "We will decide who from NPR will go into space. Besides, John, I think we can agree that NASA will not be sending a paraplegic as the first journalist to go into space. Right?"

I did agree, at first. Then I began to think about the problem. Was it really such a lost cause to think that even as a paraplegic one might be able to train and compete for a slot on a space shuttle mission? There was no denying the sentiments in the voice of my editor. It was a lost cause. "I'm sure it would be a good experience for you to apply, anyway," she said with the conviction that we have not reached the point in human evolution when paraplegics are sent into space.

Would the space program actually be crazy enough to send a crip into space? If NASA would not consider such a thing, then it was a lost cause, a waste of time. But this was not the real issue. The real issue was to look at the problem on its merits, independent of whether or not some institution would give me permission. What would a disabled person do on the shuttle? Was there any intrinsic value in sending paraplegics into space separate from the number of parking spaces this would free up on earth?

As I began to think about the problem it became clear that if all I tried to show was that NASA had no reason not to send a paraplegic into space, then I had no chance. Paraplegics in space? Maybe someday. Just as electing an African-American president of the United States was a lost cause as long as no one seriously believed it would ever happen. Black president? Maybe someday. These are American homegrown lost causes where "maybe some day" becomes a substitute for actual freedom and access.

The fact that I was in a wheelchair did not instantly cause me to argue the premise. I too could believe it was ridiculous to suggest that a person in a wheelchair might travel into space. I too wondered if I was wasting the application. The tone of my editor seemed to suggest, don't rock the boat, don't attract attention. Today we're doing journalists in space, John, maybe someday we'll do disabled people in space. That could take a long time. For the last 230 years we've been doing the white guys in the White House program.

Maybe someday . . . But to address this issue of space travel on its merits I would have to completely reevaluate how I thought of myself. Paraplegic, Paralyzed, Disabled Guy, Wheelchair User: all of these categories became suspect. For instance, the word "paralysis." I have always hated this word. It seems to suggest that a person cannot move at all, when actually even the most disabled person can move. It really depends on how you look at things. Compared to birds, we have lost the use of our wings, and compared to fish, we have lost the use of our gills. I'm sure that to fish, humans all decked out in scuba gear look pretty much like marine animals from some particularly tragic special education class. To birds, humans flying by peering out of the tiny windows of pressurized jetliners must look as odd and tragic as a busload of people in iron lungs.

To deal with the tragedy of not being able to live underwater or in the air humans invent a less humiliating way of thinking about it. It is not we who are flawed by not being able to survive in water or fly through the air. It is they who are underwater creatures, it is they who are winged, their physical assets redefined as rungs of evolution's ladder. Fish below birds, all of them below humans. But when we are not slaughtering them with rifles, jet engines, and nets, birds and fish must view us as the slow group.

To address whether or not paraplegics should become part of the space program you had to confront the real problem with paralysis, the physics, not the sociology. Is it the wheelchair? Is it the curbs? Is it the stairs? It's the gravity. Think about it. Paralyzed people live in an excess of gravity. So much gravity, in fact, that they often need to use wheelchairs or other gravity-assist devices. Far from being a problem, an environment where one could float around instead of walking would be just perfect. Lose the gravity . . . no need for wheelchairs. In outer space, with everyone floating around, it would be difficult to tell the paralyzed people from the nonparalyzed people. Perhaps this was NASA's problem. Like the issue of gays in the military, if paraplegics were allowed into space people would think that all astronauts were paralyzed . . . (or secretly wanted to be).

So when I described the mission I would pursue if given the opportunity to travel into space, I emphasized these issues. It began to seem as though I had a distinct advantage over the rest of the pack. How better to demonstrate the features of a gravity-free environment than to see disabled and nondisabled people working in space together? "Besides," I would tell the selection committee, "I have already experienced significant G forces hurtling through space in an out-of-control car." That put me ahead of the other journalists. As for the astronauts, even they had physical difficulty with the awkward space suits they wore, which required them to be attached to various tubes and machines. "I am way ahead of NASA in the urinary catheter department," I told the committee. "I could train the astronauts."

There were other advantages. A journalist who was also a paraplegic would undoubtedly have something to say besides "gee whiz" when he looked out the window. A voyage into earth orbit would become a voyage from literal confinement to weightless freedom. There would be no better way to convey the reality of space travel than to have this be part of the story. The image of six able-bodied astronauts working side by side with an orbiting crip would be a powerful by-product of the space program that until now has not given society at large much more than some Tang, Teflon, and a few really fabulous pictures. If the most profound image of the first space missions was seeing the earth as a fragile teardrop in space, then the image of human adaptability conveyed through the experiences of astronauts and a crip who have all had to adapt to survive would extend that original lesson. If the fragile earth shows what can be lost by humanity if it is not careful, then this new image would show what can be gained by putting a few preconceived notions aside.

The argument was persuasive enough for me to be selected as part of the pool of 100 semifinalists, along with Walter Cronkite, Tom Brokaw, and Geraldo Rivera. Cronkite and I made it into the next round of forty. No one besides me from NPR made it past the application stage. Far from feeling that I had triumphed over my editor's original skepticism, I felt guilty about using the chair to go to the front of the line once again. This feeling was only compounded when the AP wire ran a story with the headline: NASA PICKS PARAPLEGIC FOR JOURNALIST IN SPACE PROGRAM. The story was picked up by CBS, which asked me to appear on the "Morning News" the next morning from Chicago. I was told the interviewer would be Forrest Sawyer. The other guest would be Walter Cronkite. It was May 5, 1986.

A little more than a month earlier I had moved out of the apartment I shared with Martha. It simply became impossible to continue trying to make a household work with someone who was fully convinced it could never work. She had become very blunt about it. She regularly let me know that she wasn't going to be able to live with someone like me. Martha was someone who could easily imagine me as an astronaut but not as her boyfriend. Being an astronaut was something I really had to think about to be convinced it would work. Compared to traveling into space, living together seemed easy. But living with me long-term was quite beyond Martha's comprehension.

It was both difficult and obvious to conclude that Martha's ambivalence had anything whatever to do with the wheelchair. Difficult because this was the ultimate spiral staircase, the cosmic unfixably broken elevator, the ultimate inaccessibility nightmare. The thought that there could be no possible ramp up into Martha's life drove me into hysterics and made me want to move heaven and earth to build one. But it was also obvious. Who would want a crip as a boyfriend, let alone as a husband? The question was torture, but also comforting. If the wheelchair was the only thing Martha couldn't deal with, then everything else about me must be perfect. I was just one teensy, weensy detail away from winning her.

I still had the keys to our apartment. Martha and I were still friends. I was convinced that she would eventually come to her senses. However guilty I felt using the wheelchair to get in front of a line, I would not hesitate to use the wheelchair where Martha was concerned. Martha loved adventures and I had plenty of those. I was the only one Martha knew who had any chance of going on the space shuttle and I was going to appear on television with Walter Cronkite. There was still something to work with here.

I had dinner with Martha the night before the appearance on CBS. Her dark, thick hair was blowing in the breeze. It was late spring in Chicago. The wind retained its chill, but the change of seasons rounded winter's sharp corners along the lake. Time was passing. We were moving apart. If I were to convince Martha that we could be together it would have to be soon. "I miss your arms, you know," she said as she placed her head on my shoulder.

Martha was a physical treasure. Her strong body was rounded like an Irish landscape and her eyes were its clear, dark nights. She was matron, devil, and angel in equal measure. She would sigh deeply as I took her in my strong arms. My powerful fingers would knead her ribs and shoulders. The strength of my hands and arms made her breathless. As she exhaled from my open palm on her breast, I believed I could shape her body inside and outside. I rode her like sunlight rides the floating leaves on a stream. Though she would tremble with the force of the tides themselves, I would never let go. In our love, what loss there was in my body could be reclaimed in celebrating hers. She would let go. I would hold on. In her pleasure was our dream.

Our greatest adventure was in this reinvention of intimacy. But in the end, it only made her long for the original. She dreamed of a physical home I could never go to. I could see that she had these dreams. I could do nothing but hope they would go away. Our love was an island. Just as Robinson Crusoe's world of ingenuity and self-sufficiency had made him want to go home, Martha wanted from my body the one simple act of sexual union it could not give. She was Robin. I was her man Friday. But I dreamed of being her Batman.

Martha could not have been more excited about my selection by NASA. She had believed it was possible all along. Now others were dreaming our dream. Far more than simply being a name on a list, the fact that I was considered at all was its own journey into uncharted frontiers. I held her close. She said, "Part of me wishes that we still lived together." Which was all that I needed to hear. "Maybe we still can," I said. Looking back, this could only be translated roughly in my own heart as "I'm desperate. Take me back. I'll try to be better. I'll get rid of the wheelchair, honey. If you want me to cover it up entirely with a burlap sack and some gaffer's tape, I would be glad to." This was the attraction—a truly lost cause. The ultimate long shot on the moronic oval racetrack of life's repetitive little tragedies. In my pocket I felt the keys to our old apartment still there.

After a long, thrilling kiss in the night breeze, I walked her home. We traded details. I had not been seeing anyone. There could be no one to compare with her, I said. She sighed and insisted that there was no one to compare with me. In passing she mentioned that there was this stage manager in town working an industrial show with her, and that she had been with him a couple of times. This could only have meant that he had been at the apartment one or more nights, and since the industrial show was still in town, it was possible he was there at the moment I was walking Martha home. In my reverie I nodded and forgot this little detail until it was too late. "Don't forget to watch tomorrow," I added. "I wouldn't miss it," she said. "You'll be great."

The call on the set at the local Chicago affiliate was 5 A.M. Chicago time. I was to be wired up in a small room and would participate in the interview by intercom. I would not be able to see Cronkite or Sawyer, though they would be able to see me in New York on their monitors. I wore a blue suit. This was to be my television audition, and I was going to try and make a good impression in addition to holding my own on the inevitable questions.

This was my chance to convince people across America that it was not just some crazy idea for paraplegics to go into space. I wanted to come across as a journalist and not a wheelchair version of Susan B. Anthony. It was important not to make this an argument over discrimination. If discrimination became the issue, viewers would just collectively yawn, and say, "We get it. First, parking spaces, now the wheelchairs have their own Malcolm X." But if I could get people to see the advantages of wheelchairs in space on the merits alone, then surely they would pay attention.

The television crew was setting up the shot, and I could see in the monitor that they were composing what seemed to be a very tight head shot. I suggested that they widen it to include the chair. "You don't want the wheelchair in the picture, do you?" asked the cameraman. I said that since this interview concerned the possibility that a paraplegic would be chosen to go on the space shuttle, that they should indicate visually who it was in the wheelchair. Otherwise, people were going to conclude that Walter Cronkite had just had a stroke and couldn't walk.

"You're sure you want the chair in the shot?" He was acting as though the wheelchair was something I had spilled on my tie that morning while eating breakfast. "Don't you think it's a part of the story to have the wheelchair in the picture?" Perhaps things were not going to go well here. The cameraman widened the shot as much as he could for the small room we were in. It looked fine. We were ready. If it was this nerve-racking to simply talk about going into space, what would it be like to actually be waiting on the launchpad?

The first time I heard Forrest Sawyer's voice was over a tinny earpiece in a cramped room in the Chicago bureau of CBS News. He spoke to me off the air during the commercial a few seconds before the interview segment was to begin. He mentioned how he had always wanted to be an astronaut, that he was going to talk to Cronkite first, then ask me some questions. There would be only a couple of minutes for the whole segment he said.

Cronkite was introduced as "someone who wanted to be the first journalist to go into space," while I was introduced as someone who wanted to be the "first paraplegic in space." The camera was on me as Forrest made this introduction. I could feel that I visibly flinched. I could not see myself, but it was quite possible that this flinch was even sneerlike. I intended to set Forrest straight when he asked me a question, but for now I just tried to stay calm.

The first question was about whether Cronkite was afraid to go on the shuttle after the *Challenger* accident. He said that he was glad NASA was dealing with some of these problems now. When a journalist goes up, he said, things will be much better. Then Forrest came to me and asked me my thoughts about fear in the aftermath of the *Challenger*. I indicated that I too was not afraid but I also noted, "Forrest, I want to be the first journalist in space just like Walter Cronkite, not the first paraplegic in space." I couldn't tell how I looked, and I couldn't see Forrest's reaction to me. But as soon as I said it, the hairs on the back of my neck tingled a little. In my earpiece Forrest paused icily. "Okay . . . yes . . . of course." Here I wanted to talk reasonably to the American people, and already in my first sentence I was sounding like Charles Manson. Forrest turned back to Walter in New York. "So, Walter Cronkite, do you think your age will be a factor up there?"

This time it was Forrest's turn to march across his own tongue. He could be forgiven for not realizing on the first go-round that I was sensi-

tive to being called the first paraplegic in space. He was, after all, read-
ing off a script handed to him by the morning TV writers. But asking
Walter Cronkite to talk about his advancing age on the network where
he had been replaced as anchorman a few years back was like asking
Ted Kennedy if he had ever thought of naming one of his children
Mary Jo.

I couldn't see it, but on the set Cronkite looked away from Forrest
and right at the monitor. He ignored the question. "I'm more interested
in what John is doing. I think it's fascinating." I completely forgot anything I was going to say about the advantages of wheelchairs in space or
about the empowerment of the disabled. I began to babble something
about how proud and honored I was that Cronkite and I were part of
this group of candidates, and that to be on the same planet, let alone TV
program, with Cronkite was a peak moment in my life. I stopped myself
before I went over the edge and began thanking him personally for
ending the Vietnam War and urging him to run for president.

A minute into the segment America knows that I am not afraid of
outer space, that I don't like to be called a paraplegic, and that I apparently worship Walter Cronkite. It was not going so well for Forrest either. At this point, the host of the "CBS Morning News" is watching his
guests conduct their own interview. Back in Minnesota my mother has
passed out because Cronkite had called me by my first name. "He called
him John. Oh, my god! Walter Cronkite and my son are on a first-name
basis." As if our whole family would now be spending our summers
abroad Cronkite's yacht.

Cronkite asked how I would handle being in space, and I replied that
as long as NASA can get me into the vehicle, I can handle everything
else. "I realize that there are no ramps up to the launchpad at Cape
Canaveral. But then I don't plan to take my wheelchair into space anyway. In a weightless environment, who needs legs?" The guys working
the camera in Chicago liked this point. They nodded and gave me a
thumbs-up. The segment ended with Cronkite and me saying how important we thought civilian space travel was no matter what setbacks
NASA had to deal with in the wake of the *Challenger* disaster. There
were thank-you's all around, and the segment was over. The soundman
took my earpiece and said, "That was great, what you said. You know, if
you think about it, who needs to have legs in space?"

"I knew it would be great," Martha said on the phone when I got
home. She had called from her apartment and said that her family in
Toledo had said they liked the suit and wondered how long I had
known Walter Cronkite. "Tell them Walter and I are like this." She said

how much she had enjoyed seeing me the night before, and that she wanted to see me again. She did not say when. I wouldn't have heard anyway. I was delirious.

The next call was from my parents' house. My father concluded that, based on that interview, I would probably be going on the shuttle before Walter Cronkite. My mother was worried about Forrest. "I thought you and Walter were kind of harsh to Forrest Sawyer. First you yelled at him about calling you a paraplegic, and I thought Walter was going to hit him when he brought up that age thing."

"I didn't yell at Forrest, I just had to correct him."

My mother knew better, as always. "Honey, I think I can tell when you want to poke someone in the eye with a dinner fork. I'm sure the rest of America thought you were perfectly polite, but I know that nice Forrest Sawyer could tell." She added, "And a mother can always tell. I think I'm going to send Forrest a thank-you card."

The rest of the day went quickly. I received a number of enthusiastic calls from around the country. There were friends, a few I hadn't spoken to in years, and a Hollywood television producer asking how much I would sell the rights to my story for if I went on an actual mission. "I'm going up there to be a journalist. My job is writing stories, not selling them." I suggested that he contact NASA, and that it was a little early to talk about movie rights. I received no calls that day from the NPR science desk.

I wanted to spend the day with Martha. She had been so encouraging about wheelchairs in space. It was as much her argument winning the day as mine. I decided to drop by the old apartment and surprise her. I rolled uptown after work as the night was falling. It was warm enough to roll without a jacket, and soon the heat inside my shirt made it seem almost like a summer night.

My arms propelled the chair in a good rhythm. It felt like flying, there along the lakeshore. I looked at the lights across the water and wondered if it would ever really be possible for me to ride into space. Everything was so abstract. Truth would be measured in actions alone. There was always such a temptation in America to redeem all of the good feelings before anything really changed. The symbol part was easy. The hard part would be to actually make it into space. I haven't made it there yet, but where I ended up later that evening was strange enough.

I rolled up to the building where I had lived with Martha, and down into the parking garage entrance, which had no stairs. The buzzer for the apartment was down the stairs, inside the main entrance, so there was no way for me to announce my arrival. I got into the elevator and went up to the twentieth floor. My heart was pounding. I knocked on the door. It seemed for the first time in a long while as though everything was going to be all right. This was where I belonged. Martha had seemed sad the night before. She needs me to hold her, I thought.

I knocked again. There was no answer. She wasn't home yet. I had my keys in my hand from opening the outer door to the building. I put the key in the lock and rolled into the apartment where I had lived just a few weeks before. The place was dark and about the same as I remembered it. I rolled into our old bedroom. Her bed was in there now. The view out the window was spectacular. I sat on the bed and put my head back. I might as well have climbed into a tank full of cobras. It had been a very long day. Feeling as though all was right with the world, I pushed my head deeply into one of the pillows Martha and I had lain down on together so many times. I smelled a familiar sweetness, closed my eyes, and fell asleep on Martha's bed.

I awoke to the sound of voices down the hall. I immediately understood what a terrible mistake I had made. I recalled that Martha had told me the night before about the stage manager she had been seeing. There was a male voice in the other room. It was talking about some of the characters in the *Lord of the Rings* trilogy. "I once had a cat that I named Bilbo," he was saying. "Bilbo is symbolic, you know, he's not just a fat guy with a pipe." I could hear Martha making conversation, saying, "Now Bilbo is one of those little guys, the Hobblettes."

"Hobbits," he corrected her. "And Bilbo is symbolic, you know." Martha did not answer. I imagined that she was nodding her head, trying to look interested. "Bilbo represents all of the conscious beings at our level in the universe. He is the questioner. You know, like in Dungeons and Dragons?"

Who was this guy? There was no time to eavesdrop. I had to get out of there. I had a few options. I could stay where I was and pretend that I was asleep. I could emerge from the bedroom and say, "Hi, everyone. Don't mind me" on my way out. I could try to make it into the other bedroom and leave after they'd gone to bed. Since it was warm out, I had worn no jacket. If I had even tossed a sweater onto the couch or something, Martha would have been tipped off and some scenario for me leaving would have presented itself by now. They clearly had no idea that I was there in the apartment.

I was getting a bit frantic. What had seemed like such a heartwarmingly great idea an hour before had become a nightmare. More than anything else, I was embarrassed. My main thought was to protect Martha. I didn't know who this guy was, but I couldn't allow my presence to ruin her evening. I decided I could not just pretend to be asleep and be discovered. I also could not roll out into the living room and chat my way out the door. The awkward pallor that a man in a wheelchair coming out of a woman's bedroom would cast on everyone else was unacceptable, I thought. The polite thing would be to hide.

I could see a light snap off down the hall. "I'll turn off the stereo," someone said. There was no time for any more planning. They were coming to bed. I was in the bedroom. It would be impossible to get into the other bedroom down the hall without them seeing me. I was sunk. But instead of just being discovered, sheepishly apologizing, and leaving the apartment, I made a shocking, and what to this day seems like a completely insane decision. I scanned the room frantically. The closet? The window? Who was the expert in discovering places where wheelchairs could go? Who had, just that morning, told a national television audience that it was possible for paraplegics to go into space? I looked at the space under the bed and made a quick visual calculation. Yes, it could be done.

Out in the apartment, things were really moving. "I'm going to brush my teeth. Go ahead and get us a glass of water," Martha called out to this little troll she had brought home. I had just a few seconds to think of something to do, and some bathroom and kitchen faucet noise to cover me doing it. I grabbed my wheelchair next to the bed and popped off the quick-release wheels. With a practiced motion I had performed thousands of times, I folded the frame of the chair. Noiselessly, I climbed down onto the floor and slid under the bed frame. I stacked the wheelchair frame and wheels into a compact little pile and pulled them under with me. I made sure that my feet weren't sticking out. I had one more instant to make sure this was a position I could hold. The footsteps were coming down the hall. If Martha didn't notice the slight rumple of the bedspread where I had been lying down, I would be safe.

I saw two sets of ankles enter the room. Would Martha notice the bedspread? "Let's get on the bed," the guy said. Martha said, "Wait." She sensed something was out of sorts somewhere. "What's wrong, baby?" I gritted my teeth to stay motionless. But this guy was persuasive, and Martha was willing. I could hear him pull back the covers. There was no longer any visible evidence of my presence in that room. Martha cooed, "Oh, nothing," and they both got into the bed. Their weight pushed the mattress down close to my face. Around me, socks and underwear, pants and shoes, began falling like the debris from a midair collision. My situation was beginning to dawn on me. It was 11 P.M. Dawn was about eight hours away.

I had spent the morning talking on national television with Walter Cronkite and Forrest Sawyer about whether Cronkite or I would be the first American journalist to travel into the vast empty frontier of outer space. Now, with my wheelchair under Martha's double bed and the mattress inches from my nose, I was about to listen to the woman I loved being bonked by a skinny-ankled *Lord of the Rings* fanatic. More than any trip to the moon, this truly felt like the final frontier where no man, let alone paraplegic man, had gone before. The bed began to move above my face. I wasn't going anywhere. If the bed slats holding the box springs held, I might not be crushed to death by morning. I hoped Martha and the Hobbit stage manager weren't planning on sleeping in.

As the activity above me continued on a steep crescendo, I had a few things of my own to do to prevent discovery. If having a man in a wheelchair roll out of a girl's bedroom could put the brakes on an evening of love, discovering an old boyfriend and his folded wheelchair under her bed was more like a bucket of ice water. This went beyond finding the vibrator or the trashy novel. Martha might just overload, claim she had never seen me before, and shoot me as an intruder. I quietly pulled my body into the smallest shape possible. I made sure that the chair's metal was not going to click up against the bed springs.

I could not tell what exactly they were doing up there. I could hear Martha's rhythmic moaning. It sounded sincere. For a moment I felt a wave of jealousy and anger, but as I looked at my predicament I could hardly blame Martha. Mostly I had to laugh. It wasn't as though I had found Martha and this guy at home on my couch, or making out at the next table in a restaurant. They were being discreet. I just happened to be six inches away.

I didn't like this guy much, but as time went on I found myself rooting for Martha as I lay under the bed. I was the coach and she was the home team. I was urging her body on as if, like old times, I was up on the bed with her. I knew her body pretty well. I also knew how to decode the little noises she made. When Martha was on, her little moans were like individual words, each with its own note, length, and cute little rattle. When she was feeling it, each cry would end with a slow fade before she would take a breath and begin the next sound. When things weren't working quite right, the cries would lose their commitment and begin to sound the same. She started out committed, but after a few minutes I could feel her drift. I could hear her say, "Down a little." He would respond, "Right here?" "Over more." "How's that?" "Just go up . . . up." "Here . . . here?" "Yes, there. Stay right there."

There was a pause as the Lord of the Rings attacked the target.

"There?" This guy was not exactly a heat-seeking missile. "No; over more." It was as if the two of them were repairing something under the street and Martha was shouting to some guy down a manhole who was wearing a hard hat. The bed began to really move above my nose now. He increased his speed and enthusiasm by making noises of his own. Grunts and "Yeah, baby's" and a lot of "Oh, yes'es." I wanted to tell him to shut up so I could hear how Martha was doing. Her voice was beginning to sound like a child being driven across railroad tracks at 70 miles an hour in a jeep.

I could hear that the moment had passed. She was flapping in the wind through another wasted window of opportunity. Finally she said, "Why don't you just go in me?" He stopped and I could hear him fumbling for something. "There it is," someone said as a foil wrapper fell to the floor near my head. "Is it on?" Martha said definitely. I chuckled to myself that this was something I did not have to bother with. Then I heard a sound come out of Martha that I had never heard before. It was high-pitched at first, then ended up in a gravelly bass gasp of pleasure.

I guess I know what that is, I thought. The big lotto jackpot, the real McCoy, the Amtrack Sunset Unlimited. I was a little scared of the shaking oak beams all around me. There was a twinge of sadness in my stomach as I listened to them howling together. This is the reason I'm under the bed and he's on top of it. Maybe this is why I wanted to go on the space shuttle. Maybe the absence of this experience is the explanation for every crazy dare I've ever taken. Just one lousy little detail, Martha, and you will dump me for a guy with a tractor mechanic's fingers and a grazing yak's tongue.

The yak began to shout, "I think I'm going to . . ." "Go!" she said. It was over in a moment. He screamed, the bed slowed down, and they stopped bouncing above my face. Martha made a loud, happy, triumphant sound, but it was not her own body's victory. It was a sound I knew, but coming from me, not her. She had faked an orgasm; he had gone over the top. They had both gotten something out of the deal. I understood. She was happy for him. Feeling him go to pieces gave her the same pleasure I would feel for her when we were together.

Spent Adonis still had a couplet to rhyme here. "That was more fun than a barrel of monkeys." After he's just finished making love to the woman of my dreams, he says more fun than a barrel of monkeys? Even Martha sounded puzzled. In her laughter I could almost hear her wondering if there was anything good on TV. "Did you come?" he asks. Martha pauses, "Yeah, couldn't you tell?" No way, I thought. That much I knew. Martha wasn't going to marry this guy either.

They made a couple more passes, which turned out about the same. When the mattress finally stopped shaking and they fell asleep, I was alone there under the bed in the dark listening to them breathe, and was in terror that I would fall asleep and snore, or that one of my legs would have a spasm and make a loud noise.

It was my warped mind that had been responsible for selecting this hiding place under her bed, and now my paralyzed body was going to betray me. It was the perfect training for the isolation and disorientation of extended space voyages. I lay there tense and completely still for about eight hours. There wasn't much to do to pass the time. I found a ballpoint pen next to some lint, and on one of Martha's bed slats I scratched out a message: "5/6/86 I was here," and then as an after-thought, "You never came."

If I had been standing on the moon I could not have been farther removed from what passes for normal life in America. The day connected in a delirious, sleep-deprived theme. From hanging out with Cronkite, to traveling into space, to staring up at Martha's bouncing bed slats—unthinkable things were possible. Lost causes could be found. They were right there under the bed. But if no one dared to believe enough to say them out loud, they would remain lost.

Lost causes are big business in the United States. There is much more effort put into curing spinal cord injuries or discussing the legal issues involved in suicide for the severely disabled than there is in integrating disabled folks into society at large. Pray to be normal no matter how impossible it seems, is the sentimental message. The alternative is too horrible to contemplate.

Morning made everything on the floor visible. Shoes, socks, under-wear, and condom wrappers had all dropped very close to the bed. It took considerable time and care, but I managed to toss each trifle a few inches or feet out from the bed, so when Martha or what's-his-name reached down to get dressed they wouldn't see me. The one item I could not reach was Martha's bra.

At about 9:30 A.M. they stirred, made one more halfhearted attempt at copulation, and got up. Ankles moved around the bed. Hands were picking things up. It seemed as if I was going to make it. In a few minutes I would have spent an entire night, undetected, under the bed of two lovers. In the real world, surely fewer people could say this than could say they had climbed Mount Everest, or orbited the earth.

The last thing Martha reached for was her bra. Her hand came down, then her hair. I could see her head. Could she see me? I held myself utterly still, without breathing. She picked up the bra and for an instant

I was relieved. Then, very slowly, her head came back down. She had put on her glasses and was staring me straight in the eyes while slowly shaking her head. I would have said something like, "I really love what you've done with the place," but her companion, whose name I never learned, was standing on the other side of the bed talking on about some concert he had gone to in high school.

Without a word, or even a flinch, Martha stood up and suggested that they both go out to the kitchen and have some coffee. The first thing she did after discovering me was to brush her teeth. It was a completely Martha thing to do. "Don't you have to get down to the auditorium before eleven?" she called from the bathroom. She seemed to be getting rid of him. But there was also the possibility that she didn't want him around while she mauled me with a boat hook and packed my body parts away in the freezer.

In about fifteen minutes the front door closed and he was gone. Martha waited about thirty seconds for him to get into the elevator and then she yelled from the kitchen while she rummaged in a cupboard. "One minute you're on TV, the next minute you are under my bed. What the fuck are you doing under there?" I pulled myself and the wheelchair out as Martha stomped into the room. Instead of a knife for carving me up, she had brought a large mayonnaise jar from the kitchen. "I imagine you'll need this right about now." I was deeply touched. My bladder was about to explode. I filled the jar and then some.

She sat on the bed and just shook her head as I tried to explain. "I came over to surprise you and came in here and fell asleep, and when I woke up you were both out in the living room."

"Why didn't you just come out?"

"I didn't want to ruin your date. Who is that jerk, anyway? 'More fun than a barrel of monkeys?' Where did he learn that line, at Toys "R" Us?" We laughed. For both of us, this was an epiphany.

"Now do you understand why I can't be with you? You're insane. But I still love you." As she hugged me, I felt the apartment keys in my pocket.

"Here, please take these. It's far too dangerous for me to have them."

As I handed back the keys, I knew it was over with Martha. A few months later, following an investigation into the *Challenger* accident, NASA concluded that there were many more things to fix at the space agency than frozen O ring seals on booster rockets. There would be no journalists in space, with wheelchairs or without. But in the summer of 1986, I learned that it was possible to fold a wheelchair and hop under a bed noiselessly in an occupied apartment in under ten seconds. I also learned to believe that it was, in theory, feasible for paraplegics to travel into space.

Today Walter Cronkite is still the famous, avuncular, semiretired newsman/megastar he was back then. Forrest Sawyer has given up CBS and is a star anchorman at ABC News. Martha is married and living happily in Chicago. Today, I am about the same, scarred for life from the experience of spending the night under her bed. I no longer work for National Public Radio. I work on TV with Forrest Sawyer.

The Point of
No Comment

*I*t took years of being in a wheelchair before I could be truly
amazed by what it could do, and what I could do with it. On a
winter night in Chicago, after a light snow, I rolled across a clean stretch
of pavement and felt the smooth frictionless glide of the icy surface. I
made a tight turn and chanced to look around and back from where I
had just come. The street lamp cast soft icicle rainbows that arched over
and highlighted the white surface with bursts of color. Tracing out from
where I sat I saw two beautiful lines etched in the snow. They began as
parallel and curved, then they crossed in an effortless knot at the place
where my wheelchair turned to look back. My chair had made those
lines. The knot was the signature of every turn I had ever made, revealed by the wintry template of newly fallen snow. It was the first time
I dared to believe that a wheelchair could make something, or even be
associated with something, so beautiful.

I float through forests of pedestrians on the sidewalks of New York,
Chicago. A wheelchair presses its advantage on the pavement, street-
smart, good with cargo, fast and smooth. While walking measures out
landmarks in running shoe bounces or high heel castanets, rolling
glimpses a city in pans and dolly shots . . . a pedestrian movie with a
soundtrack of breathing. The spaces in the pedestrian traffic are liquid
passageways that open and close. I weave my way through the people as

sunlight passes through a crowd of sky divers on its way to the ground. I live in the blank spaces between the business suits and the gridlock.

On America's pavement there is a rough coexistence between wheels and legs. Between intersections, battles are lost and won every minute of every day. Scores are calculated, rules are kept and broken. It's a finesse game of bowling where speed and precision rule, but the object in this contest is never to knock down any pins. Points are acquired for continuous motion, for never having to say excuse me, for weaving from sidewalk to road and back without stopping for a light. Points are lost for causing elderly people to jump, and for running over anyone's feet. The only way to shoot a strike is to roll from point A to point B at top speed without stopping. There are at least two ways to shoot a gutter ball. You lose if you scare someone so badly that they fall down, or if someone asks if you need a push or tries to push you. This is the worst of all.

These days, more than just wheelchairs roll down the alley. Wheels are everywhere. Whether they be other wheelchairs, stroller wheels, or Rollerblades, a whole civilization inhabits the pedestrian strip. Vendors throw their nets and homeless beggars cast their palms into the current. The river yields only with difficulty. There is no simple fitting of a wheelchair into the pedestrian world. The ramped curb cuts built for wheelchairs are now clogged with mothers and governesses pushing carriages. People stand in the curb ramps, sucked intuitively to the lowest point in the channel of traffic. They yield only when a chair comes straight toward them, and only then at the last minute.

It is quite difficult to get a mother with a stroller to yield a wheelchair ramp, but it can be done. Often, approaching with speed alone from the front can move the stroller back or to the side. But scaring the mother is strictly forbidden. From behind, when a stroller is present all you can do is leap the curb or say excuse me. Leaping the curb acknowledges that the ramp is shared territory. Some chairs always need the ramps, and have no option. The real pavement hogs are the Rollerbladers. They weave in and out between the people where I once rolled unchallenged. They always seek the strip of pavement at the center of a road, the smooth pavement fillet road engineers call the crown. Bladers are intruders in a ramped world. In the manifesto of crips, four wheels good, eight wheels bad. Some wheels are more equal than others.

In Chicago, on Michigan Avenue, there is a wide sidewalk on the west side of the street. From the Chicago river to Lake Shore Drive the sidewalk descends steeply at one point. It is ramped on the west side on virtually every block. During 1987 I lived in an apartment at the bottom of that hill and worked in an office at the top. Rolling to work every morning was a character-building, hand-over-hand, rope climb. Coming home in the evenings was flat-out, downhill, and effortless.

Though I rolled in rhythm and wove my way with precision, the presence of a wheelchair in the crowd never seemed as natural to the crowd as it did to me. Where I saw beauty and grace gliding down, others, particularly those walking toward me, saw terror, collisions and serious injury. Going up, where I saw a bracing physical challenge, others saw pain and suffering. On the uphill leg the pedestrian comment was, "Here, let me push." The downhill caption was, "Hey, watch out! You're going to get a speeding ticket." Up and down the sidewalk hill in Chicago I imagined that there was a way of rolling in the chair between fast coasting and slow climbing where people would not be compelled to remark either that I needed a push or a speeding ticket. I took the unwanted closed captioning as a physical challange. Somewhere between fast and slow, between deliberate and headlong was this mythical point of no comment.

On the streets every day as I reach a cruising speed virtually anyone in my path will say, "Excuse me," or "Watch out," to the person next to them. Mothers who see me look around for their wandering toddlers, and scream, "Look out!" The child runs to Mommy and stares fearfully as I go by. It always seems so odd to hear it, yet to dwell on it seems neurotic too. I can steer. I truly can negotiate my way down the street. But the impulse of pedestrians is to imagine collisions, to presume that there is something wrong. The people who'd rather be safe than sorry, without realizing it, erect walls of chilly exclusion as I pass. I cannot control the impression that my physical shape and presence is foreign.

When I described this to an African-American friend of mine he responded with a knowing nod. "It's like the power locks. And the toddler grabbing." When he walks down the streets in a white neighborhood he can hear the power locks click. He can see the mothers grab the children. Perhaps it's all very innocent and tiny. Yet it delivers an unmistakable message: "You're in the wrong place. I always wondered if I looked too angry or too . . . something. But it was just that I was there."

Rolling isn't as different from walking as you might imagine. The speed at which I travel is a function of rhythm. Inside my paralyzed soul the pendulum of walking still swings. Beat . . . Beat . . . Step . . . Step . . . A wheelchair with standard 20-inch wheels requires a stroke in cut time. Step . . . Step . . . Step . . . becomes

Roll Roll Roll Roll RollRollRollRollRollRollRoll Roll Roll Roll.

Because I still feel the old rhythms of walking, I have large, bicycle-

sized wheels on my chair and small diameter hand rims for pushing.
They slow down my stroke and flatten out the rhythm of rolling. They
also allow me to go faster, but with large-diameter wheels the beat of
rolling is that same centered rhythm of walking, at a speed about twice
as fast as a normal walking pace.

Roll . . . Roll . . . Roll . . . Push . . . Push . . . Glide . . .

Rhythm is something that must be felt. Rhythm breaks down the menacing foreign threat of wheelchairs into the fluid motion of rolling,
which anyone can see if they look. There are places where the rhythm
comes through to everyone. The joggers and tourists on the wide paved
trail along Lake Michigan in Chicago would watch me roll toward them,
in some places for half a mile as I made my way from the hill at the
Shedd Aquarium to where the path curves around Lake Point Tower. To
them what I was doing looked like fun. A runner might catch the rhythm
of my arms and at that exact moment we would be racing. Two runner's
steps to each rolling push of mine. The adrenaline would surge in each
of us. We would pace each other for a while and either an uphill grade
would slow me and the runner would pull ahead, or a downhill would
allow me to surge forward. If we were on the flats, it was a joyous battle
of physical wills. I might pass the runner or the runner might pass me.
In each case, the rhythms of forward motion, legs and spokes, were in-
tertwined.

At the top of the hill on Michigan Avenue, just beyond the white stone
Wrigley Building, a bridge leads over the Chicago river and intersects
with Wacker Drive running east to west. Wacker follows the river all the
way into the financial district. The corner of Michigan and Wacker is a
crowded, busy intersection as well as a major bus route. The buses make
right turns from Michigan Ave onto Wacker. In the afternoon rush hour,
on a clear day when the sun shines out of the west, the drivers make
their right turns into the blinding sunset, which shines directly in their
faces until they find the shadow of one of the tall buildings farther down
the street.

One of the chief joys of rolling is passing pedestrians on the uphill.
At rush hour you can surge past dozens of pedestrians at a time and
easily beat the street traffic on the uphill. I had stayed ahead of a bus
for five intersections as I approached the top of the hill and the Wacker
crossing. The light was green and the pedestrian sign said WALK. There
were some pedestrians in the street, but the road was cleared of the
first wave of people, and the anxious drivers waiting to turn right were
eager to be off. Two or three cars turned as I reached the intersection.

I was still ahead of the bus. I rolled forward into the street as the bus started its turn.

Almost immediately I realized that the bus driver could not see me. At four feet eleven I was just about the height of the bus wheel now coming straight toward me as it made the sharp right turn. The bus was going to hit me. The wheel rushed at me like a black demon with truck treads for teeth. The bus blocked out the sunlight as its own shadow covered me, a prelude to being squashed by five tons of glass and steel. People standing on the corner began to scream. I veered off, but the wheel kept coming. There was nothing to do. I jumped free of the wheelchair and with my gloved hands slid back quickly across the pavement, out of the reach of the wheel.

The last thing I saw before I hit the ground were my legs. I could not move them, but it was up to me to save them from the bus. In the momentum of my jump I tried to ensure that they too were thrown clear of the wheels and not stuck in the wheelchair to be crushed. The bus wheel hit the chair and tipped it as I sailed backward. I couldn't feel my legs. I couldn't be sure that they weren't trapped like the chair. To myself I said, Come on, guys, fly, as I vaulted with my arms away from the chair being consumed by the bus's wheel.

As the bus slowed, people everywhere were screaming. I could hear the sounds of people banging on the windows inside the bus, people who had seen me crossing the street and had then seen me disappear. There were two sharp popping sounds as the bus tire crushed and destroyed my wheelchair. My thin, high-pressure tires exploded as the bus came to a complete stop. The chair was directly under the right front tire of the bus. I was sitting on the pavement a few feet back. I was staring at my legs to confirm in a way no sensation could that they were still connected to me. I pulled them toward me into a cross-legged position, hugging my ankles like children. I was unhurt and helpless. There was something completely incongruous about the scene. I couldn't walk, but that was true before the bus hit me.

I looked at the crumpled pile of twisted spokes and broken tubing that I had been moving in so effortlessly just a moment before. The wheelchair was destroyed. I had no sensation in my legs, but I was sad for the chair. It had died to save me. It was a deeply emotional moment. I longed to move the bus off the chair, my old friend on the uphills and downhills. The late afternoon sun glinted off the silvery jagged remains of the crushed aluminum tubing. I had not received a scratch. I thought of Rick, after the accident, unscathed and looking through the wreckage of a crushed automobile at someone he loved deeply, now changed forever. He had been unable to move then, I was unable to move now. I watched. The tears streamed down my face as I laughed at the ridiculousness of the situation.

"Are you okay?" Someone from the crowd spoke. Most people stayed back, not quite knowing what to do. I was unharmed, the wheelchair was crushed, should they call an ambulance or just keep walking? I couldn't help them. The door to the bus opened slowly, and the one person in all this who most wondered what had happened but was surely the most terrified to find out, the bus driver, leaned her head out of the door. She knew she had run over something. The screaming people in her bus and on the street indicated that there was a person down there somewhere. Until she saw me waving at her, and my tear-streaked smiling face, she looked like a person who expected to see some pretty grim remains under her bus. "I'm fine," I said. "Is that your bike?" she pointed to the wheelchair. "It used to be a wheelchair," I said. "Jesus Christ," she said.

An ambulance arrived. Two paramedics ran over to me and asked if I had been hit by the bus. "Yes," I said. "Can you walk?" they asked. "No," I said. "Get the stretcher," one yelled. "Can you feel your legs?" he asked. "No," I said. There didn't seem to be a way into this conversation. "Look, I'm a paraplegic," I tried to explain. "Not necessarily, son," the paramedic said hopefully. "Now lie back while we put a brace on you." It seemed cruel of me to tell them the truth. They were trying so hard to make me walk again. "That's my wheelchair, there under the bus wheel," I told them. "I couldn't walk even before the bus hit me."

The paramedics had never encountered anything like this. Someone who was unhurt in a collision with a city bus was telling them it was okay that he couldn't walk. "Do you need the ambulance?" It was hard for me to answer the question. My first impulse was to say, "No way, man, I'll just take a cab. There's nothing wrong with me. I don't need an ambulance." I said that I would be happy to take a ride to my apartment, where I had a spare wheelchair. "I can't go anywhere like this." I wasn't hurt, but I also had been rendered unable to move because of the destruction of my chair just as surely as if it had been me pinned under the bus wheel instead of my chair. I was injured, I was unharmed, it had been a close call. It was all of the above.

The bus driver backed the bus up and revealed my broken chair. I asked the paramedics to put it in the ambulance with me. The driver said that that was not possible. "We have to take this to the bus station for inspection. That's the rule in any accident." The paramedics said that they were required to take me to the hospital even if it was for a routine exam. "It's for insurance reasons, you know." I was sad to be separated from the wheelchair even if it was just a broken heap. I didn't like the way the driver threw it into the bus. I was still sitting on the ground waiting for the paramedics to bring a stretcher to carry me over to the ambulance. One of the passengers stepped up to me and winked.

"You're going to be a millionaire now, buddy. You should get a lawyer and sue the pants off the CTA. Guy in a wheelchair, run over by a bus, pain and suffering, the light was green, we all saw it. You're going to be a millionaire." The American attitude toward disability was never so perfectly expressed as in the sentiments of this very enthusiastic man standing at the corner of Michigan Avenue and Wacker Drive. He saw advantages to being a paraplegic as I sat cross-legged on the pavement, my wheelchair a useless hulk under the wheel of a bus; advantages that were hidden away as long as I was rolling. Perhaps this guy would have shaken his head with a hint of sorrow as he watched me pass him, rolling, a few minutes before on my way up the hill. Now that I was immobilized on the pavement, he wanted my autograph. To him, I had just won the lottery.

So is there a point of no comment? I found it one day on the way down the Michigan Avenue hill. It had been a long day. I was tired and I stopped worrying about speed and pedestrians: a dreamy dissolve and the walking people became moving posts in a paved slalom course. I pushed ahead, and the territory between the bodies became an ether, a river of space into which I could glide while they, like cattails in the current, could not.

Gravity pushed the chair ahead, and with the smoothness of curves etched on a lathe, I carved a trajectory around the pedestrians at a speed far above that of walking. Fingers touched the wheel rims, trimming to the right and left. I was trailing a thread on a windless slope, drifting around briefcases and suits and ankles and dress shoes. Speed became a test of the limits of the fabric of the space itself. The only appropriate speed was the fastest possible. The space between people became my space, and the whole scene unfolded as a postulate: Can this be done? Can the staccato pedestrian rhythms blend with the reedy line of effortless rolling descent? Wheel jazz.

When the fear of collision vanished, I ceased to look like a piano rolling down a hill. The chair and the legs joined for all to see in an unsolicited statement of grace. There was no suggestion that I was speeding. I glided by faster than it took to think of comments about speeding tickets, but this was no mad dash of escape; for once, I was not trying to outrun their preconceived notions. The spaces between pedestrians were made for wheelchairs, and I belonged there. Pedestrians saw it as well. On their faces was: "That looks like fun." When had they ever yearned to be in a wheelchair before?

The promise of art and revolution is that people might discard their preconceptions and truly understand what is in the mind of another. What would a world look like in which people dare to wish to know what it is like not to walk? The point of no comment exists. It has a signature. It is the smooth curve a wheelchair makes in cold snow.

It is beautiful.

I never sued the bus company. I suggested that they buy me a new wheelchair. They did.

Beat Reporter

As the sole journalist in a wheelchair during my years at NPR, I was determined that I not get handed all of the disability stories. For some reason, I feared that I would get typecast and end up doing all the stories about Baby Doe, Steven Hawking, Vietnam veterans, wheelchair basketball games, and the Special Olympics. As I discovered over the years, being assigned stories about disability was not something I ever needed to fear. My own lack of enthusiasm about disability stories fit right in.

There was no disability beat for a reporter in the early eighties. NPR and the rest of the media seemed to care very little about disability stories regardless of who was doing them. Today the only sure way to get an editor interested in disability is to work Dr. Kevorkian into the lead; otherwise, forget it. Disability is a difficult sell unless the subject is in intensive care clinging to life after a sports injury, terminally ill, obsessed with suicide, or taking up hang gliding from a wheelchair. None of those stories speaks to the day-to-day realities of crips. But then, America apparently doesn't think of disability as having much day-to-day reality. The disability experience for the media is part Frank Capra, part Vincent Price, with nothing but the occasional Vietnam movie in between.

In 1983 a woman in Riverside, California, named Elizabeth Bouvia went on a hunger strike to kill herself. She claimed that as a woman with cerebral palsy, which rendered her a quadriplegic, her life was not worth living. Her doctors indicated that they would forcibly feed her the moment she was too weak to resist, and Ms. Bouvia had gone to court to prevent their intervention. NPR thought the legal issue of whether she could decide to kill herself, even though she was physically incapable of taking her own life by any other means than starvation, was worth regular coverage.

My crip friends and I followed this case with great interest. Quadriplegics were offended that Elizabeth Bouvia could get national attention for insisting on killing herself while the lives of quadriplegics who went to work and had families were invisible. Crips weren't asked to comment publicly about Elizabeth Bouvia. My quadriplegic friends said that she was not really suicidal. "She just wants a new TV, you wait and see." The coverage at NPR was typical of the rest of the media. It made me angry that NPR accepted, without questioning, Elizabeth Bouvia's assumption that her life was not worth living because she was a quadriplegic.

If it had been some obvious omission solely on the part of NPR rather than a lockstep consensus of the media at large, it would have been easier to voice my criticism. I could not point to another treatment of the story in the mainstream media that reflected my concerns that Elizabeth Bouvia's declaration of her First Amendment rights came at a cost to the lives of other quadriplegics who did not share her conviction of hopelessness.

I told the national desk editor that I felt that the NPR coverage of Elizabeth Bouvia did not reflect the views of other quadriplegics. While she might want to take her own life, I argued, the idea that being a quadriplegic was an understandable reason for doing so was profoundly offensive to people with disabilities.

I was told that under no circumstances was NPR saying in its coverage that quadriplegics' lives were not worth living. It was a question of free choice and individual liberty. Some quadriplegics wanted to live, some wanted to die. Should doctors help those people who wanted to die, but could not? That was the question. I was told that because I was in a wheelchair I might not be completely objective in this matter.

The idea that I was biased and that they were being objective in their coverage was an outrage, but acting outraged only underscored their suspicion that I was "biased." I argued that the legal issue was only a small part of the story. By letting Elizabeth Bouvia's assumptions about the value of her life go unchallenged, NPR was losing an opportunity to explore what made the story interesting: that one person's concept of the value of life might not apply to others in the exact same circumstances.

This, I was told, was irrelevant. The story was not about Elizabeth Bouvia's life, it was about the law and the First Amendment; that's why the courts were involved. It had nothing to do with Elizabeth Bouvia's, or anyone else's, experience. That was a medical detail. That Elizabeth Bouvia's medical condition was a detail, when her possible suicide was perceived to be a national news story, pushed the limit of credulity. I was arguing with Martians about the rules of baseball.

In the end, Elizabeth Bouvia decided not to kill herself. When I asked the national desk editors about this, they said that she was obviously a disturbed woman. How would they know? Their stories had always been about the law and the courts, never about her life, and why she had once thought it so worthless. As far as I was concerned, they had missed the whole story. If she had filed her case today, Dr. Kevorkian could have saved Elizabeth Bouvia the trouble of a hunger strike. Progress.

I generally avoided the issue of disability at NPR because the reaction from people if you brought it up too often reminded me of how blacks described what happened to uppity niggers in the early days of the civil rights movement. To be branded as a dangerous "uppity nigger" trying to "stir things up," people told me, was as easy as bringing up the subject of race in public. To whites, people who brought up the issue of race were violating the rules in some way, and betraying an inability to deal with the way things were. Blacks who stayed quiet were celebrated as pillars of strength and leaders in some liberated society of the distant future. In my world, "uppity crips" were called by a different name: people with a "bad attitude" who were to be distinguished from the people with good attitudes. If my non-crip friends ever discussed the issue of disability with me, it was to comment on my attitude. "John doesn't let anything stop him," they would say. "Disability? Why that's the last thing you ever think of when you are with John."

There was always something wrong with the idea that because of some attitude I had, people wouldn't see something that was such a large part of my life. I was anxious not to let things get in my way so that I could get where I was going. I didn't think of it as an attitude. My friends were grateful for the fact that I acted in such a way that they didn't have to think much about wheelchairs. I wasn't so sure that I was responsible for that. Wheelchairs, and the obstacles in their way, are things people just didn't want to think about, period.

I spent very little time with other crips. Some people would ask me if this was because of some problem I had with being disabled. I could never tell. The two worlds, crip and non-crip, were so different. There didn't seem to be any overlap. You were either in one world or the other.

In 1986 I got a call at the NPR bureau in Chicago asking me if I would like to come to New Hampshire for the weekend and see what disabled winter sports were all about. It was the first time since leaving a hospital that I would be spending any significant time with a large number of other disabled folks. There would be snow and instructors, ski poles and prosthetic legs, wheelchairs and chairlifts.

Each year, organized groups of disabled athletes gather to enjoy the winter. Crips love to hurl themselves over icy precipices. But ski resort communities with a tourist trade have a realistic economic interest in seeing that springtime does not bring with it the discovery of partially thawed disabled skiers who, while coming down the slopes, went off to that great telethon in the sky. So when the crips ski, they generally organize gatherings that come with plenty of supervision in the form of instructors and ski pros. One week each winter somewhere in America, the crips take over the mountain.

I was on the next plane from Chicago to Portland, Maine. A driver would take me to Attitash, New Hampshire, an hour away. I was to be instructed in the use of a sit ski, a little plastic bucket/toboggan for paraplegics. I was hauled up a mountain, and using metal wrist grippers, I sailed down, the quiet winter air rushing past my ears. Out of the wheelchair, my body was like a bag of baseball bats and Jell-O riding a dessertspoon down a mountainside. Close to the snow, the horizon slips easily from sight. It feels like falling.

The hiss of winter erupted like a jet from beneath the path I etched into the powder. Each bank of a curve in the wide slaloms sloshed gravity up against my bones like buckets of thick paint. I held on as the speed increased, and I began to master the rhythm of moving from side to side and not tumbling over. Flat-out and downhill I was a brain pan bowled over the edge of a glacier. From above I still looked like a guy in a weird little toboggan. The form was clumsy, the farthest thing from the spiny ballet of spandex Olympians, but at ground level on the way down it was all motion, exhilaration, and grace. On the way up, from the chairlift, I could just make out voices on the edge of the trees.

"To the right. To the right . . . To the left, to the left . . . Right, right . . . To the left."

Blind skiers. It was the voices of the instructors tethered to their sightless companions. I listened to them in the echoless snow cushion of the mountain. The blind skiers were tethered by the gossamer thread of a trust I could not imagine—what if the sighted one made a mistake? The blind skier would smash right into a tree. But there was no mistake. Faith in the truth of another human being's voice freed them to ride the flourishes of gravity with their feet and legs alone, skis reading the mountain's topographical braille. From my little toboggan, the sight of going over the edge was frightening enough, but to feel the ground slip away in the dark, sensing the earth's curves with only the fluids of your body—what could that be like? I imagined piloting a small canoe on the little bubble of water inside a carpenter's level that had been hurled out a window.

The wind rushed past my face. In exhilaration I lifted my body up with my arms, swinging the chair lift over the trees. There was just the oddity of two skiers, one sighted and one blind. Tethered together gracefully they superseded form in a pure headlong state of motion where anything seemed possible. At that moment on the mountain I dared to wish for blindness so as to share in the exhilaration of pure gravity. It was a crip utopia on the mountain. Some people skied in little plastic buckets as I did. Other were strapped into fiberglass cases that were bolted to a single ski. They gave the impression of riding a winter sport unicycle. There were the amputees on two limbs, one prosthetic, the other super-formed. There were other amputees with their prosthetic arms affixed to ski poles for balance; then there were the hot dogs, the armless torsos on legs whose balance was adjusted with a move of the head or shoulder. At the top of the heap were the leg amputees who skied solo on a single limb. Some of these folks used poles with ski outriggers to compensate for having only half the surface area touching the snow. One even forwent the outriggers and skied on a single hip, knee, and ankle, using poles alone for guidance. On these slopes in New Hampshire, she was pushing her single blade down the mountain, using the stump of bone at her waist as a counterweight, making the most of her slim contacts with the snow. It made her go faster.

Here, each mode of hurtling was different, constituting a unique sport in itself. On the same mountain and in the same snow, people everywhere were defying form and technique. There was none of the blandness of the usual trip to the slopes, where contrasts are in the Gore-Tex, sunglasses and car keys. Here, each implausible headlong plunge overflowed with breathless physical adventure far beyond speed.

At the lobster feed that night, back at the lodge, I wandered among all the people I had seen on the slopes. It was a fashion show, like any other Saturday night. Crip skiware and other ornaments of crip chic adorned the benches of a large cafeteria. Empty pants legs were cut to fit muscular stumps. Some stumps had bold striped or patterned socks pulled over them. A particularly shapely torso concluded in a bright turquoise stump of pure thigh. Assertive and defiant, the wheelchairs were decked out in colored spandex regalia and high-tech splendor.

At one end of the room they were serving lobsters and corn on big, sturdy paper plates. The whole lobsters drained oily puddles of juice onto laps and tables as diners rolled, hobbled, or hopped to tables to eat. The blind sat with the blind. The paraplegic wheelchairs sat with the paraplegic wheelchairs. Quadriplegics with other quads. Amputees with like amputees . . . no leg and arm combinations. It was leg to leg, arm to arm, crutch to crutch, prosthesis to prosthesis, like a Balkan convention of the war wounded. I scanned from table to table, a crutch here, a chair there. The one thing they had found to do together was to tear the limbs from lobster bodies and stuff them in their mouths. I stared. It was something to stare at.

None of this was news, and it didn't fit into any of the constructs that the media had for exploring disability. There was no "issue" here. There were no "critics of disabled skiers" to talk to, no experts, no lawsuit, no one trying to commit suicide, just people enjoying lobster after a day on the slopes.

I asked my editors only once at NPR if I could do a story about a disabled person. It was a "triumph over adversity" story with what I thought was a spectacularly bizarre twist. It was about a young disabled man who had made it in radio against all odds. "That sounds like your story, John," the editor said. I told him that I hadn't made it against all odds, and besides, there was nothing about being in a wheelchair that made it difficult to talk on the radio. "This guy is really disabled," I said without revealing any details about the story. It was about a young man with Tourette's syndrome, Saul Lubaroff, a DJ in Iowa City, Iowa.

His day job was the Saturday morning pre-football, easy listening show. His music came off a tape or a satellite. All Saul did was the weather and a little local news. Each hour he announced the "KCJJ Money Wheel," a caller contest that was a cross between a Vegas roulette wheel and a carnival beanbag toss. The prize was a jackpot, usually an odd number, like eighty-four dollars and thirty-five cents.

Saul's night job was as rock DJ Dave Desmond at a station on the other side of town. I discovered him in a small story on the inside pages of *The Des Moines Register*. It was about how Saul was working as a DJ, even though he had an unusual disease that caused him to blurt out things uncontrollably in the presence of others. How this worked with a live broadcast microphone present was not explained. Saul kept control of himself when the microphone was on. How he could do that and not control himself at other times was also a mystery. The story did explain that what Saul blurted out were not just noises and shrieks: Saul's outbursts were almost always obscene.

If Saul really was a guy who would talk normally one minute and be shouting the next with no way to predict what was going to happen, I would need an engineer to watch the sound carefully. The brilliant and unflappable Chicago bureau engineer, Flawn Williams, said he would go. Our assignment was to record and interview a "D" list part-time DJ in an "Z" list radio market at a nearly automated easy listening station. I told Flawn to pay particular attention to any obscene things Saul might suddenly scream out. "Is this a story about Tourette's syndrome?" he asked. I showed him the article in *The Des Moines Register*. "I'll need a good limiter then," he said, and began poking around in the equipment cabinet.

We arrived on a Saturday morning and pulled up to a concrete block building in the middle of a field next to a tall, steel antenna tower. Saul was inside doing his shift. It was a few minutes before his news break. We had time to get acquainted. Flawn set up his microphones. The large reels of tape which contained the music slowly turned: a Whitney Houston tune was playing.

Saul was a stocky redhead who bounced around, laughed a lot, and had not shaved in several days. "You the guys from NPR?" he asked. I introduced myself and Flawn. Saul started to say something about the station when, all of a sudden, he yelled, "I masturbate." He rolled his eyes and tried to act nonchalant about this involuntary commentary. Flawn immediately grasped the audio challenge here. He looked at his meters and up at me as if to say, "Ask him to scream 'I masturbate' one more time." We didn't have long to wait. To break the ice, in between screams about masturbation, I spoke with him about some of the details of Tourette's syndrome that I had learned from my research.

"Are you taking Haldol?" I asked him about the powerful tranquilizer that doctors prescribe to Tourette's syndrome patients to calm their outbursts. It does not control them. "I'm on Haldol right now, babe." Then, without a pause, he screamed. "I love you. I love you. I smell like come . . . I smell . . . I smell like come."

Flawn and I looked at each other again. He nodded that he was getting the sound at a proper, undistorted level. I was not someone who had ever had much difficulty in finding a question to ask, but Saul had really shut me down. "So . . . Gee, uh . . . Saul. How exactly did you get into radio?" Saul glanced at the clock and then back at me. "It's the only thing I have ever wanted to do." Saul loved radio even more than I did. "Radio is me. It's who I am inside. Listen to me. You can hear me . . . who I am." Listening to Saul was quite an adventure.

He picked up a piece of cardboard from his microphone table, placed it into his mouth and bit down. "I love you, I love you," he screamed again. He winked at me and said, "Here we go. Two-minute break." The second hand on the clock was approaching the top of the hour. Flawn moved his microphone into position next to the station's live mike. Five seconds before air, Saul screamed once more. "I masturbate, I masturbate, I smell . . ." The last words he swallowed. He shook himself, took a deep breath, and flicked the switch that opened the microphone and put us all on the air.

As Flawn and I watched, Saul read the local news, gave the correct time, and delivered the weather report off a wrinkled piece of torn newsprint paper. His voice was even, smooth, and medium-pitched, just like other commercial radio voices. He read the copy with the proper cadences and all of the right feeling. He stumbled once, on the name of the coach of the University of Iowa Hawkeyes' football team, Hayden Frey. He got out on time. The first song up on the tape was Gordon Lightfoot's "If You Could Read My Mind." He announced the song and said he'd be back in the next hour. "This is Saul Lubaroff, KCJJ news."

It was an utterly forgettable AM radio break. For Flawn and I in the studio it was two of the most harrowing, electrifying minutes of radio we had ever experienced. As Saul shut off the mike, Flawn and I exhaled as though we had just driven a motorcycle off a waterfall and made it to the shore alive.

"I love you!!!" Saul immediately began screaming again. "I masturbate, I masturbate!!" The pent-up energy from his few minutes of control on live radio crashed over him in a wave of deadly candor. What Saul could restrain on the radio, he could not control for our microphones. Saul knew we were going to put his recorded voice on the radio, but he also knew that our microphones weren't live, so for some reason he couldn't make the magic work for him.

Of course, if he had been able to control himself for us we would have no story. We developed a lurid split loyalty to Saul and his Tourette's syndrome self. Each time he would speak I would cross imaginary fingers and pray that he stay in control. He never could; but each time he exploded into a self-destructive obscene shout I would look at Flawn as if to say, "That was a good one. Let's have a couple more like that."

Saul also understood that we were there to witness his disease as much as we were to interview him. When his Tourette's self stepped up to perform, Saul stepped back, exhausted. "What's going on inside you?" I asked. "Is there some little troll shaking the cage, trying to trip you up?" He told us about someone inside him he called Tony.

"Tony Tourette is in there. Think of whatever you wouldn't want to do or say. That's what Tony is going to say. If you see a girl with large breasts and dirty hair, what is the one thing you don't want to say? That's what I'm going to say." Then he looked at me and yelled, "You're a cripple. You're a cripple!!"

On the one hand, Saul was exhibiting the rarest and most disturbing feature of his disability; on the other hand, he was confirming what I often suspected, that behind their smiling faces, people looking at me were thinking what Saul had just yelled. Whenever I had this thought, I always chalked it up to my own paranoia; now I was not so sure.

Saul was a great guy with a big problem. The days we were with him he met someone who became his girlfriend. She called up to say that his voice was sexy. Only after she met him did she learn of his Tourette's syndrome. Saul said that on their first date, one of the things he blurted out at her was, "I want to squeeze your tits." I could imagine this as a far more serious problem than wetting your pants on the first date, as I had done when I met my wife.

The piece we produced on Saul aired as a twenty-minute spot on NPR's Saturday morning program "Weekend Edition." In the course of editing the story there were heated debates about whether to let Saul's outbursts go out on the air uncensored. His mother, a nice Jewish mom who had watched with horror as her oldest son grew up and began to scream the most unthinkable things at her friends in their living room, insisted that we air his outbursts uncensored so people could get the full impact of what Tourette's syndrome means.

At NPR we had editorial meetings about how to deal with the outbursts. "I want to fuck you" was out. "I love you!" was in. "I smell like come" was the most awful sentence NPR's editors could imagine going out over the air on a Saturday morning at breakfast time. But we insisted that if properly produced it would go by so fast that no one would know what he had said. In the end there were five "I smell like come'" and seven "I love you's." There was one "I'm a virgin up the asshole" (where Saul garbled the last word so that only we knew what he had really said) and two "You're a cripples'." It was all a disability rights issue. Airing Saul's outbursts was as much a matter of civil rights as the width of the bathroom door in the NPR offices. It also meant a lot to me that the first mention of my disability in a national broadcast was made by another disabled person. His disability was being mentally unable to stop himself from pointing out that I was a cripple. Normal in America meant keeping such a thought to yourself.

Here was a guy who came as close as was physiologically possible to saying the most tasteless, obscene things on the air. He was paid minimum wage. On the other hand, Howard Stern, who does the same thing every morning on his coast-to-coast radio show, has no medically defined syndrome. He would not call himself disabled, yet he comes as close as he can to crossing the legal line between obscene and appropriate while the microphone is live. Howard Stern makes millions of dollars. If there were a disability beat, Saul would be one of my regular pundits; maybe I would make him an entertainment reporter. Imagine Saul interviewing the same people Barbara Walters profiles in her specials. With Saul you would be assured of that extra level of candor that nondisabled correspondents simply could not deliver.

If there were a disability beat, I would include a story about another man I once met, Abdul Haq, the most fearless general from the Afghan Mujiheddin, Afghanistan's resistance movement of holy warriors who defeated the Soviets on their last battlefield and sounded the death knell to nearly a century of communist rule. Abdul Haq told me a story about his disability and said that during the 1980s it was a closely guarded secret he told to no one. One indication that the Afghan war was long over and that his command was very much in the past was the fact that General Abdul Haq even dared to tell the story about his unfortunate trip to New York City in 1986.

"I was a big commander then," he said in the backyard of his house in Peshawar, Pakistan. "If anyone had found out, it would be very bad for me." We sat in the relentless biblical torpor of the Hindu Kush, 121 degrees Fahrenheit. Each of his visitors lived in New York, or had at one time, and when Abdul Haq told his story we each felt that sympathy unique to New Yorkers when they meet someone fallen prey to the city's unstoppable reality.

You had to know that Abdul Haq's foot was blown off to realize that it was a piece of wood that he walked on whenever he took a step. Even with his limp, it was difficult to imagine Abdul Haq out of his depth. He commanded the holy warriors of Kabul, Afghanistan's capital city, during the decade-long war with the Soviets. Today he lives in exile, in Peshawar, where he hastens to tell you that in his country it is not nearly so bloody hot.

If you collected footnotes to the war in Afghanistan, Abdul Haq's name would be there in a dusty old shoe box, among the detritus of the cold war's last battlefield. He collects such footnotes himself; his shoe boxes contain letters from former presidents, State Department officials, the United Nations, and the CIA. His larger boxes contain videotapes of the war. They are fuzzy but unmistakable footage of a forgotten finest hour. The war with the Soviets has been replaced by a factional standoff between Muslim fanatics who have divided Kabul into a half-dozen Sarajevos. The nights of Kabul resemble the shimmering incendiary finery of the Gulf War, and its days the miserable triage of Bosnia.

It is perhaps a mistake to call the latest trials of Afghanistan forgotten. Largely unreported and unseen, there is little to recall in the first place. Since the Soviet retreat and the end of the cold war, Afghanistan's carnage has been off-the-record, which is where Abdul Haq's New York story begins.

"It was always off-the-record during the war. But now it is just a funny story." He glanced around to see who of his household staff might be listening. "You have to understand that I just have a problem with New York. I had an awful experience there." His voice trailed off as he slowly shook his head. We began with the usual disclaimers about how New York gets a bad rap, or that more bad happens in New York because more of everything happens in New York, or that the city is safe if you know what you are doing. "Maybe this was the problem," he interrupted with a wave of the hand. "What did I know? I had only been to the White House before this."

Abdul Haq was on somebody's "A" list during the eighties. His friends included Ronald Reagan, who toasted him at a state dinner in 1985 by saying "Abdul Haq, we are with you." "We" gave Abdul Haq and the Mujaheddin some of our most advanced guerrilla weapons, including advanced handheld Stinger missiles, which the U.S. government is now trying to buy back. Abdul Haq has no stingers today. He fired all of his at Soviet aircraft years ago. His more fundamentalist allies stockpiled their Stingers for the post–cold war era.

All told, three billion U.S. dollars flowed into Afghanistan during the eighties, and along with it, U.S. officials, senior and not so, bound for the glory of the Khyber Pass, or at least the twentieth-century equivalent of getting your picture taken with an authentic Mujaheddin warrior. There are pictures of Abdul Haq with congressmen, State Department people, CIA officers, and countless other hangers-on in the struggle of the Reagan administration's central Asian contras. Some of these pictures hang on walls in Washington, the rest are stashed away in Abdul Haq's shoe boxes.

"I got off of the plane at JFK airport and I was the first time in New York," he began. "I went to my hotel, maybe Hyatt, maybe Hilton, I don't remember. I was there, it was a minute only, and I left to walk outside. I was carrying five thousand dollars in cash in one pocket and my wallet in the other, and I was going to meet someone. Outside my hotel was a man showing this game with three cards and another man was playing and some people were watching. It was clear to me what was going on." Abdul Haq began to shake his head, as though this was the moment when all had gone wrong. "I could tell that the man was being tricked, so I said to the man which card he should pick."

In a scam that was at least as old as the Khyber Pass, the man playing the game pretended to be amazed and insisted that Abdul Haq play the game to prove he knew how to win, while the man running the game pretended to be angry at being found out by this "clever tourist." Abdul Haq bought the whole routine. "I reached into my pocket and pulled out this large wad of five thousand dollars cash and took one hundred and placed it on the table." Abdul Haq saw that our faces expressed a certain fatalism about what happens to people with wads of cash who stand around Grand Central Station playing three-card monte. He waved his hand. "I know what you are thinking," he said. "But I did not lose at the game, you see."

When they saw the wad of cash, the two men at the card table dropped the pretense that they were strangers. One grabbed the cards, the other folded the table. Just before they sprinted away, a hand reached into Abdul Haq's jacket as he watched, too amazed to move, grabbed his wad of money, and disappeared down the street into a crowd of midtown pedestrians. "I had been in New York for three minutes exactly," he said. He ran after the men, but on his wooden foot he could not catch them and would never be able to recognize them even if he had. He stopped at a phone booth to try and call a friend who could direct him to a bank where he might get cash even for cab fare.

"I set my wallet with all of the credit cards by the telephone, and after I hung up the phone I walked away and forgot my wallet." A minute or so later he realized this second mistake, and when he went back to the phone booth, it was gone. "I know what you are thinking, that here is this general of the Mujaheddin who is in New York for three minutes and is robbed of everything but his clothes." We told him it could have happened to anyone.

Because Abdul Haq received a good chunk of the billions of dollars the U.S. was sending to the Afghan resistance, he was able to call Washington and his money and credit card problems were over as quickly as they had begun. "But I was very worried and scared about what had happened," he said. I said that five thousand dollars was indeed a lot of money. "No, no, no," he said. "It wasn't the money. I was worried that other leaders in the Afghan resistance would find out. If they knew that two men stole five thousand dollars right off of my body and that I didn't catch and kill them it would mean that someone in Kabul would try to overthrow me." The people in Kabul played more serious games than three-card monte. "But people in Afghanistan know that you have a wooden foot and can't run fast," I said. "Yes, yes, but they wouldn't understand. They don't know New York. I would have had to kill those two men, or else it would have been me who would have died in Kabul."

Hiding a disability, and how powerless it made him on the streets of New York City, was a matter of life and death to Abdul Haq. I couldn't argue. I also couldn't help thinking about those two thieves outside Grand Central Station, who in nabbing five thousand dollars from a limping crip, without knowing it had gotten something much more valuable. The CIA claimed that it was Abdul Haq's wiley genius as a commander in Kabul that had made it possible to completely defeat the Soviets. According to Abdul Haq, the war in Afghanistan, the fate of the most powerful resistance leader in Kabul, even the billion-dollar U.S. policy of aiding the Afghan rebels against the Soviet army, had depended on what two thieves in midtown Manhattan knew. They knew that he was something of a sucker for three-card monte, that he could be fleeced of his money, and that he couldn't run for shit. Perhaps the KGB would have paid a lot more than five thousand dollars to find this out.

The assumption that disability is something that can be defined by a reporter's beat, that it is some separate category independent of other news, or that disability rights stories, by themselves, reveal anything of the people they claim to be about, are two equal and opposite fallacies. They would have us believe that the experiences of the disabled are not universal, and that people with disabilities have little or no life outside their struggles and strangeness.

Such assumptions exclude consideration of the special qualities someone like Saul Lubaroff might bring to the job of, say . . . weatherman. They prevent us from seeing that blind skiing is an experience anyone might find thrilling. They tell us to pay attention to Elizabeth

Bouvia's lawyers and not to her own struggles with quadriplegia. Finally, they keep us from seeing that even a tough Afghan general, who can count U.S. presidents among his friends, needs a little help sometimes, and that the key to winning the cold war involved a secret even the CIA didn't know about.

Getting Past
Security

*M*y first foreign assignment for NPR was to cover the Palestinian uprising against Israel, which erupted in the West Bank and Gaza Strip in the final weeks of 1987. I departed for Jerusalem in the spring of 1988.

The Palestinian uprising exploded onto the headlines during the last sleepy years of the eighties, but it ended with a whimper, lost in the footnotes of the cold war's collapse and George Bush's war with Iraq. In the midst of the brutality of 1988, Palestinians and Israelis had no inkling that it would take six years for the Palestinian flag to fly officially over occupied territory, as it does uneasily in the West Bank town of Jericho and the Gaza Strip today. More popular scenarios, depending on your point of view, would have been now or never, with no middle ground.

But in the late eighties, after more than a generation of wars conducted under cold war sponsorship, invasions by neighbors united by hatred, and an arms race that filled the warehouses in the Middle East with every conceivable advanced and heavy weapon, the Israelis and Palestinians were finally confronting each other in the crowded sliver of land that they would eventually have to share. With stones and rifles, flags and graffiti, tear gas and gasoline bombs, a vast, global-scale conflict was suddenly reduced to a series of deadly pranks in the rocky, craggy schoolyard where western civilization had grown up thousands of years ago.

In 1988 Israel and the occupied territories looked like an exotic Disneyland in disrepair, overrun by street gangs, unruly soldiers, and journalists, one of whom was in a wheelchair. In the three short years I was in Jerusalem I confronted most of my theories and assumptions about independence, disability, journalism, and America. The Middle East was where I learned how to keep a wheelchair moving regardless of weather, geography, and national politics.

Imperfect as it was in America, wheelchair access felt like one of those coveted luxuries of western modernity, along with working telephones, automatic teller machines, and supermarkets. In the places I would need to go in the Middle East, I expected to leave accessibility behind. In such places, I imagined I would truly be on my own. I had been assured that Israel would be more accessible than most places. The Arab-Israeli wars had produced thousands of crips, American Jews told me. I would find Israel with plenty of ramps. The geopolitical barbarity that had made Israeli society terrified and bellicose for much of its existence was supposed to make me feel right at home.

I had brought two extra wheelchairs, an enormous box of parts, three additional sets of wheels, two cases of hydrogen peroxide to keep catheters sterile, and twenty pairs of my standard-issue, white handball gloves for serious out-of-doors-all-weather wheelchair work. There were two-dozen tire patch kits, three sets of all-terrain tires, a heavy-duty power reversing drill with bits for titanium, aluminum, and hardened steel. I had a tool kit which apparently fit the airport X-ray profile of a grenade launcher. Security inspectors gathered around the screen, whispering and pointing.

I had to explain to the young female Israeli security officers at Heathrow Airport boarding the flight to Tel Aviv why I needed more than one set of wheels. I also had to explain about the gloves and the bags of inner tubes and tools. I told her that I was a reporter on my way to the Middle East. This was my job, but the idea seemed ridiculous, some kind of scam for getting through customs, and it wasn't working. The agent thought I was lying, and I was holding up the line in the departure lounge.

She took me into a little room away from the other passengers. Here the young female agents were replaced by brown-skinned men with open shirts, walkie-talkies, and curly hair. They also asked about the gloves, the tools, the inner tubes, and this story about how I was a re-porter on my way to the Middle East. It still sounded like a lie. They inspected every tool, the oddly shaped ones and the familiar. "You can buy tools in Israel, you know," the security chief in London said. "Do you think only Americans know about tools?"

When some people heard that I was going away to the Middle East, they immediately thought of Leon Klinghoffer, the man in the wheel-chair who was killed by PLO terrorists on the *Achille Lauro* cruise ship in 1987. People said, "You're in a wheelchair, aren't you worried?" It was as though people assumed that the PLO went for the *Achille Lauro* cruise ship *because* Klinghoffer was on it; a campaign of terror that be-gan with the Munich Olympics in 1976 and then moved on to the Spe-cial Olympics. So, of course I should be worried.

I arrived in Israel in April 1988 at the height of the Intifada. The Palestinian uprising had many rules and players from countless factions, Jewish and Palestinian, but unlike some other Middle East conflicts that preceded it, few pieces of equipment were required. All that was needed was two peoples, two histories, one army, and an ample supply of rocks. There was plenty of all three in Israel and the occupied territo-ries. Mostly, there were rocks everywhere, which was why the Palestin-ians seemed to be doing so well.

It would take two years for the overwhelming force of the Israeli military to hammer the very fashionable and newsworthy Intifada into just another stalemate. But when that stalemate broke in 1993, the chair-man of the PLO would be shaking hands at the White House with the prime minister of Israel. The man who would be shaking Yasir Arafat's hand, Yitzhak Rabin, in 1987 as minister of defense had given the Israeli army orders to break the bones of Palestinians caught in rock-throwing demonstrations. Disabling demonstrators was preferable to killing them until the bone breaking appeared on television around the world and disability was suddenly far more shocking than the rising death toll from the uprising. A "CBS News" camera caught soldiers using large rocks to break the bones of a Palestinian man on a rocky hill in the occupied West Bank. The world would watch the news footage of hundreds of Intifada funerals, but these pictures provoked an unprecedented outrage against Israel.

The Palestinian uprising was the biggest story in the region since the war in Lebanon ended in 1983. At the beginning of the Intifada, the world press arrived for its latest fix of Middle East destiny. To see the show one needed an Israeli press pass available only at the Israeli Government Press Office, Beit Agron, which in Hebrew means, roughly, "the house on Agron Street." On the day I arrived in Israel, I rolled from Arab East Jerusalem and the American Colony Hotel to the Jewish west side to get my pass.

Nothing ever says that you are now entering or leaving THE ARAB SECTOR. But it would be a delusion to conclude that there is any lack of seriousness about this separation of two peoples. There are no checkpoints in the city denoting the green line from the 1948 Israeli war of independence. An Israeli friend once suggested to me that this absence of checkpoints and border posts is a sign of just how seriously Arabs and Jews take Jerusalem's internal borders. My friend liked to compare it to Berlin and its green line from the same period of history. "They needed a wall. There they needed checkpoints, they needed police to keep them apart. If they really hated each other, they would not have needed these things. You see that their wall came down. They did not have enough hatred. Here we have no wall. It would be a waste of money." As in no other place in the world, in Jerusalem the real borders are in the mind.

Even though Jerusalem was fully annexed by Israel following the Six-Day War of 1967, the unification of the city apparent on maps eludes residents who live with the old borders every day. Israeli sovereignty has failed to end any number of Jewish exiles from Jerusalem. The various exiles of the Jewish people are enforced in checkpoints of history and hatred as Jews and Arabs travel the streets of a city they both call their capital. Jerusalem is an orphanage to all those who would dare to claim the city solely as their own. The faces in its corridors are uniform, like the bricks and stones in a cathedral. In Jerusalem, I was to learn that it is those who would make no claim on the city, who claim no membership in its history, who stand out.

The road from my hotel to Jerusalem's walled old city was called the Nablus road, named for the city of Nablus, which Jews call Shechem, located some two hours away on winding roads through the West Bank. It also runs along the edge of East Jerusalem through a narrow, seemingly aimless corridor surrounded by walls. Behind the walls are famous houses of the rich scions of Jerusalem's long history, the houses of the Nusseibehs, the Dijanis, the Husseinis. There are houses from the colonial past, and some from the Arab patrician past. Here also are properties dating from the proud Jewish history that preceded the establishment of the modern state of Israel.

I turned the corner and an entire street full of commerce stopped and stared. As I entered the narrow streets of the neighborhood of Mea Sharim I could see why. This was the most famous orthodox Jewish neighborhood in Jerusalem, save the small community inside the walls of the old city. The checkpoint was guarded only one day a week, on Friday evenings and Saturdays, the Jewish Sabbath, when cars and other impious objects were barred from Mea Sharim's warren of synagogues, apartments, and shops. This border inside Jerusalem had more to do with Babylon and the Romans who had exiled Jews from this city over its 4,000-year history than with Zionism, the PLO, and the Intifada. It had nothing to do with Palestinians, except that if a Palestinian car strayed into Mea Sharim during Shabbas, it would be stoned just as swiftly and angrily as an errant, impious, Jewish car.

Everyone looked me up and down. The pairs of men standing together could be seen talking openly about me in Yiddish. One unabashedly pointed at the wheels of my chair and continued to talk, as though I were a Polaroid snapshot on a bulletin board. The children stopped their playing and joined the pointing. Their chattering mothers didn't stop talking to each other, but their eyes continued to follow my movements. There was no fear. I was out of place, not them. On each face the same look of amazement. "What planet are you from? Where did you park your spaceship?"

I might have looked unusual in a T-shirt and black jeans, rolling in a wheelchair with hard, knobby, tank-tread tires. But here on these streets, the concept of unusual seemed a little loose, to say the least. It was an April day and sunny. The noontime temperature was already about 80 degrees. All of the men were in fur hats or black wide-brimmed hats, full-length black coats over vests, shirts, slacks, and black, round shoes. The women were covered from head to toe in misshapen wigs, cotton tops, and long skirts. The ramps in this neighborhood were for the strollers, and there were many of them. Most strollers carried two kids, with a few toddlers tagging along behind. The youngest children were uncovered, but the boys all looked like smaller versions of their bearded and scowling fathers.

The image of an Orthodox Jewish family was certainly not new to me. There were ample occasions to see the black-hatted men and their wigged wives at New York City airports and on the city's streets, and behind the counter at 47th Street Photo, the electronics market run out of midtown Manhattan. But here was a whole community of people in a hot, sunny, Middle Eastern city dressed for a Polish blizzard. *They* looked like a colony from the outer planets. But because I was on their planet, I had no more reason to stare than they did; so we stared at each other.

Here, within sight of the Temple Mount in the old city of Jerusalem, the rituals and dress of a 1,900-year exile were preserved and carried out. The historical fact of exile from the destroyed Jewish temple, and the building of a pious life around waiting for a promised Messiah to lead the prophetic return, was so central to the Orthodox Jews of Mea Sharim that an actual exile was irrelevant. You didn't need to leave the City of David to enter the Jewish Diaspora.

I waved my hands in friendship. Some of the children waved back. I knew something about their way of life. I presumed that they knew nothing about me. Plenty of people in Israel speak English, but I wanted to communicate in Hebrew, thinking that it would dispel any presumptions about my being a tourist. I had learned some tentative Hebrew from an Israeli teacher. My command of grammar and vocabulary was pretty bad, but I had mastered her Moroccan, south Tel Aviv accent.

I thought one good reason for learning Hebrew and Arabic would be to explain what I was doing at the bottom of stairs, or anywhere else, before people called the ambulance. I wanted to be able to tell people that I was a reporter so that they wouldn't think I had lost my parents in a refugee camp. In deciding which Hebrew phrase would be most useful to me, in Israel I settled on *Efshar Ha Lazor li*. ("Is it possible for you to help me?") With the rejoinder, *Ein Beyah*. ("No problem.") I presumed that I would need to ask for help. I presumed even more certainly that, from time to time, I would need to tell people that I needed no assistance.

I would never consider asking for help in the United States. It was not until I realized that I would need occasionally to ask for assistance if I ever hoped to succeed as a journalist in Israel that I understood the consequences of never doing so back home, where it was a sign of failure. It was customary in America for utterly lost males to drive around looking for a street, adamant about not asking for directions. In Israel, asking for help was nothing to be embarrassed about. Among Palestinians it was virtually a national pastime. No one ever worried about getting lost in Israel or the occupied territories. A driver would think nothing of stopping every quarter-mile or so and asking directions of everyone, and getting a different reply from each person. Often, groups of people would crowd around the car shouting and arguing different suggestions. It made for the appearance of a more open and welcoming society. It did not mean that drivers in Israel were more likely to get where they were going.

I chose to speak with a round man and his brood on the street in Mea Sharim. "Could you help me find Agron Street, please?" I delivered this in overloud neophyte Hebrew. My vocabulary may have been bad, but my accent, I thought, was pure south Tel Aviv.

"You are from United States, right?" He walked up to me with his two children tagging close behind. Crestfallen that he would answer me in English, I told him I was born in Ohio. "Ha, ha. Ohio, Cleveland Indians." His knowledge of Ohio was about as extensive as my Hebrew. "I think that you are not Jewish. But where do you learn to talk?" He was impressed by the accent. "Most American Jews are speaking Hebrew like Alan Alda." He made a face and said a few words I couldn't understand but were apparently an Orthodox rabbi's imitation of Alan Alda speaking Hebrew. It made the people around him laugh. I had never been much of a fan of Alan Alda's even in English. Now I wanted to avoid sounding like him in Hebrew. But if my accent was not bad, then what had tipped him off about my national origin? "How could you tell I was from the United States?" I asked.

"Who else could you be? If you were Israeli, you would be in a car. If you were religious, you would be in the house. If you were Palestinian, you would not be in Mea Sharim. Only an American would be on the street in this wheelchair." He answered as though he was reciting a theorem in geometry. "But I am a reporter," I said. "So . . . A reporter in a wheelchair coming to Israel in the middle of this Intifada? You must be American. Who else would do something like this?" I had never before been stared at for being an American.

For residents of Jerusalem, the disability experience depended largely on what side of the 1948 green line you lived. I would be spending time on both sides of that line, in all kinds of terrain. Spinal-cord-injured Israelis, like most Israelis, did not spend a lot of time in the West Bank or in Gaza. Israeli crips prided themselves on their advanced, lightweight, American-style wheelchairs, their high-tech athletic training center outside Tel Aviv where they honed wheelchair basketball and tennis skills, and their government-supplied vehicles. Israeli crips could most easily be spotted in their cars, which were equipped with Israeli government-supplied, roof-mounted wheelchair carriers.

The racks would allow a driver to place a folded wheelchair in a metal box on the roof of a car. A driver would transfer into the front seat of his or her car, fold the wheelchair, then attach it to the rack. It would electrically or manually retract with the chair and close into a box on top of the car. These carriers were only rarely used by American crips. They were more identifiable than a handicapped parking sticker, and in Israel they looked like they had been designed in an industrial arts class. The government subsidized the cars, the army supplied the racks. Everyone had one.

Israeli crips had lots of gadgets. Their chairs were very light for running on gymnasium floors and flat pavement. They were low to the ground. Israeli crips were not into marathons or distance running. They were more into basketball, tennis, and driving around. Israeli crips didn't act like somber nostalgic war veterans as much as they acted like a secret paraplegic and quadriplegic strike force. Most spinal-cord injuries in Israel are not from any war. As in the United States, they are casualties from traffic accidents. But the culture of disability in Israel is distinctly military in nature. Wheelchairs are technology. Israeli crips look at their chairs like they look at advanced jet fighters. And like F-16's, they needed good pavement for takeoff and landing.

The best pavement in Israel is in Tel Aviv. Most Israeli crips did their rehabilitation at Tel Hashomer Hospital outside Tel Aviv, which was also Israel's most famous acute trauma facility. The worst Israeli war wounds are treated here. The neighborhoods around Tel Hashomer were specially designed for wheelchairs. They were nice-looking, with newly built wide doors, ramped entrances, and freshly paved driveways, each with a parked vehicle equipped with the telltale wheelchair luggage rack on the roof. The houses were absolutely accessible, and the neighborhood was something of a crip ghetto, the only place in Israel where I would ever regularly see people in wheelchairs on the street. It was the Mea Sharim of disability. Unlike the bookish overweight rabbis of Mea Sharim, the orthodoxy here was athletic; it was also still distinctly male.

On a visit to Tel Hashomer I encountered Dr. Avi, who could show you computer-assisted electric nerve stimulators that would trigger leg movement. These leg movements did not replace walking; they were a kind of controlled spasticity, and once you were wired into Dr. Avi's special seat and plugged into his computer, he could have you pedaling away like a robot come to life. Dr. Avi urged me to play basketball. I told him I had no time. He showed me dozens of special grabbers and reaching devices and dozens of clamp-on gadgets for a wheelchair. "Here you can put your drinking glasses, and here you can put your Sony Walkman, and here you can put your clicker for the video. The cell phone is going right here. This clamp is for your tennis racket." "Tennis racket?" I asked. "You said that you didn't play basketball, so you are from the tennis?" The possibility that I did neither was a little unnerving to Dr. Avi. "Do you think you need to see a counselor?" I said no.

He spent a lot of time looking at my chair, which did not meet the profile of the paraplegics he usually encountered. He particularly noticed the wide, knobby tires. "What happened to your wheelchair? I think it is too heavy, and you are sitting too high up." I told him it was for moving around in places where there was no pavement, in the West Bank and Gaza. He said not to go to those places, that it was too dirty. "You could get an infection, and you could get a flat tire."

Finally I told him that I was just looking for a doctor to run the occasional kidney test to make sure my plumbing was okay. "You are worried about your plumbing?" He nodded with a smile of recognition, as if he finally understood the reason for why I had come. He stood up and motioned for me to come with him over to a supply drawer. He opened the drawer, and inside it were a number of white- and flesh-colored plastic rods. He picked one up and bent it. It apparently had some kind of wire inside, for it stayed bent. "Would you like me to put one of these in your penis?"

I could not have been more shocked if Dr. Avi had been wearing a trench coat. "Many of the paraplegics have these in Israel," he said. "What size are you?" I suppose that penile implants have more medical credibility than the plastic dildos available over-the-counter in sex shops on Times Square. But Dr. Avi's idea of curing impotence was to surgically turn my organ into a flexible stand-up Gumby toy. For a moment I thought of Martha back in Chicago, and what her reaction to Dr. Avi might have been. Perhaps she would have become a real fan of Gumby's. "Doc, I'm not worried about that right now." He nodded and asked me if I was sure I didn't want to see a counselor, or get a new chair. "No, thanks," I said, and left.

On the way out, a couple of Israeli paraplegics rolled up to me. After talking with Dr. Avi I expected to see signs of a tent pole in these young men's sweatpants. They were intently examining the scratches and modifications on my chair. The large rubber knobby wheels attracted the most attention. "That chair is not good for tennis, you know," one of them said. "I know, I know," I said, quite accustomed by this time to having my chair criticized, my lack of sports training ridiculed, and hearing suggestions for counseling and surgery on my penis. "Did you have to make this chair yourself?" I replied that I did not make it myself, that it was a chair designed for heavy use in my job. "What is your job?" they asked with some doubt on their faces that I could ever show up in a chair that scratched and dented and get work. "I am a reporter." They thought for a minute and then smiled. "You are American, right?"

If hanging with Israeli crips was like watching a scene from the movie

Top Gun, visiting spinal-cord-injured Palestinians was like reliving the valley of the lepers scene from *Ben Hur.* Palestinian men and boys were just as swaggering and boastful as Israelis, but Palestinian crips were not big on either pride or swagger. The Palestinian office for the physically disabled dispensed big, clunky, low-tech, mostly used wheelchairs from the basement of someone's old house down a steep flight of stairs.

"I would like you to come and visit and see our many programs, but it will be difficult for you." The head of the organization wore thick-lensed glasses and was partially paralyzed from polio. He hauled his considerable weight up and down the stairs to his office and phone using wrist crutches. He received few calls. Mine was the first call he had received from a disabled person from the U.S., or any journalist. "Perhaps you should get a new office with no stairs," I suggested. He shook his head and said, "It has always been here. We should change it someday. But it is easy for us to call the crippled people on the telephone for their needs."

It was, if anything, more of a rarity to see Palestinian crips on the street, even though there were thousands of disabled Arabs in Israel and the occupied territories. As among Jews, the oldest and most numerous of the disabled were from polio and the familiar road accidents and other injuries. The most recently disabled, constituting by far the youngest group of crips, stemmed from the violence of the Intifada.

Their needs, according to the Arab rehabilitation organizations, typically involved institutionalization for the most acutely disabled. Disabled people who might achieve some measure of independence could expect to obtain a used or occasionally new mass-produced, cut-rate wheelchair bought in bulk by poorly funded institutions with no thought of custom fitting chairs to individual crips. Wheelchairs were the servants of cold war policy, like anything else in the Middle East. Israelis with the F-16 fighter jets in their air force had American Quickies, Quadras, and other ultralight-model chairs. The Arabs flew Soviet MIG's, and their wheelchairs came from eastern bloc industries which stamped out thousands of identical, marginally functional chairs in a single factory run.

Medical treatment was also different on either side of the green line. The rehabilitation organizations in the West Bank and Gaza would make it their business to send families the latest Arabic magazine articles on medical operations you could have performed in Jordan or Saudi Arabia, which claimed to restore a paralyzed person's ability to walk. The fathers and mothers who avidly followed these medical developments on behalf of their disabled children could be found in town after town throughout the occupied West Bank and Gaza. Their idea of rehabilitation was to pray for their child to walk again some day. Many would save thousands of dollars for the trip across the Allenby Bridge over the Jordan River to Arab hospitals to receive miracle treatments in Amman or the Gulf states.

Until the family prayers were answered, these disabled young people were on display to journalists and other visitors as martyrs, while a father or brother described the awful crimes of the Israelis that they said had caused the injury. They were the ornament of their family's collective sacrifice in the struggle against Israel, their physical independence postponed or lost in geopolitics.

Jutting out of the confusion of Jewish gravestones covering every square foot of the Mount of Olives sits the main Palestinian Hospital in Jerusalem. Mokassad Hospital is a five-story building at the summit of the Mount which casts its shadow each morning on graves that the Bible says are quietly awaiting the arrival of the Messiah. From its top floors to the west you can see the sun-baked whirlpool of religion and politics that is Jerusalem; the picture that has served as the frontispiece of history since before the Crusades stretches to the horizon. The walls of the old city, its prophetic gates, the valley of Gethsemane below, the domes of ancient mosques above covering the ruins of even more ancient Jewish shrines can be seen from Mokassad's many patient rooms. The busy people inside rarely have time to look out the window. In 1988, the hospital was the main trauma unit for casualties of the Intifada. In the center of the emergency room area was Dr. Dijani, a short, bald man with gray-green eyes and a tender face. I saw him a dozen or so times during my three years in Israel. Each time he was splattered with blood and iodine solution. Each time he was exhausted and shouting for family members to stay out of the operating room. When young people would start to give speeches and shout at the reporters gathered to cover the latest casualties, Dr. Dijani would break them up.

"Where did you get that chair, in Israel?" Dijani asked me, as though Israel was a suburb of faraway Kazakhstan rather than the place where he paid his taxes. He looked at my tires in the same way the Israelis did, but his questions were different. "Do those wheels move in the sand?" I assured him they did, but whatever kind of wheels you used, sand was still difficult. "We have only these old chairs you see here," he said. I asked him why the chairs were of such poor quality when so many of the spinal-cord-injured Palestinians were so young. He said that the good wheelchairs cost a lot. Parents were reluctant to spend money on a wheelchair for a son or daughter, he said, if they were praying to send them to Jordan for an operation to be cured. "What operation?" I asked.

"There is no such operation for spinal-cord injuries like these." In bullet wound cases the injury to the nerves is usually more decisive and localized than in the blunt trauma of auto crashes and other catastrophic accidents. "I know," he said, and shrugged. "But what can I tell them? They want a cure."

There was a whole corridor of such patients on the top floor of Mokassad Hospital. The dim halls of the building and its rattling elevator were as old as the rehabilitation hospital I had gone to in Michigan. The resemblance ended there. There was no physical therapy on this floor. Patients were warehoused. They were not pursuing some plodding, nightmarishly boring rehabilitation goal. My quadriplegic friend Roger would not have lasted long here. But he would have been able to sleep in for as long as he wanted. The patients were mostly medically stable, and were staying at Mokassad for different reasons. Some were waiting for a surgical procedure usually related to the intestines. Bullets were particularly fiendish to the abdomen. Concern over wheelchair skills and the building of compensatory muscles in the arms and shoulders would wait while patients learned if they would ever be able to eat normally again. Some of the patients stayed at Mokassad because there was simply no place for them in their home villages, often rugged communities built on the sides of rocky hills where it would be impossible to move. It was no better in the flat lands along the Mediterranean. Off the pavement in the Gaza Strip there was nothing but thick, dry, white, wheel-numbing sand. Some spinal-cord injured remained at Mokassad Hospital because their homes were in some of the worst, most crowded refugee camps. These places were so filthy it would literally be dangerous for someone with a urinary catheter to stay for any length of time.

On one bed a thin young man smoked cigarettes and talked and laughed with a crowd of other young men in the room with him. His name was Radwan. A nurse told me that he had been at Mokassad for some months. His parents, she said, wanted to send him to a hospital in Riyadh. "They have doctors from Houston there," she said. When I entered Radwan's room and said hello, our eyes locked.

My presence was puzzling at first. The young men in the room were wary and awkward until they learned that I was a reporter. A friend of Radwan's who spoke English began to tell me the story of Radwan and his injury, and the other young men in the room joined in. Radwan was nineteen years old and was injured at the Jebaliyah refugee camp, the largest camp in the Gaza Strip, the place where Palestinians liked to say the Intifada began. He had taken a gunshot from a soldier on the second day of the uprising in a giant chaotic demonstration in Gaza during which dozens of people were seriously injured or killed.

Radwan did not tell me these things. Radwan could not speak English back then, and I could not communicate at all in Arabic at the time, so we just stared at each other. Radwan's mind and my own were far away from the Intifada at that moment. Radwan had many questions. He had been lying in his bed for six months, hearing the stories of his injury told by others. As I listened, Radwan spoke less. His colleagues were giving the speeches. Radwan's little crumb of martyrdom belonged to the Palestinian nation. He watched it going by like a distant parade. I did not dispute those crimes. I did not doubt the lopsided exchange of a thrown rock for an Israeli bullet to the chest. But what did the Palestinian nation have now for Radwan?

Radwan's eyes looked up and down my chair while a young religious student named Abdel Hadi, who appeared to be his closest friend, gave an emotional speech about the bravery of his sacrifice in the fight against Israel. Down by the side of Radwan's bed was a bag of draining urine. Radwan was looking at my leg for such a bag. While his friends recounted the Intifada's glory I lifted my pants leg to show Radwan that I carried no bag. He looked astounded and pointed questioningly to his groin. I reached into my canvas backpack and pulled out my clear plastic catheter in its bottle of hydrogen peroxide. I pantomimed the four times daily task of removing the tube, inserting it, filling the dingy urine bottle, and then dumping it and putting everything away. Radwan smiled, he understood. I wanted to know how he got out of bed, so I pointed to him and then pointed to the junky looking wheelchair beside his bed. He nodded and said something to his friends. They immediately jumped into action, surrounding the bed to lift Radwan up and set him in the chair.

I waved them off and motioned for Radwan to pay attention. I lifted myself off my chair and onto the edge of his bed. Then, with an even swifter move I hopped back into the chair. I repeated the move more slowly. Radwan's intense interest crashed up against our language barriers. He raised his hands and tried to say something, then just sighed and laughed. He spoke to his friends and one of them translated. He said that Radwan was very interested in the moves I was making. I could see that without knowing Arabic. Radwan knew before I arrived that it was possible to move from chair to bed and back again independently. But watching me was the first moment he believed it was possible for such a move to be a trivial physical event, absent the risk of falling and profound humiliation. Radwan was quick, but he had never been encouraged.

His arms showed this lack of encouragement. He had, no doubt, been strong six months before, but in bed now he looked frail. He was thin and smoked heavily. I placed my hand around his biceps and showed him the rock-solid muscles around my arm. His friends bragged about the strength of their friend, but both Radwan and I could see that his arms were weak. I showed him some rudimentary wheelchair moves, wheelies and a midair turn. I transferred onto the plastic chair in his room and back into my own chair.

Wordlessly we communicated as I climbed down onto the floor. The religious student, Abdel Hadi, who was standing closest to Radwan and had his hand on Radwan's shoulder, abruptly jumped up and moved toward me as though I had fallen. "Mister, please, take your time. We can help you?" This time Radwan waved his friend with the worried look away, and watched from the bed as I pulled myself back into the chair with a quick two-arm lift. This move took me a long time to learn back in rehab, where I had never been very good at it. I was nervous as I tried it on the floor of Radwan's room. If I missed getting my backside up onto the chair the first time, Radwan's friends would not let me refuse their help the second time. I was proud to have nailed the two-arm-floor-to-wheelchair-lift on the first try, without losing my pants. I wished my physical therapist Donna could have seen me.

Radwan Abu Smaish had lived in Nusirat refugee camps in the Gaza Strip. Nusirat is in the middle of Gaza and is one of the smaller of the Gaza camps. Its residents became refugees in 1948 as waves of Arab residents fled south away from the population centers of Haifa, Jaffa, and Ashkelon. Today, you could not find a place on earth more densely populated with people who insist that their real homes are someplace other than the Gaza Strip. Of the Gaza refugee camps, Nusirat is among the most inaccessible. Its streets are unpaved. Deep white sand is everywhere.

The wheelchair in Radwan's room was lame, creaky, and primitive, with solid rubber wheels. Its vinyl maroon-colored upholstery was stretched and torn in places, making it impossible to sit straight in the chair. Its tall armrests were not removable, significantly complicating the business of transferring from chair to bed or from a vehicle to the chair. Its footrests were removable, but their mechanism for clamping on and off had worn away, and one footrest was stuck in place, while the other one was bent and jammed with black, oily dirt.

Radwan was the same age I was when I had my accident. His injury was from a bullet, but it was at the same level as mine. He was a T-5. His level of paralysis was identical to mine. In his case it was much more of a miracle that he was alive. A bullet entering the back at mid-chest level usually proceeds on to penetrate the heart or the aorta, causing virtually instant death. Radwan's original injury had surprisingly few complications. His complications came from lying in a hospital bed at Mokassad for months. If he had been in the U.S. he would have been up and around by this time. He also would not have had an in-dwelling urinary catheter. The fact that he had been fully catheterized for months meant that Radwan had probably lost the ability to function without one. It would greatly complicate Radwan's ability to survive in a place like Gaza, where sand and filth were impossible to avoid.

Radwan had no choice but to survive in Gaza, as it was his only home. The road he would have to take back to the Gaza Strip from Jerusalem was a difficult one. He would have to make it there without any organized rehabilitation. There would be no one around him who would give him encouragement to do anything but stay in his home and wait for Israel to disappear so that they could return to Haifa, or Jaffa, like the rest of the Gaza Strip had been doing for more than four decades. In the emasculated world of a refugee camp, Radwan would find few handholds.

Radwan had been engaged to be married. After his injury, he voluntarily ended the engagement. It was perceived as the manly thing to do. Radwan received more encouragement for unilaterally breaking his engagement than for getting a new wheelchair, or even getting up out of bed. He was one of the *shebab,* "the young men" of the uprising. He was on display. He was the PLO's version of Jerry's kids. "Radwan is one of the first of the *shebab* to take the Israeli bullet," Radwan's friend, Abdel Hadi, said, beginning another speech. "You have met one of the most famous *shebab* of the Intifada."

In Radwan's eyes was the question I had seen before in the face of my quadriplegic friend Roger: What will happen to me? I had no answer. But for Radwan it seemed as though there were ways of introducing him to a different way of thinking. He had some advantages. It was at least flat terrain in Gaza as long as you avoided the sand, and as a Palestinian, Radwan would never need to learn the shocking truth about Gumby, or have his lack of interest in tennis criticized by Dr. Avi. Radwan wanted to know more. He was no charity case. He was not a Jerry's kid. There were things I could tell him. I would see him again.

As I left to go, one of Radwan's friends asked me during what month of the Intifada I had been shot. "The Israelis shot you?" In the Palestinian teenage boy's concept of melodrama and martyrdom it would have been another historic chapter in the chronicle of the Intifada if a journalist had been shot by the Israelis. "I was not shot," I told them. "I am an American. I was injured long ago." They spoke in Arabic for a while, looking at each other, then back at me. After a moment one of them turned and said, "Then you are from the Vietnam War?"

For Radwan's existence as a paraplegic to make sense among his peers he would have to become a martyr for the PLO, for me to make sense to the Palestinian boys in Radwan's room I would have to become a Vietnam veteran. To elude such categories is the great adventure and the great tragedy of human life on earth. To leave the expected is to swim out into a void. You see the eyes watching you on the way out, and if you make it, you see them again on the way back. To elude the categories and expectations of his peers, Radwan had his work cut out for him. He would need a decent wheelchair, and importing a good one would cost double the selling price in Israeli import taxes. The same taxes would have been levied on my wheelchairs but for my special journalist work-visa exemption. I could help Radwan with wheelchair maintenance. My own paranoia about failing and flat tires in the Middle East meant that I had more than enough extra parts with me in Israel to make a complete wheelchair for him. The security people at the airport had been right to suspect me, not as a terrorist but, as it would later turn out, a wheelchair smuggler for Radwan.

Cheating

*F*acing the 1948 green line from the east, the old city is the poem of stones and tears that most embodies Jerusalem's past and present. It is predominantly Arab Muslims and Christians who live within its walls and among its domes. Its markets of livestock, produce, and dry goods are crowded and noisy. That virtually all of the young Palestinian men are wearing oversized homeboy stonewashed jeans and Ralph Lauren knockoff shirts cannot erase the feeling of antiquity here. Everything about the markets, from the hanging goat carcasses outside the meat shops to the trays of green pistachio confections dripping with honey, seems medieval. There are also a few stairs.

To enter the old city gates in a wheelchair is to go down a rabbit hole. Without warning, streets become staircases and tunnels. There are maps, but topography is not something anyone typically cares about in Jerusalem. There are thousand-year-old ramps inside Jerusalem's walls, but they are not for wheelchairs. They were made for the two-wheeled wooden pushcarts that have been a fixture for hauling goods around the inside of the city for centuries. They were strips of stone and masonry spaced wide apart on the stairs to match the width of the pushcarts' axles. They were of no use to a wheelchair, which fits perfectly between the ramps. I descended on two wheels, bouncing down one step at a time, knowing that there was no way back up the way I had come.

The two-wheeled descent in a chair is a spectacular attention getter. All the way from the Damascus gate to the bottom of the Bab el Wad, the road leading into the center of the city, each doorway filled with watchers. As I descended, details about who I was floated along the narrow streets. At the top of the hill I was a tourist. "Mister, would you like to see special holy land crafts?" One flight down and the pitch changed. "Where are you going? For a special price I can be your guide for the day?" He insisted, as did everyone who made the offer, that he knew every inch of the place. In broken Arabic I asked if he could show me the ramped areas of the old city. One by one, each would-be guide backed away with a befuddled look. I explained that I was a reporter visiting the city. A crowd gathered around me, and a group of little boys triumphantly escorted me past each shop. "Safahi al Koorsimutaharrak," they would shout in Arabic. "The Journalist of the Wheelchair" was how they boiled down my identity from the halting introductory conversations I had at each landing as I made my descent.

Three millennia after the advent of monotheism, and after countless parades of conquerors, governors, viziers, crusaders, and would-be messiahs, the people of the Damascus gate rolled it all out for the "Journalist of the Wheelchair's" arrival in Jerusalem. Heads poked from second- and third-story windows. People waved. The heads called down for an explanation. The boys shouted up to them, "The Journalist of the Wheelchair." I passed beneath Arab Christians and Muslims who all welcomed me with the enthusiasm of fulfilled prophecy. They were glad to see me. I was just looking for some wheelchair ramps. It was enough. I could not imagine that someone at some time had not scouted the old city for ramps, but here in the theater of Jerusalem it was as though the search for wheelchair ramps was one pilgrimage that had never before been attempted in this city of ancient pilgrimages.

In peace or war, in this century or in any of the last thirty, Jerusalem, Israel, and the occupied territories together constitute history's oldest and most popular theme park. There are rides for all ages, religions, and cultures. Frontier settlements and Iron Age villages, folk-singing Zionist outposts, shrines to Muslim empires past, Jewish ruins, military monuments, and all of the richly ornamented Christian sites dedicated to the assumption that Jesus slept here (we think). Or was it over here?

Without question, the Christian rides in Jerusalem are the most forgettable. They have the worst special effects, and are crowded with German pilgrims and TV evangelists wearing baggy shorts and clutching their Bibles. The Christian churches are, with few exceptions, showpieces, charitable works supported with money from the outside, having much more to do with a Christian experience in Europe than the Middle East. Most of the Christian landmarks are dormant shrines to old arguments between popes and Orthodox patriarchs and caliphs having little to do with the time or place where Jesus grew up and died. There are a handful of historically dubious places for Christian pilgrims. The dingy grottoes, tombs, and street corners where Jesus was thrown, dragged, bled, drank some vinegar, was condemned and then nailed to a post one spring day 2,000 years ago are mobbed with tourists and souvenir salesmen today.

The Church of the Holy Sepulchre itself is a sprawling trophy from the Byzantine Empire administered grumpily by representatives of the Catholic and Orthodox churches. Seventeen centuries ago they argued about whether Christ had three aspects or just one, whether he was poor or rich, whether he needed a spokesman or just a book. Today these same churches argue over who will repair the leaky roof over the place where an angel allegedly told the first Christians, "Seek ye not the living among the dead." It was the last time that advice was heeded.

The Christian sites cannot compare with the Dome of the Rock Mosque, where you can stand in line to view an actual hoofprint of Mohammed's horse on the rock inside where Mohammed ascended to heaven on his never-to-be-repeated night ride to Mecca, or the site of the old Jewish temple with the actual stones excavated to reveal places David hung out after dropping Goliath with a significantly smaller rock.

Muslims and Jews expected God to visit them, and they arranged their lives and prayers accordingly. With time-honored fatalism, followers of the Koran and the Torah presumed that among the reasons God spent so much time in Jerusalem was that there would always be plenty of Jews and Muslims there to irritate, torture, teach, or save. A rabbi and biblical scholar from the West Bank insisted to me that his presence in Israel had more to do with love of the land and history than with God. "I don't need to look for God. He knows where to find me," he said "God understands that we Jews will always be here. Maybe that's why he has spent so much time over the centuries kicking us out of this place."

Among the millions of pilgrims in Jerusalem, it was the Christians who came looking for God as if to confirm a juicy rumor they had heard. Christians have been trolling and casting for God since before the crucifixion. Just as Jesus found some sympathetic anglers right off the bat and convinced them to join the coming Christian hordes, Christians approach the question of finding God with the gusto of a fisherman working a trout stream. Each denomination has its own strategy for hooking the big one. Catholics go for the shiny lures with lots of ugly, dangling hooks. Protestants like live bait.

Shortly after my arrival in Jerusalem, I got a telephone call from someone who said cheerfully in unaccented American English, "Hi, John, it's your mother." I knew the voice, but it was not my mother's. If it had been any place other than Jerusalem I would have recognized it. But the last person I expected to hear from out of the blue like that was my born-again Christian, former mother-in-law, Hallie. Hallie had made it to Jerusalem before me by nearly a year. She was working for an evangelical group in the old city, where she lived a stone's throw from the Church of the Holy Sepulchre. Hallie and I were always the odd ones in the crowd of Alice's family. Looking at her happy, round face under a Jerusalem lemon tree, I felt that if anyone I knew would ever have come here to find me, it would have been Hallie.

She had come to Jerusalem because she was convinced that Christ was on his way back and saw my presence as further confirmation. "I expect that you are in Jerusalem to report on the big things that are happening here," she said confidently. "It is amazing, isn't it," I said. I told her I had heard that ABC's "Nightline" was going to be broadcasting from Jerusalem in a few weeks. Her face nodded as though everything I was saying confirmed some theory that she had. But when I began to tell her that I had already been quite busy reporting the daily violence of the uprising and the Israeli military's attempts to deal with chaos in the West Bank and the Gaza Strip, she looked puzzled. "You're here to cover that stuff," she said, as if the Palestinian uprising was nothing more than a dispute over a city zoning ordinance. To Hallie, steadfastly waiting for Jesus, that was precisely all it was. Jerusalem was like that. You could see whatever you wanted: whatever history, whatever news, whatever future.

When it was in their interest, each group in Jerusalem could be keenly aware of the rituals and rhythms of the other. During the early months of the Intifada there were two weekly rituals in Jerusalem guaranteed to make news. One was on the Christian day of worship and the other was on Friday, the Jewish Sabbath eve and Muslim Friday prayers. On Sunday mornings the Israeli government would hold its most important cabinet meeting of the week. It was an opportunity for the Israelis to reclaim control over the uprising story by timing government announcements for the slowest news day of the U.S. and European week. On Friday afternoon, while the Israeli government shut down for the Jewish holy day, regular Muslim prayers at the Al Aqsa mosque on the

Haram Esh Sherif were the week's other scheduled political headline event. The Palestinians would use this event to reclaim the attention of the West, and week to week throughout the spring and summer of 1988, back and forth it would go.

Haram Esh Sherif is Islam's "Noble Sanctuary," once the site of the ancient Jewish temple in Jerusalem. Upon the ground of Haram Esh Sharif, Muslims pray to the east and south where Mecca, the birthplace of Mohammed, lies. To the west the Jews gather at the remains of the temple's western wall to pray. For them this noble sanctuary is the Temple Mount or simply ha-Kotel: The Wall.

The religious sheiks who administer the Islamic shrines on the Haram forbid non-Muslims from entering the grounds of the Haram on Friday prayer days. According to some interpretations of Jewish law, Jews are forbidden to enter the Temple Mount at all, because they might stumble over the sacred (and misplaced) Ark of the Covenant (which they are not supposed to touch until the Messiah arrives). There are plenty of waivers and loopholes, so nothing prevents the occasional Jewish demonstration from parading around the Temple Mount calling for the bulldozing of the Islamic shrines. Likewise, Palestinians were happy enough to allow infidel reporters to witness any organized call for the destruction of Israel, so for the largest planned demonstrations Arabs would smuggle Westerners and their cameras into the area.

There is only one way to get from the Muslim quarter of Jerusalem to the Jewish quarter in the old city in a wheelchair. You roll into the Jaffa gate on the western side of the city. Past the shops and restaurants of the Citadel you make your way through the Armenian patriarchate houses with their archways and sunny porches. A road takes you to the southwestern corner of the city, where the road turns east and takes a steep downward descent toward the Jewish quarter. The road is so steep that, like the stairs at the Damascus gate, it is a one-way, down-only route. The speeding traffic alone is treacherous. The gloves holding back my wheels were hot from friction. I would remove my hands from my wheels to cool them every few moments, and the chair would surge forward from gravity's pull down the hill. Grabbing the wheels, the chair would slow once again and my gloves would heat up. In this lurching, clumsy way I made my way past the edge of the Armenian quarter, down past the religious institutes and apartments of yeshiva students that make up the Jewish neighborhoods overlooking the Temple Mount.

On the right, just outside the main wall, is the abandoned, excavated City of David, which makes the architecture of the functioning old city look modern. The white stones of the renovated Jewish quarter have been laid as they have always been in Jerusalem. Here the stones are new, all from construction begun since the 1967 Six-Day War; brilliantly they reflect the city's much fabled sunlight. Their sharply cut corners betray their young age.

Rolling down the hill, the Temple Mount comes spectacularly into view. The domes of Al Aqsa mosque and the Dome of the Rock monument protrude from the gentle, waving branches of trees planted in the wide-open spaces of the Haram. The walled-in sanctuary inside a walled city is glimpsed in mid-descent. As I roll forward, the Islamic domes sink down inside the Jewish walls built by King Herod. At the bottom of the hills, weaving around parked tour buses and police vans, I pass under a chain barrier and through a checkpoint and roll up the gentle grade toward the Western Wall. On the left, crowds of Orthodox boys stand around smoking, talking, and staring. On the right, tourists in brightly colored hats look from the stone buildings to their open guidebooks and scratch their heads. At the wall itself, hundreds separated by sex pray quietly. Near the wall, the harsh sounds of the city are muffled into the corner of old stone. It is a crowded, frenetic, and completely sacred place.

Through the arch at the southern corner of the Temple Wall, where the praying takes place, is a paved road leading into the Muslim quarter. It is the Wilson Arch, and around it elaborate archeological excavations have unearthed stones dating back to the first Jewish temple in 1000 B.C. The road was cut by Muslims in 1920 to allow easier passage from the Muslim quarter out of the city by way of the Dung gate on the city's southern approach. It was a calculated irritation to the Jews who prayed along the wall to find Muslims using it as a roadway for commerce.

For most of this century Muslims and Jews have fought over what could be done on this road. There have been riots and political crises over the placement of benches, the blowing of horns, the herding of livestock. This road is the one path with no stairs directly connecting the Muslim quarter with the Jewish. It is the way out of the city. The one wheelchair-accessible way to complete the circuit is to descend the steps at the Damascus gate, roll around to the Chain gate, reenter the city at the Jaffa gate, and come upon the Jewish quarter from the hill out of the Armenian Christian quarter. After 1967, the Wilson Arch road was closed, the Muslim prank concluded by the victorious Israeli army.

There is a door there now, and a locked iron gate. I asked to be allowed to go through. The Israeli guard laughed and said to go away. I said in an outraged voice that there were only stairs along the other passages. He shrugged. In Jerusalem doors are not functional. They are, like every other object in the city, symbolic. Their face value cannot be redeemed here on earth. The door remained shut. The guard ushered me away. There would never be an Americans with Disabilities Act dispute over wheelchairs on this little stretch of road.

The Western Wall lies at the base of three stone staircases. One long and very old one leads directly on to the Temple Mount through the Mugrabi gate. Another sharp, steep, new one leads back into the shops and residences of the Jewish quarter to the west, and the Muslim quarter to the north. The third leads up to the Israeli police station, where blue uniformed sentries monitor this tense confluence of history, culture, and religion.

Most reporters observed Friday prayers from the roof of the Israeli police station. On my first visit a giant, bald officer named Moshe carried me up to the top of the station on his back. I had rolled along toward the staircase with other reporters, knowing that at some point it would be just me and the stairs. I would have to come up with a way of getting up the stairs or turn back. Each Friday, and many other times during the week, when violence brought the media to a police security barrier, Moshe would face the grumpy press corps. The reporters would make their demands and try jumping police lines and Moshe would stare them down, shout them down, or throw them back over the line in a classic display of Israeli bluster. These confrontations would usually end with Moshe screaming and red-faced and the reporters yelling back every word and phrase they were not permitted to print back home.

It was my first encounter with Moshe and his gallery of media contrarians, and I was back in the crowd worried about running over people's feet and trying to keep from being left behind. With tension high in the city, and with a dangerous demonstration expected where civilians might be injured or killed, Israeli soldiers would be at their most aggressive. I feared the embarrassment of being in the way, although exactly how I might be *in the way* of two groups bent on killing and maiming each other was unclear. I was all ready to turn back and try to recruit some reluctant reporters to haul me up the stairs, when Moshe, seeing an opportunity to further infuriate the press corps said, "I will take you up." He motioned for two of his junior officers to lift me onto his back and to carry my chair up the steps. The rest of the press corps were told to wait below. Reporters who had awkwardly tried not to notice my predicament suddenly insisted that they were my friends and colleagues and had to be permitted up on the roof. Moshe laughed and ordered his guards to block the way behind him as he proceeded to carry me, like a banner of righteousness, up to the police post which looked directly down onto the plaza in front of Al Aqsa mosque.

Thousands of Palestinian worshipers had already gathered in front of the mosque. The prayers proceeded peacefully until just before the end of the customary short speech by the sheik. A demonstration by women calling for "Death to Israel" and an "End to the Occupation" began the confrontation. A crowd of young men then appeared and, as if on cue, the Israeli police and the young Palestinian boys began to battle. The Israelis used their rifles and tear gas while the young men threw rocks. The chaos continued until a squad of soldiers stormed the Temple Mount and a number of arrests were made. The Palestinian casualties were carried out to ambulances waiting to take them to Mokassad Hospital and Dr. Dijani.

In just a few moments, the quiet reverie of prayer under the broad oak and cedar trees on the Temple Mount had dissolved into chaos, obscenities, tear gas, and death. What was horrible about this demonstration and all of the ones I witnessed after that was how all of the fights between Israeli soldiers and Palestinians seemed to have a script. There was none of the random violence of war in the Intifada. It was a game of skill and wit, equal parts prank for a lazy afternoon and revenge killing. The fight between the Palestinians and the Israelis had all been worked out so very long ago.

Once in the Gaza Strip, surrounded by a crowd of Palestinian children and mothers, an Israeli armored truck rumbled up the street. In a flash, the crowd vanished into the narrow labyrinth of the adjacent refugee camp. I was stuck there in the sand holding a microphone, staring at the barrel end of a truck full of Israeli soldiers. The soldiers sighted me through their assault rifles as their truck drove around a corner. They didn't fire. I was in no danger. The Israelis and Palestinians were set on killing each other. Under the Intifada's rules, there was no score for hitting me, no way for an American in a wheelchair to be in the way of its injuries and death.

Slowly, the old men and women worshipers on the Temple Mount coughed the stinging tear gas out of their lungs and regained the strength to walk back through the old city to their homes. Moshe allowed the rest of the reporters to see the end of the riot. They rushed to learn the details, casualties and the number of arrests, like baseball fans arriving late to the game. Two people were reported to have died in this demonstration. More than two dozen were taken away by the police. The news story sent back to NPR consisted of those casualty numbers, the sound of guns popping on my tape recorder, and the detail that ". . . this was the first time Israeli police had stormed the Temple Mount since the beginning of the Intifada."

This demonstration on the Temple Mount was immediately overtaken by far more prominent and bloody milestones of the Palestinian uprising's first two years. I never forgot the trip up the stairs on Moshe's back. His interest in helping me that day created problems for me with the press corps after that because they concluded that I was somehow beholden to the cops, like a teacher's pet or team mascot. I never went to the old city police station to watch Friday Muslim prayers again, but every time I encountered Moshe at other stakeouts and violent news events I could count on him to push me to the front of the line and to make a big point of letting me into places, and just as big a point of refusing others.

Palestinians who observed this, when they weren't suspecting me of being an Israeli collaborator, were impressed by what they assumed was my strategy for outwitting my colleagues and the Israelis. Israelis also thought the wheelchair was a clever gimmick. Some members of the press corps resented this as a new way to be stiffed by the Israelis. I alone felt guilty. Even though all I was doing was showing up, being pushed to the front of the line made me feel like some international affirmative action case. Being left behind because I couldn't walk made me want to apologize to my editors back in Washington, while getting this royal wheelchair treatment from the Israeli police made me want to apologize to everyone in the press corps. Succeeding on the merits of reporting skills alone seemed impossible.

It is very American to make these ironclad distinctions between the individual merit of a person and opportunities for advancement that have to do with family connections, wealth, wheelchairs, race, and other intangibles. Palestinians and Israelis would declare how impressed they were that I had found a way to turn something as obviously humiliating as a wheelchair to my advantage. It was just this impression that, as an American, I found humiliating. In America the primary virtue is in doing something "despite the wheelchair," or "even though you are black or a woman." Succeed by incorporating what makes you different into your goal and you are perceived as having cheated. Success that feels like failure. It is a feeling that runs quite deep in the American psyche, as I had the occasion to learn a few months after my arrival.

I had met a West Bank settler who seemed to know more about what was going on in the extreme right wing of the Israeli settlement movement than the average homeowner/gunowner you might encounter there. His job was to drive people around and show them the West Bank's many biblical/historical sights. His name was Yehuda, and he had a contract with some of the Israeli nationalist foundations, which were nearly always based in the United States, Canada, or Europe, and which funded settlements in the occupied territories. Yehuda was often the VIP tour guide for potential benefactors who came through the West Bank. He was very skilled in finding just those roads which best illustrated the myth that Jews were occupying a land that was mostly empty. On Yehuda's tours you would overlook breathtaking valleys and canyons that contained a few Jewish settlements, which he described as "outposts of a prophetic return to an ancient land." The roads Yehuda avoided led directly through the teeming urban markets of the impoverished Palestinian cities and villages along the Nablus road. He called the Arab roads "shortcuts" which he wouldn't hesitate to take if he was in a hurry and had his M-16 rifle with him. The Palestinian uprising did not concern him, and Yehuda was angry at the Israeli government for being so upset about it. "The Arabs know how easy it is to get Jews to feel guilty," he said. "They just throw a few stones."

In spite of his politics, Yehuda and I hit it off. He knew quite a lot besides biblical history. I wanted to talk to him about any people he might know who were buying up land in the old city of Jerusalem. The extreme right wing of the settlement movement was attempting to use large amounts of outside money and a sympathetic Israeli court system to coerce the sale of land by Arabs near the Temple Mount. This had been going on for quite some time, but now there was evidence that a well-financed effort planned to build a so-called Third Temple on the site of where the last two had been torn down nearly two thousand years ago, and where Arab Muslim shrines have stood for more than ten centuries.

It was a ridiculous idea in practice. The Israeli government was not about to start a war with the Islamic world over some scheme to build a Third Temple, but the existence of a fringe group dedicated to this goal was highly inflammatory at a time of serious unrest in Jerusalem. It was an important story, and I thought Yehuda might know some of the people involved. I had broached the subject with him before, and although he liked me, he was deeply suspicious of the media and wasn't talking.

I decided to accept an invitation to have lunch at Yehuda's house in the settlement of Beit El, where I suspected he might feel more comfortable being candid than behind the wheel of his tour bus. I had been in Jerusalem for a few months, staying at the American Colony Hotel, each night eating its food. I was happy for the opportunity to eat a real home-cooked meal.

Once, in the rehab hospital back in 1976, a doctor offered the following in response to a question I had about how my newly paralyzed body was going to function: "If we ripped your large intestine out of you and placed it in a dish it would just continue working all by itself." This was supposed to make me feel better about my bodily functions. Instead, for more than a decade I had feared that deep inside my body a time bomb was ticking. Total loss of intestinal control without warning was my own personal doomsday scenario, the kind of event after which life itself hardly seemed possible. In the nuclear winter of this total physical humiliation I imagined I would wander the earth confused and dazed, begging for clean laundry until my early death.

In my years as a paraplegic this scenario had never even come close to happening. But eating hotel food for weeks on end in a place halfway around the world would test my more than decade-old notion of intestinal control. The abstract fear of this doomsday scenario had to be balanced against the very real fear of missing a story. In the beginning, I was afraid to say no to anything: There was no deadline I wouldn't meet, no stairway I wouldn't be carried up, no elevator too small for me to get out of my chair and slide into, no terrain too daunting to avoid if there was news. Proceeding, even though my body might be on shaky ground, was the only option in the competitive pressure cooker of the Middle East press corps.

Lunch started out simply enough. Yehuda's house was large and of a stone and masonry design that he said was an Arab style. Yehuda was not fond of the cheap, homogeneous socialist architecture of Tel Aviv, a city I was surprised to learn that he would happily push, along with its square blocks of apartments, commercial sprawl, and uninspired houses, into the Mediterranean. Yehuda's house had a spectacular view of the canyon surrounding Beit El, where in Genesis it says that Abraham, the patriarch of Judaism, built an altar to God after passing through Shechem, the city that Arabs call Nablus.

We sat in the living room and spoke of the Old Testament. I was in one of Yehuda's reclining sofa chairs, having transferred out of my wheelchair. Confidence and professionalism was what I wanted him to see in me. We ate olives for more than an hour. We must have consumed nearly three dozen. Yehuda was speaking to me intently about how each trip to the synagogue for a Jew was a ritual moment of the long-lost temple of Jerusalem that Jews mourned along with their beloved land of Israel.

I felt a curious little wave of sensation down in the fog of my body's numbness. I shifted in Yehuda's living room chair and casually reached back to tuck my shirt into the back of my pants and discovered that my doomsday scenario was well along, in the worst possible way, and getting worse by the second. I never expected that I would come face-to-face with the abyss in a Naugahyde recliner in a living room overlooking the cradle of Judeo-Christian civilization. The very fabric of reality seemed to have torn, and blowing through it was some cold galactic wind.

In this moment, Yehuda's face appeared to be at the end of a long tunnel. I could see his lips moving, but I couldn't hear his voice. He didn't know that everything had changed. Only I knew that. Soon all discussion of Jewish theology would be forgotten. I imagined that the chair I was sitting in would have to be hauled outside in the yard and doused with gasoline for a bonfire. Perhaps the Talmud had a commentary on this situation, that I had rendered his entire Orthodox household non-Kosher and it would have to be burned along with the chair. Would Yehuda and his family have to move? Maybe they could just throw me over the side of the cliff in flames, where I couldn't harm anyone else's furniture. I sat in the recliner thinking of ways to end my life. If I never moved from that spot, I wondered if life could go on forever with Yehuda endlessly discussing the Old Testament, and me with the same dumb smile frozen for eternity on my face.

At first Yehuda did not seem to like having his commentary on Isaiah interrupted, then when he understood what had happened, he snapped his household into action. A bunch of little boys appeared, carrying newspapers, towels, and buckets. Yehuda was the general at the head of a parade of forelocks, little yarmulkes, and plastic garbage bags. Yehuda's wife handed me a thermos of what she said was her family's reliable antidote for inclement intestines. In a few minutes I was in Yehuda's van headed back to the hotel. My nightmare had become just another adventure. Even though I felt pretty awful, there was something liberating about having the darkest imagined fear of your existence, quite literally, hosed off as harmless reality.

The idea that humiliation is some capital crime of the spirit is a fiction. The sentences we hand down for losing control and succumbing to physical limits in life are arbitrary acts of self-loathing. All human beings have bodies that define their existence and which can veto the best-laid plans of the mind and soul. We are taught to view our physical life as the edicts from some committee of biological saboteurs who were once our allies in youth, but as we age or physically change, only conspire to depose the mind from its throne as President for Life.

Physical limits are a natural binding force in society, bringing people together. The arrogance of presuming that physical limits are somehow in opposition to life and to be hidden away is tragic. When people succeed "despite their physical limitations," just as when crips "have the courage to go on despite their disability," they are celebrated by the group. But when people's physical limits become obvious, they expect to be shunned and left to their solitary self-hatred. It should be just the other way around. Separating oneself through personal triumph over some physical limitation is an act of isolation that repudiates the influences of family and community; openly acknowledging limitations binds and draws people together, as an emblem and reminder of just how similar we all are.

My mind had told me that there would be no way to survive the humiliation of my body's very public loss of control. Reality was quite different. My tragedy was simply one of the household chores that day at Yehuda's house on the West Bank. I presumed that I would need a brain transplant; Yehuda proved that all I needed were some towels and a mop. I smiled out the window on the trip home. Yehuda and I were friends now. "I can tell that you are not a Jew," Yehuda said to me as he dropped me off at the hotel. "It takes a lot for you to feel guilty, more than throwing some stones." Yehuda said he would call me sometime.

The next day Yehuda gave me the names of people he said it would be very interesting for me to talk to. They were all members of the Third Temple movement he had convinced to speak with me. My story about the preparations for the building of a Third Jewish Temple and the Israeli government's concern about unrest in the old city was small but it was well ahead of the major U.S. papers. Now I did feel guilty. None of the other reporters had used their intestines to gain access to the Israeli ultranationalist inner circle as I had with Yehuda. I had an unfair advantage because of my disability. I had rolled in front of the line, used one of the handicapped parking spaces, paid for lunch with food stamps. I had used my wheelchair as a crutch, my father might say. I had cheated.

After enough experiences with the chair in this new place I discovered that having a disability offered an advantage in seeing some of the more subtle differences and similarities between Arabs and Jews. There were vast differences in how Palestinians and Israelis reacted to disability. The simplest tasks were rich with cultural commentary. Far from disabling me, being in a wheelchair allowed me to discover deep truths about Arabs and Jews much more quickly than from the sole vantage point of a journalist outsider. Those truths were not news, but they did allow me to acquire a familiarity with both Israelis and Palestinians that I never imagined achieving when I first arrived.

For example, among Palestinians it was risky to roll too near a doorway or a set of stairs. A crowd would soon gather, and I would be carried to the top of the stairs whether I wanted to go there or not. Often, if I said I did not want to go to the top of the stairs, the assumption would be that I was too shy to actually ask. "No, thank you," was not nearly emphatic enough to keep from being lifted.

Among Israelis there was no danger of being lifted up unexpectedly. That's not to say that Israelis were callous and uncaring, just a bit brusque like Moshe, the police lieutenant. An Israeli encountering a man in a wheelchair at the bottom of some stairs would more than likely shout up to the top, "Hey, Itzik, there's a crippled guy down here." Then he might ask if you wanted to speak with someone up above. There was a bookstore in downtown Jerusalem that I would visit regularly to buy English magazines to keep up with news outside the Middle East. One day I asked the owner to pass something down to me from one of the upper shelves. He was happy to do it, but added, "What you need is a grabber like my cousin has. Where is your grabber?" Israelis would love to tell you about the one relative or friend they knew in a wheelchair, and all about their various grabbers and gadgets.

My favorite gadget story involved renting cars. I could rent from Israelis who did a brisk business all over the country supplying cars to tourists, or I could rent from Palestinians who operated a couple of rental agencies on the road to Ramallah north of Jerusalem. I tried the Israelis first. At the major dealer in Jerusalem nearest my hotel I asked to rent a medium-sized vehicle. "But you can't use the pedals. How are you going to drive?" The manager of the office came out from behind a tall counter. I showed him my valid American driver's license. He turned it over and said, "Look, you still can't use your feet. Didn't the army give you a car?" He assumed that I was an American Jew with Israeli citizenship who would indeed, if disabled, be eligible for a government-subsidized, specially equipped car.

I told him that I had no interest in renting a car I could not drive. I said I wanted to rent a car equipped with hand controls. I told him that I was not an Israeli citizen and needed the car for my work as a reporter. "How are you going to put the chair in the trunk?" he asked with a jolly, unflappable skepticism. "I put it in the backseat." "How will you stop without your feet?" he asked. "How will you go?" He acted as though I were trying to pull a fast one of some kind. "Look," I said, "if you put hand controls on one of your cars, I will be able to drive it. If I can drive it, you can rent it. If you rent it to me, I will give you money. So there you go." He paused to think about this.

It is possible in the United States to rent a vehicle equipped with hand controls from any of the major rental car companies. This was not always the case, but today if you find an experienced enough dealer you can even rent hand controls on demand on the same day, although most places require some kind of crip advance notice. The controls are bolted onto the steering shaft and then removed by mechanics at the rental agency so that the car can be rented without controls for other drivers.

In Israel the demand for hand-control rental cars was nonexistent in 1988. I was expecting my request to be unusual but not impossible, since there were plenty of disabled people in Israel. The rental manager said that he would check into it and call me back. I had hoped to rent a car that day, but I was familiar enough by this time with how things were done in Israel that I was not surprised by the wait.

When he called back, his plan was to rent me a car at the top rate, equipped with hand controls that would be specially installed just for me. "For the controls it will cost sixteen hundred shekels. I can buy them from two guys from the army, Ehud and Itzik from Haifa." This was about eight hundred dollars, which was way over my NPR allowance. "What do you mean, this will cost sixteen hundred shekels?" He said the controls would be permanently installed, and that I could have them for my own when I was done. "But what if I don't want to buy a pair of hand controls for eight hundred dollars?" I asked, knowing even the most expensive controls in the U.S. cost about two hundred fifty dollars, maximum. "You have to have them. How can you drive? You can't move your feet."

"I know I need the controls. I asked for them. I just don't want to buy these. I'll rent them, but when I give you back the car, you keep them." He exploded. "That's ridiculous! I can use my feet." The discussion quickly became about why I was trying to force a nondisabled person to buy a set of hand controls that he obviously didn't need. This was an unexpected turn. I did discover that in Israel hand controls were either on or off a vehicle. There was no bolt-on, bolt-off option as in the States. When I looked at the Israeli design I could see that they were quite permanent. I was told that all of the Israeli hand controls were manufactured by two crips who lived in Haifa and built hand controls to the specifications of the Israeli army. Everyone went to see Itzik and Ehud.

I proposed an alternative that took into account my special circumstances as a disabled foreign reporter who did not own his own vehicle. I suggested that I purchase one of the many U.S.-manufactured models of bolt-on hand controls. I would bring them to the rental agency. I would install them and remove them when I was finished with the car. I would keep the controls to use on other cars I would rent. Since they could be used by me in any car, they would be worth buying. They also cost about forty dollars, compared with the eight hundred dollars in Israel for a one-time-only design. Since they did not require major mechanical work to install, they wouldn't tie up one of his vehicles just for me.

It seemed like the perfect solution, but as I explained it, he just kept shaking his head. "What about the insurance?" He said that for me to use the U.S.-manufactured controls I would need a permit to use them in Israel. "Fine," I said. "Get the permit. I'll get the controls." He said he would call me.

When he called back he seemed very excited. "I found the permit. We can rent you a car as soon as you get these hand controls from the States." I said that I would get the controls the following week. He explained that all I needed to do then was to install the controls and have them inspected for the permit. "Where do I do that?" I asked. "You go to Haifa and speak with Ehud or Itzik. They will look at everything and you can buy your permit from them the same day." With Ehud and Itzik involved again, the nature of this scam was beginning to dawn on me "How much is the permit?" I suspected that I could make a wild guess and be very close. He rustled some papers over the phone and said, "Yes, I have it right here. Ehud and Itzik said that it would be no problem." The insurance permit would cost about sixteen hundred shekels.

"Right. I pay forty bucks for the hand controls and the permit costs eight hundred dollars." The rental manager thought that this was perfectly normal and even acted a little exasperated that I would suggest such a crazy roundabout way of getting this done. "It would be easier, I think, to just buy the hand controls, like I told you the first time. It costs about the same. You would be saving forty bucks, I think." That was the end of that. "Isn't it funny how it works out that way," I said to him. "This is Israel," he said back. I told him thank you and hung up. I received the hand controls from the States the following week and even went to another Israeli agency where no one knew me. The response was familiar. "But you can't use the pedals." The manager said from the counter, shaking his head. "How will you drive?"

As a last resort I went to one of the Palestinian rental companies. I wasn't expecting much. My request of the Palestinian agency would be at least as unusual as it had been for the Israelis. Certainly, the same rules applied under Israeli law. Salim greeted me at the door of the agency. I had rolled to the office, which was just up the road from my hotel in East Jerusalem. There was sweat on my brow. It was a hot day.

Salim was eager to push me away from the road. I told him that everything was fine. I rolled into his office. "Would you like some coffee . . . some tea?" He snapped his fingers and a group of boys appeared with wooden stools for sitting and a table for cups and saucers. I was so convinced of the futility of this pursuit that I didn't even bring the hand controls with me. I explained that I was a journalist and an American and that I wished to rent a vehicle. Salim stood up and rushed into his office as he barked more commands to the boys, who swirled around with cups of tea and plates of cookies.

I assumed that he was calling Abdul and Omar, the Palestinian equivalents of Ehud and Itzik. But when Salim returned, he had a standard contract for car rental. He wanted to see my license and to know what kind of car I preferred. I told him. He handed me the papers and said that I could pay at the end of each week. He showed me the daily rate, suggested a place where I could get cheap fuel, and pointed to the place on the contract where I would sign.

I was a little confused. That this transaction would be simpler in a place under Israeli occupation compared with Israel itself didn't make any sense. "Don't you want to see me drive or anything? I can't move my feet, you know." Salim looked horrified, and as he translated the remarks for the others present they also looked dismayed. An old man came forward and said, "There is no problem, Mr. John." Salim told me that he and his entire family wanted me to know that they wouldn't think of questioning my ability to drive and that if I thought they were questioning me, then they were very sorry. He offered to reduce the rental rate as compensation for the misunderstanding. I told him that there was no misunderstanding, but that I wanted him to know that I planned to put some metal hand controls in the rental car so that I could work the pedals.

The older man now began to speak sharply to Salim. He was Salim's father, and he had gotten the impression that his son was badgering me. Salim looked even more horrified and said, "No problem, Mr. John, we are sorry that our cars are not quite right for you." Again he offered to reduce the rental rate, and as his father barked at him in Arabic, Salim said that one of his brothers would drive me around anywhere I wanted to go if I did not want to use the hand controls.

At this rate I would end up with a free fleet of cars and a staff of drivers. I thanked Salim and said that I would be happy to pay the original rental rate, which was half of the Israeli rate, with no special charge for Ehud and Itzik. My only hardship here at Salim's agency was having to eat a full-course dinner of chicken and rice. Salim's father insisted that I be his guest to allow him to make amends for his rude son. As the chicken was served, one of Salim's brothers handed me the keys to a mid-sized Subaru. In broken English he asked, "You are journalist?" I said yes. The young man tiptoed forward and I could see that he was about to ask a question. His friends stood behind him. They were quiet and in a state of some suspense that I recognized. They were waiting, like my brothers and I would in the presence of my grandfather, waiting to see if he would actually tie his shoe with his good arm.

The young man stated the question on everyone's mind. All eyes were on me. "You were shot by Israeli soldiers?" This little committee of the nation of Palestine sitting around a table of chicken and rice in a little town on the West Bank stared, silently waiting for my answer. "No," I said. It was something of a disappointment. I rented cars from Salim for the next two years. It was the last time Salim's family ever mentioned the fact that I couldn't walk.

The surprise about working in the Middle East was just how much easier it was in so many ways than living in America. In America access is always about architecture and never about human beings. Among Israelis and Palestinians, access was rarely about anything but people. While in the U.S. a wheelchair stands out as an explicitly separate experience from the mainstream, in the Israel and Arab worlds it is just another thing that can go wrong in a place where things go wrong all the time.

It would be wrong to conclude too much about any nation solely from its approach to one man in a wheelchair, although in the history of anthropology it is undoubtedly the case that much more has been concluded about whole races on the basis of far less information. In the Middle East, day-to-day life was close to the experience of living in a wheelchair. This was not to say that being in the Third World was a crippling injury; rather, it was to go through life with the presumption that things were not going to go your way, an experience relatively rare in America and the industrialized world, but extremely common almost everywhere else. Whether it was taxes, the weather, a war, neighbors, or the infrastructure, no one in the Third World expected such things to go well. This presumption of physical adversity was widespread among Israelis and Palestinians faced with their relentless conflicts. The belief that around the next corner there was going to be some obstacle fit well into my own sense of the world acquired from a wheelchair.

Americans expect things to work. It is one of the consequences of being a superpower. Disabled people expect things not to work whether they are Americans or not. In Israel and the occupied territories I shared no language or religion with the people I met. To my surprise, I discovered that we shared a world view that had always isolated me in the United States.

Once, long after returning from the Middle East, I asked a manager of a Broadway theater in New York City to help me up a set of stairs to the seat I had paid sixty dollars for at the box office. He looked shocked and told me to leave. If I hadn't brought some attendant to help me up stairs, I could not attend the show. "We're not allowed to touch you, sir. We're not allowed to do that," he said angrily. No amount of insisting that it was possible for me to be carried up the stairs, or to haul myself up and have an usher carry my chair would convince him to let me into that show. I missed it. I sued the theater. More than eighteen months later, after a judge ordered it, the theater had a lift for wheelchairs, but the show, *Jelly's Last Jam* (about racism and how a light-skinned black tried to pass for white in American show business), had closed long before. This is how things are done in America. In the Middle East, among Arabs or Jews, I would have encountered more steps and fewer lawyers, judges and wheelchair lifts, but I have no doubt that in Jerusalem I would have seen the show.

Footnotes and
Checkpoints

*I*n November 1988 a small historic landmark came and went for the Palestinians. In Algiers, before a meeting of the PLO's National Council, PLO Chairman Yasir Arafat declared the nation of Palestine independent. Arafat was a ceremonial leader of a ceremonial government in exile ruling over a fictitious national entity located in an all-too-real spot on the globe: Israel and the occupied territories. Declaring independence was one of those events intended to transform Arafat and the PLO into global villagers from their perennial role as Israel's Most Wanted. Branded as ruthless Arab villains and the world's most cinematic bad guys, by declaring their own state in the community of nations Arafat and company hoped they might be seen as Third World visionaries seeking planetary peace. Instead, they looked more like participants at a grumpy family reunion, with feuding clans bickering and threatening to blow each other up over how to share a long-lost trust fund called Palestine. The Algiers meeting was televised throughout Israel, the West Bank, and Gaza. It was watched by Palestinians, Israelis, and hundreds of journalists; I watched from a living room in the Gaza Strip.

The Israeli army had closed Gaza to any traffic and had placed a curfew on its six hundred thousand residents. They had done the same over most of the West Bank. For four days, the duration of the Algiers conference, it was all to be a "closed military area," an Israeli spokesman explained. Reporters would be banned from the occupied territories. The Israelis did not want any news coverage of reaction to the declaration of an independent State of Palestine from the place where that state was supposed to be. On its first "Fourth of July Weekend," the territory of Palestine would look about as independent as cold war East Berlin, with armed guards, armored vehicles, and closed borders. Ironically, Berlin would be free of Soviet occupation within the year, while for Gaza it would take nearly six years for anything to change.

To get into Gaza's closed military zone, I had smuggled myself past the Israeli army that morning in an Arab taxi with a wheelchair strapped on top of the car, as camouflage. At Erez, the main military checkpoint between Israel and the Gaza Strip, the driver explained that I was just a poor cripple coming from an Arab hospital in Jerusalem bound for home in Gaza before the curfew. The soldiers didn't even look to see the man with the blond hair asleep in the backseat of the taxi.

My pragmatism about the wheelchair made sense. There were precious few advantages to be had as NPR's correspondent; I might as well use this one, especially since there appeared to be no reward for waiting patiently in the Middle East. The chair could get me into places others would be barred from even as it made my visibility greater. I was far better known than other journalists who had spent the same amount of time working in Gaza.

This higher profile meant that I had found many important friends quickly. When I suggested to Taher Shreiteh, a Gaza stringer who worked for many news agencies and was a longtime friend of CBS correspondent Bob Simon, that I wanted to find a place to stay in Gaza under curfew during the Algiers conference and the expected independence declaration, Taher and his brothers happily insisted that I stay with them.

The day before Arafat's speech in Algiers we sat around Taher's house off Mugrabi Street in Gaza City watching television, playing backgammon, and waiting for the sun to go down. Every household had a stash of fireworks for celebrating Arafat's expected announcement. The decorations were to be strung through the neighborhood after dark, this being the only way to elude Israeli patrols, and though his address was scheduled for early evening, no one expected the PLO chairman to say anything worth celebrating much before two in the morning. Every Palestinian (and every journalist who has ever had an appointment with him) understood that Yasir Arafat never did anything on time.

It did not much matter that this event was to be very long on symbolism and very short on substance for the people in the occupied territories. For Taher's neighborhood in Gaza it was an excuse to have a rousing good party, dream about the future, and piss off the Israelis. Some people would die and others would be injured, but to hear a declaration of independence broadcast live and see the red glare of a few Egyptian bottle rockets was worth a demonstration and a whiff of tear gas, even if morning came with the same political hangover Gaza had been experiencing since Israel's first independence day back in 1948.

Taher had been given an expensive miniature video camera by CBS News for recording the historic celebrations. Since all network crews were banned from the territories, Taher would get the pictures for the "Evening News." I would conduct radio interviews, record the sound of the celebrations, and then on the morning of the day of the independence declaration I would smuggle myself back out of Gaza with Taher's CBS videotape, meet a waiting CBS car to whisk me to the Tel Aviv bureau to drop off the pictures, then go home to Jerusalem to file my own stories for NPR. I had no idea how I was going to get out of Gaza under curfew, or even move around, with Israeli military patrols everywhere. The humanitarian agencies had already made it clear that they would obey Israeli rules and not give journalists any unauthorized rides.

I thought at first that I might be stuck in one house for the whole weekend and have no story except how much money I had lost playing backgammon with Taher's brothers. For the trip to Gaza to be worth anything I would have to move around Gaza City. The streets were not completely deserted. Like all Israeli restrictions, there was a certain looseness to this curfew. Old men and women with pots of rice and beans on their heads could apparently move unimpeded. But no vehicles were allowed to move, and adult Palestinian men were strictly confined to their houses. It was understood that anyone found on the street shooting videotape would be arrested, and any foreign journalists would have their credentials pulled, or worse. But the rest of the curfew seemed to be only haphazardly enforced.

I set off from Taher's house for the United Nations Refugee Agency, UNRWA. I would go to Shiffa Hospital on the other side of town to check on casualties. Finally, I would visit the Marna House hotel in the rich Gaza City neighborhood of Rimal. Alya Shaawa, who ran the hotel, was always good for some stimulating conversation, a decent sandwich, and she served the best cup of coffee to be had between Tel Aviv and Cairo.

I began by sneaking along the backstreets and smelly alleys, avoiding the well-paved main roads where Gaza's level topography made rolling a breeze. Gaza's main intersections were blocked with burning tires and debris, and boys in ski masks were busy painting graffiti on the walls. I rolled by one intersection and no one even noticed me. An Israeli patrol suddenly turned the corner, and while the masked boys vanished, I could do nothing but sit there and watch them pass by. I got no notice from the soldiers, either. With their rifles at the ready, they hauled barricades out of the road and doused burning tires, and then drove on. They looked right through me. As one patrol stopped to put out a fire, I pulled out a microphone and began recording. Still, no one noticed. I felt like a ghost.

Under curfew, Gaza's street life moves to its rooftops. Planks laid from roof to roof form an alternate street map for moving around the city and refugee camps out of sight and range of Israeli patrols. As I rolled through the neighborhood, the people on the rooftops watched me and called ahead to the next block to let them know I was coming. As I came around each corner, I could hear the whispering from above. *Sahafi Koorsimutaharrik,* "Journalist in the Wheelchair." After a few blocks I was rolling without any fear of being stopped, either by soldiers or the Palestinian boys with their masks and gasoline bombs. Down on the streets, among the combatants, I was as invisible as the old men pulling their donkey carts, part of Gaza's wallpaper, but from the roofs of Gaza I was something new to watch.

The rooftop network had notified the United Nations that I was coming long before I arrived. When I rolled up to the door of the UN compound it opened and I was whisked in. The Palestinian workers thought it was an act of bravery to have come through the streets in broad daylight in a wheelchair. I couldn't convey how easy it had been. Each time I tried to say that the reason I had no fear of being stopped was because no one was paying any attention to me, the workers applauded. "You are speaking with great courage," one of the doctors said. It was the same at Shiffa Hospital, where my arrival was applauded in the halls. The young male patients in their filthy hospital wheelchairs gathered around to inspect my chair and tape recorder while the doctors asked me what I had seen on the streets.

I arrived at the Marna House hotel, and Alia greeted me at the gate. "We knew that you would come. The boys called from the roofs to say that you were defying the curfew." She turned to one of her guests, an academic type working on a project who'd been stranded in Gaza by the Israeli restrictions. "He is one of our bravest journalists," Alia said, as if describing one of her own sons.

The fact that I was out in the open at all was its own marvel to the Palestinians that weekend. Although there were many Gazans in wheelchairs from auto accidents and the daily confrontations with Israeli bullets, the crips from Gaza did not show themselves except to occasionally beg in the market. It was an unwritten rule, a line everyone agreed not to cross, a barrier of shame that was as invisible to me as I was to the Intifada's combatants on Gaza's deserted streets.

The curfew itself was a kind of invisible wall in the mind, tended by Israelis and Palestinians in a bizarre ritual of agreement. If everyone in Gaza refused to stay home—if even a fraction refused—there would be no curfew and no way for the Israelis to enforce it. Guns were not needed to enforce a curfew if people believed it to be in effect. Years of Israeli occupation and the considerable violence that came along with it had built these walls. The stateless limbo of the people of Gaza had turned them into a demoralized society of the politically disabled, surrounded by what they believed to be insurmountable barriers.

Just as there was no need to lock crips up to confine them to their houses if they believed there was no point in going outside, the Palestinians of Gaza only needed to be told that they couldn't go out. The Intifada itself was about the breakdown of such barriers and the rewriting of all these rules. Because I didn't see the walls and the combatants didn't see me, I moved about freely. From their rooftops, the Gazans under curfew saw this freedom and called it bravery for lack of a better name.

I returned to Taher's house just as the sun went down and the young men were preparing the fireworks for Yasir Arafat's speech. The radio was blaring the endless preliminary remarks of every PLO faction leader and the background hubbub of the organization's attempt to achieve a consensus on the two main issues at the conference: declaring a Palestinian state and renouncing the armed struggle against Israel. The incoming Bush administration had made it clear to the Arab world that an explicit renunciation of violence by Arafat would result in a major concession from the U.S. government: direct talks between the PLO and Washington.

Taher was checking his CBS camera to make sure it was working. Outside, the boys began to string PLO flags across the roofs and utility lines. Younger boys collected piles of rocks to throw at the soldiers. Taher's mother and sisters prepared a big meal of bread, olives, and a greasy lamb stew with piles of tomato salad. It was many hours before Arafat made the announcement. Shortly before midnight, an Israeli patrol surrounded Taher's house and ordered one of his uncles to paint over some anti-Israeli graffiti on a nearby wall.

An officer demanded to search the house. He'd had a report that a journalist was inside. Even with my poor Arabic, I could tell that they were having some kind of argument about a journalist. I slid out of my chair and across the floor just as one of Taher's brothers rushed into the room. He pointed to a small closet door behind a bed and I got in. I listened through the wall to the banging of the soldiers threatening to arrest Taher and his brothers, and the wailing and angry tirades of Taher's mother. In the background I could still hear the Arabic speeches on the radio from Algiers getting ready to announce the independence of Palestine for the first time since 1948. In the dark I felt confused echoes of history. Was I like Anne Frank, boxed away behind a wall in my own unseen world, while men in uniform stomped around below, convinced I was nearby? Or was the confused history all my own? In Taher's closet I resembled only myself, hidden in another peculiar crawl space like the floor under Martha's bed, hoping no one would find me.

Arafat's radio announcement was followed by fireworks on the rooftops all over Gaza City. Within an hour, every intersection had a burning tire and the Israeli armored patrols were going to each tire one by one, hosing off the more dangerous blazes and ordering people out of their houses to douse the smaller ones. The night was peppered with gunshots and chanting. The sharp reports of rifles were answered by the breathy pops of firecrackers. The red lights of the ambulances taking casualties to the hospital wrapped the streets and alleys in oversized, menacing shadows. The Israeli army trucks rumbled by all night, their crackling radios filled with the shouting of military orders. From the inside of buildings, the bluish glow of fluorescent lights and the sound of Yasir Arafat on the radio drifted out on to the street. I sat invisible in the middle of it all, holding a microphone.

As roman candles lit up the area around Taher's building you could just catch a glimpse of little PLO flags flapping in the night breeze; then they would disappear into the darkness. When Taher lit his last bottle rocket he looked sad, and said, "There will be one more day of curfew, then back to work on Monday." His Fourth of July weekend was almost over. It would be six years before there was another.

I packed up Taher's camera in the morning, along with my tapes and notebooks. I had high hopes of getting a ride to Erez checkpoint in a Red Cross car, but reports of violence through the night had made the relief agencies nervous about breaking the rules. They, too, had heard of my defiance of the curfew and considered my presence to be a highly risky provocation. After rolling around openly reporting for two days and going unnoticed by the Israelis, this bravery business was getting a little tiresome. All I had gotten on tape was the sound of some fireworks popping; Taher's shaky video of boys standing around in the dark clapping; some eloquent, but hardly unique, interviews of Palestinians talking about the meaning of their nonexistent independent state, and the sound of some Israeli soldiers banging on the door to Taher's house with their rifle butts. These tapes would hardly bring down a government or threaten national security. "Look, just give me a ride halfway. The checkpoint is seven miles away." They were so convinced of my fearlessness that it made them scared to talk to me. They apologized and drove away. I told Taher that I would roll out to the checkpoint on my own. Taher said he would call Bob Simon at CBS and make sure the car would wait.

On the way out of town, I had the pavement to myself. Gaza City looked deserted; each street had an echo, each building a muffled hum from the sound of the people inside. The utility poles were draped with the remains of the Palestine independence day celebration. Colored streamers flapped in the light afternoon breeze along with pictures of Yasir Arafat, PLO flags, and balloons in the national colors of Palestine: red, green, white, and black. Black balloons were particularly hard to get in any quantity, and Taher had mentioned his source in careful whispers the night before, as though he were describing the underground arms trade. "We get the black ones from a party shop in Jerusalem, from the religious people," he said, referring to the Orthodox Mea Sharim neighborhood, with its long-standing reputation for conducting commerce out of the reach of the heavy-handed Israeli government.

I passed under the balloons and flags and alongside shuttered iron gates in front of the houses and shops lining Nasser Street, the main road out of the city. Faces could be seen peering through apartment windows and the cracks in metal doors. The word was out that I was rolling to Erez, and from the rooftops in Gaza City boys waved to me and then passed my location along to the people on the next block who knew to expect me as I came around each corner.

Just beyond the big rusted archway that said WELCOME TO GAZA in English, Hebrew, and Arabic, a man had emerged from his house with a little table and a chair. *"Inta Sahafai Koorsimuttaharak aiwah,"* he said. He then asked, "You are the Journalist in the Wheelchair, yes?" I was getting used to this title. I said yes. He set the chair down and motioned for me to sit with him for a moment. He gestured to the crowd of children looking down at us from the roof of his house and they jumped into action. A young boy appeared with a pot of tea and two small glasses. "You can drink something," said the man, whose name I learned was Fayez. I looked around and the houses were all crowned with their own contingents of spectators and lookouts.

Fayez proudly pointed out the decorations on his house as a plate of small cookies arrived. A boy called down from above, and Fayez reported to me in halting English that an Israeli patrol had been spotted three blocks away, but that we had a few minutes to speak. "The soldiers are busy with all of the balloons," he said. We sat calmly, as though there was no curfew, no occupation, and no Israeli patrol just down the street. The morning air was a rancid mélange of bread oven smells and burned rubber from the hundreds of tires sacrificed to Palestine the night before. The colorful paper litter from used fireworks was scattered over Gaza's many garbage piles. On the first full day of Palestine's era of independence, the citizens of Gaza were confined to their homes, while Israeli troops spent the day collecting party decorations.

I finished the glass of tea and said good-bye to Fayez and waved to his family. I rolled back out into the center of the road and continued toward the Israeli border. At each house along the way I was asked to stop again and have more tea. "You must come and drink something," the man of each household addressed me while his family watched from the roof, rooting for their father's powers of persuasion, hoping to get me to stop. I turned down each offer with an apology and picked up my pace, rolling past the row of tire repair shops on the edge of the city to where it forked, one path leading to the village of Beit Hanoun and the other to the Erez checkpoint.

I turned to the left and rolled right in front of two Israeli soldiers slowly going from house to house tearing down streamers and balloons. They looked bored and slightly at a loss to explain their mission that day. Each of them had two colored balloons tied to their M-16 rifles. "Where did you come from?" one of the young soldiers addressed me in Hebrew. I answered in the halting Alan Alda accent, hoping it would identify me as an American Jew on a school field trip. "I am going to the Erez checkpoint."

"It is closed here." The soldier immediately switched to English. "Where did you come from?" he asked.

"Detroit," I said with a big smile. "Actually, right outside Detroit. We live in the suburbs." The soldiers shook their heads, and the one who had not yet spoken added, "But where did you come from? This is Gaza and it is a closed area today."

Still smiling, I pointed back down the road. "It's a closed area all around here. That's why I'm going to the checkpoint. It's a closed military area. I can't stay here," I said.

"We know it's a closed military area. We are the army. Where did you come from?" They began speaking in Hebrew to each other, speculating about who I might be. They concluded that I was another mishugenah

(nut) from the Jewish settlement a few miles back down the road beyond Gaza City.

"I was visiting people back down there, and now I'm going to the
checkpoint. I had better get moving," I said and started to roll away.

The soldiers smiled and shrugged. "It's a long way to Detroit. Here,
have a balloon," one of them said. "Haven't you heard? This is an independent country today." The soldier's sarcasm was halfhearted, as if he
wished it were true and not such a joke. Standing in the Gaza Strip
holding a black balloon, he looked lost. Only about an hour's drive from
downtown Tel Aviv, he seemed much farther from home than I.

The last miles to Erez were solitary and free, with the hills of Israel
to my right off to the east and the lowlands of Gaza to the west, ending
in its forlorn Mediterranean beaches. The road wound around to the
green military checkpoint and staging area that served to mark the end
of Gaza and the beginning of Israel. The pavement here is well-main-
tained as a matter of Israeli security. Although it would also make a
fabulous route for a wheelchair marathon, this is the northern military
corridor down which tanks would roll in the event of another war with
Egypt. They had rolled this way before.

The lookout tower was visible for two miles as I approached the
checkpoint. Watching it as I pushed the chair, I imagined the officers in
the tower speculating on why I was approaching the base with such
energy. I would not pause. I would roll straight through. If I looked
calm, they would not think I was some kind of bomber or that I had
buried my audiotape and microphones deep inside my leather backpack. Only a thorough search would reveal that I was a journalist.

Up ahead, I could see that there was activity at the checkpoint. A
quarter-mile back there had been shooting and the sounds of a demonstration. Plumes of gray smoke rose above the Jebaliya refugee camp. I
had seen enough violence to make a story for Washington, but as I
rolled along, I felt as though I was abandoning the people in the camp.
I could do nothing for them. The approaching checkpoint made me
nervous. It was heavily fortified with guns and barbed wire and large
steel roadblocks that could be raised or lowered from the lookout tower
in the event of attack. Playing dumb as I had done with the soldiers back
in the city probably wouldn't work here.

I vowed that I would continue rolling no matter what, and concocted
a plan for saying, if challenged, that I was sick and had to get to a waiting
car for the drive to a Tel Aviv hospital. This seemed a dubious plan
given that I had just rolled six miles and was not even out of breath. No
matter what, I thought, I would not allow them to stop me. The skin on

my scalp tingled with anticipation of the confrontation I was sure was ahead. I could see that the roadblocks were down. I could roll right through as long as they didn't sound the alarm and raise them.

I was pushing now as hard as I could, thinking of all the times I had sprinted down Lake Shore Drive in Chicago. The curfew-cleared streets reminded me of the marathons I had run, but in Gaza the attentive crowds watched from behind closed and locked doors. The feeling of physical integrity with the aluminum and steel of my chair was like being invulnerable. The checkpoint came fully into view. There would be no Martha to greet me at this finish line. I could see people walking around, and I could make out the faces in the lookout tower. Around me were a large number of armored vehicles and heavily armed soldiers being resupplied to relieve the balloon-picking patrols already inside Gaza.

It took about fifteen seconds to roll past the checkpoint in broad view of everyone. No one noticed. I rolled toward the parking lot, and I could see the CBS car waiting patiently. The driver waved and got out of the car to open the trunk for my chair. "How did you manage?" he said. "It was a closed military zone in Gaza. When they told me to pick you up, I didn't believe it."

"It was no problem," I said sadly. I wished I could tell him something daring and dramatic. I wanted to turn around and roll back through the checkpoint again and make it worthwhile. "Hey! You missed this guy in a wheelchair rolling into Israel. Don't you want to search me?" I would yell up to the tower. "I could be a mad bomber, you know." I looked back at the officers going about their business. They wouldn't have believed me, and they would have been right.

The news story that day was the deaths from clashes in the occupied territories. In spite of the independence declaration from Algiers, there was less violence than normal. It was the top story around the world, although the notion of an independent state of Palestine was greeted with some scepticism, especially in Israel, where commentators called it a mapmaker's fantasy. The PLO might be attempting to show itself as a moderate political force, the reports said, but in 1988 Israel wasn't buying it.

Perhaps in hindsight, the real story was that by 1988 the Israelis and Palestinians were already simply going through the motions of their long conflict. The military checkpoints had become props in a show; the Palestinians were using balloons they had bought from Jews as weapons against Israel. Israeli patrols were ordered to capture the balloons and neutralize them. There was much violence to come, and many Israelis and Palestinians were to die before Gaza would be independent, or very tentatively autonomous, as it became in 1994. But looking back, as a ghost with a microphone, rolling brazenly in defiance of a curfew in what both sides called a war zone, it was clear that the war for the Gaza Strip had ended long before. All that remained was for someone to say it.

Radwan

*T*he cliché about the Middle East is that the conflicts are all 2,000 years old, and I went there fully expecting to find people tyrannized by questions left unresolved for centuries. But Arabs and Jews spend more time arguing about and acting on their contemporary history on a day-to-day basis than with anything from their ancient past. The most emotionally powerful places are also the most recent monuments: Yad Vashem, the Israeli Holocaust memorial; the simple tragic memorials to the young Arabs who died during the Intifada, scattered throughout the occupied territories; the place in the old Jewish quarter where the Israeli army soldiers reached the Western Wall during the Six-Day War; the silent, rusted Israeli war memorials from the forties. It is largely the present and very recent past that drive the conflicts between Jews and Arabs.

There is a place on the road from Tel Aviv to Jerusalem where the hills rising off the coastal plain open out into a wide basin of trees and stone. The Jerusalem road creeps along on an ascending ridge between two enormous valleys. On either side of the road is a precipitous drop to the bottom of a canyon, and all around there is a spectacular view of the ancient mountain range upon which the city of Jerusalem, a bit younger than civilization itself, is perched. Dotting the walls of the canyon are houses and apartments, some of which are about as old as modern Israel. From them, you can observe the road and the heavy traffic between Israel's two largest cities.

On the right side of the road, just before it plunges back into the twisty forest switchbacks for the last miles to Jerusalem, is a little memorial to sixteen people, Arabs and Jews, who died on July 6, 1989. Upon that spot, shortly after twelve noon, the regular Israeli "EGGED" Jerusalem-Tel Aviv bus number 405 lurched from the road and crashed into the ravine on the southern edge of the canyon. An Israeli housewife in one of the valley houses watched the crash from a distance and remarked on how the bus seemed to bounce in slow motion. It came to rest long before the sound of the crash and the screams of those inside reached her window.

One of the last times I saw my paraplegic friend, Radwan Abu Smaish, was a few days before the crash of that bus. I had seen him many times since our first encounter. Our relationship had grown since I had shown him a few wheelchair tricks at Mokassad Hospital. Gradually, Radwan learned English, and I learned to communicate crudely in Arabic. His wheelchair skills improved even more dramatically, but he was more or less permanently housed at Mokassad Hospital, away from the sand and filth of the Nusirat refugee camp, his family's home in Gaza. While I spent each day covering the Intifada, he missed most of it. When we would meet, I would tell him about what I had seen in the occupied territories, and he would tell me the new physical skills he had learned.

Radwan's possessive friend, Abdel Hadi, whom I recalled from that first day at Mokassad, still visited regularly. He and others from Gaza would keep their friend up-to-date on who had been arrested, expelled, injured, or killed. As time went on though, Radwan seemed to lose interest in the Intifada's day-to-day trade in blood, hatred, and insults. He was gaining instead a deeper passion for the challenges of his new life. It was a passion that set him apart from his Palestinian brothers fighting on the front lines against Israel. Radwan's political ideas and support for the PLO did not change, but his new life divided him from the others in ways that would, in time, become clear.

More and more young people had gotten spinal-cord injuries from the fighting, and on Radwan's ward there was now a gang of little boys in wheelchairs. On the outside they were tough, loud martyrs who made sure you knew which faction of the PLO they had given up their legs for, and would happily die for even now. They raced up and down the halls in their noisy, creaking chairs, but when Radwan appeared they looked more like the vulnerable young men they were, fearful of what kind of life they now faced. Radwan led them around like a coach. I would arrive for a visit and we would hold impromptu workshops, with Radwan asking me to demonstrate something he knew I could do, but the other boys didn't believe possible. I would go from the floor to my chair and Radwan would say, *"Na'am, kol mumpkin."* "It's all possible."

Not a lot was possible for Radwan and his boys as long as they used the dreadful wheelchairs supplied by the hospital and the Palestinian rehab organizations. Radwan had acquired a serviceable but still fairly primitive wheelchair and was spending considerable time out of bed. But going back to his home in the Gaza Strip was out. Compared to my own, Radwan's chair was maneuverable only with difficulty even on linoleum. In the sands of his home of the Nusirat refugee camp, it would be impossible.

I had decided months before to give Radwan a new chair from the extra components and spare wheelchair I had at my home in Jerusalem. I got around to bolting it together that July. I narrowed the frame to fit Radwan and raised the seat up in a more standard position rather than the steeply raked angle I preferred. The chair was a Quadra ultralight with two sets of wheels, twenty-four-inch and twenty-seven-inch. I gave Radwan the chair with the twenty-seven-inch thin, high-pressure bicycle wheels installed. I told him that the wider twenty-fours would work better in sand, but that at Mokassad and around Jerusalem these thin tires worked fine. With its black aluminum frame, its wheels cambered outward in the provocative slant preferred by American crips, and its black nylon upholstery, Radwan's chair was one of a kind at Mokassad. It had no armrests. It put the heavy Eastern European models to shame with their cheap, flaky chrome, boxy suspension, and ugly car seat upholstery.

The chair had one problem. I had spares of every part except for front caster wheels. My two swiveling casters were six inches in diameter, and fully pneumatic; they were the most specialized parts on my wheelchair. While the larger rear wheels and much of the frame were standard bicycle components and easily available, the caster wheels, tires, inner tubes, axles, and bearings were available only by special order from the wheelchair company back in California. I had brought only one set of air-filled casters to Israel. Just in case of a big emergency, I had some neoprene solid wheels that were for use on hard, flat surfaces and were made for playing basketball on gymnasium floors. The neoprene wheels were small in diameter and sank like table legs into any soft surface. But they were all I had for Radwan's chair.

I brought the chair for Radwan to Mokassad one sunny afternoon along with a full set of tools for adjusting it to Radwan's body. I placed the tools in my lap and pushed the empty chair along next to me through the hospital hallways on the way to his room. Two young boys saw me get out of the elevator and rushed to get Radwan, who emerged in a blue sleeveless T-shirt that showed his developing arms. The frail bony limbs of just a few months ago were gone.

Radwan was a real crip now. He inspected the chair as a competitor in the Tour de France might look over a new bicycle. He did a smart, swift transfer from his chair into the new black one. Radwan's legs were long and his footrests needed to be adjusted. When it looked like the chair fit him, Radwan took off down the hall for a test run. The boys followed. He came back smiling.

"It is so very light, John," he exclaimed, going up on two wheels. "It makes everything that is difficult very easy." He threw his long arms wide and twisted his upper body from side to side in a gesture of physical freedom. "It is better," he said, nodding. "No armrests." Radwan said something in Arabic to the boys in the hall and they removed their armrests and set them all in a pile on the floor. One of the boys in a particularly bad chair with nonremovable armrests pointed to Radwan's now-empty chair. Together Radwan and I picked him up and placed him in the chair, where he immediately removed its armrests and smiled. We were all on the same team now.

Radwan noticed that the casters on his new chair were different from the air-filled ones on my chair. "I think yours are better," he said. "These are not good for sand." He looked doubtfully at them. I told him that I would order new casters as soon as I could. "I just wanted you to start using the chair right away while you are here at Mokassad."

"I am going home to Gaza at the end of the week," he said. It would be his first trip home in a wheelchair. I told him that until he got the new casters he should try to take heavy sand on two wheels, keeping the small, solid wheels from touching the ground. "That will keep you going for now." Before I left, we took the twenty-seven-inch wheels off and put the wider twenty-fours on for the sand in Nusirat refugee camp. The late afternoon sun made long, spiny shadows through the spokes of all the wheelchairs as we laughed and compared tricks in the lounge at the end of the hall. I spent a few hours with my tools, tightening bolts and straightening spokes. We had an arm-wrestling contest that I won, and a hallway race that I lost. We didn't speak of the Israelis or the PLO once. The last thing I saw when I left in the elevator were the caster wheels on Radwan's new chair. I thought about all the sand I had seen in Gaza.

The red "EGGED" public buses that crisscross Israel every day are not wheelchair-accessible. Israeli crips have their own government-supplied cars, and so accessibility for the buses is not seen as a pressing need. My first view of the inside of an EGGED bus was the twisted metal and burned upholstery inside EGGED number 105 when it was hauled back up the side of the canyon where it crashed on July 6. It must have been a horrible burning ride down to the bottom of the canyon. The impact had peeled back the roof, and rescue workers had cut wide, square holes that looked like new doors in the body. The bus looked flimsy, like something made from papier mâché. In one of those strange moments in which the oddest of thoughts pops into your head, as it was hauled away for salvage it occurred to me that it wouldn't be so difficult to make the buses accessible.

Sixteen people died on EGGED number 105. If it had been just another of the hundreds of road accidents in Israel that each year kill an Intifada's worth of people, it would have been forgotten. The Israeli media reported the crash as a bus attack. The first stories said that a Palestinian terrorist had stabbed the driver. Later stories made no mention of a knife, instead, survivors on the bus said that a young Palestinian man stood up as the bus entered the canyon road, grabbed the steering wheel, and pulled it hard to the right, causing the driver to lose control of the bus. As I was on my way to meet the incoming casualties at Hadassah Hospital in Jerusalem I heard that the police were claiming that the suspect, who survived the crash, was an Islamic fundamentalist because he had a beard, was apparently carrying a Koran, and was said to have yelled in Arabic as he grabbed the steering wheel, "Allahu Akbar"; "God is Great" is what the police claimed he had yelled.

The Jews and the Palestinians all agreed that a man had stood up and yelled something as he grabbed the steering wheel. The Jews claimed that he was crazy and had been a threatening presence from the moment he got on the bus. The Palestinians, who were just as shaken by the trip over the cliff, said that he seemed to be a weak, sad young man who looked lost when he stood up to grab the steering wheel. They were sure he had not yelled Allahu Akbar. "It was a name," one man said to me from his bed. "Marwan or Radwan." He could not remember.

The suspect's name was released the day after the crash. Abdel Hadi Ghneim was a religious student from Nusirat refugee camp, according to the police. The Israeli reports were dominated by calls for the death penalty in the Knesset. Government officials said the bus killings were a new strategy by the PLO to hit Israelis across the green line, where they were most vulnerable. The PLO's outward face of moderation that had led to a renewed dialogue with the United States was false, they said. The U.S. State Department condemned the incident and called once again for an end to violence. After just a few days, the bus crash and its sixteen dead took its place on the vast scorecard of the Arab-Israeli conflict where brutality was ranked and classified, but where no single act of violence could ever be decisive.

A friend of mine obtained a copy of the official Israeli police report of the bus incident. The report speculated on Abdel Hadi's ties to religious fundamentalist radicals in the Gaza Strip. The report said that Abdel Hadi had admitted to causing the bus crash, but unlike most Islamic fundamentalists who survive their attacks to be interrogated, he did not claim that it was all for the glory of Islam. The report noted without comment that he had been depressed over the crippling injury suffered by his best friend, whom he had seen a few days before. My blood ran cold as I stared at the paper scribbled with translation marks. The friend was another young man from Nusirat refugee camp: Radwan Abu Smaish.

I knew both the killer and the man in whose name he had killed. I had felt my own personal outrage from the ceaseless violence in the Middle East on other occasions, but nothing could compare to the feeling I had as I stared at the police report and thought of Radwan, and the face of Abdel Hadi standing so close to his friend at the hospital, beaming with pride at his sacrifice and injury. I thought of Radwan in Gaza the weekend before. I thought of Abdel Hadi on the bus shouting Radwan's name at the terrified riders. Most of all, I thought of the red neoprene casters on the chair I had given to Radwan.

The motives of a distant foreign crime far removed from my life, my country of birth, and the people and places I knew suddenly revealed themselves to me with perfect clarity in a language I knew very well. From the detached perspective of a journalist reporting on a passing incident of violence, I was transformed into an accomplice to the deaths of sixteen people. I knew without asking a question that Abdel Hadi had seen Radwan trying to get through the sands of Gaza with those hard caster wheels, that he had seen how impossible it had been for his friend to move. He did not see that Radwan was out of bed, physically stronger, and exploring a world that he hadn't even imagined from his hospital bed a year earlier. Abdel Hadi could not see that Radwan saw the inappropriate caster wheels as a simple mechanical problem that he would fix with some wrenches and a new set of wheels when he got back to Jerusalem. Abdel Hadi could only see Radwan's injury and subsequent difficulties as a form of torture inflicted by the Israelis.

"Abdel Hadi saw me in that chair for the first time in Gaza," Radwan told me, "and he became crazy."

"But Abdel Hadi knew you were a paraplegic for more than a year." I was angry. It seemed an insult to everything I had lived for since my accident in 1976 that someone could find an excuse to kill sixteen people because of what he felt after seeing someone in a wheelchair. "Did he like you better lying there sick in bed at Mokassad Hospital?" I asked. "Why did he suddenly decide to kill a busload of people?"

Radwan looked puzzled. There was so much he had learned from me. It was odd to him that I had to ask him these questions about his friend Abdel Hadi. "It is a very bad thing that Abdel Hadi did. He was wrong." In his broken English Radwan explained that as long as he was in a hospital bed, Abdel Hadi could imagine that he, Radwan,, would eventually get well and walk out of the hospital, and they would both go on with their lives.

"Did you ever think Abdel Hadi would do what he did?"

Radwan lowered his head, and it was clear he understood why I was so offended and angry by what had happened. But Radwan also knew how upset his friend had been seeing him back at home in the black aluminum chair. Radwan had wanted Abdel Hadi to know that he could make a life for himself in the chair, but that was not what he saw when Radwan went to Gaza. "In the chair, Abdel Hadi could only see my legs not working. In the chair, he knew that I would never stand up. It was too much pain," Radwan said, and then he asked me a question. "Don't you know someone like this?" I closed my eyes. I was still disgusted at Abdel Hadi, guilty over why those people had died, and angry with myself for not having the right caster wheels for Radwan. But for the first time in years I thought of my friend Ricky, who was with me in 1976 when I had walked for the last time. That the pain Ricky had felt after my accident, and the changes that had taken place between us in the years after, was something like Abdel Hadi's anger I could not fathom. But like the memorial on the Jerusalem-Tel Aviv highway to the dead from EGGED number 105, I could not deny that it was very real.

Today Radwan helps run a wheelchair basketball league in Gaza. There are five teams and they travel throughout the Middle East to compete. They won a tournament in Iran in 1994. Today it is Radwan who regularly visits Abdel Hadi. He is serving a life sentence for murder in Gaza Central Prison. When I last spoke to him, he told me that the prison was accessible, and that Israelis made sure it was easy for him to move about there. "The Israelis are very respectful of the disabled people," he said. I asked him about Yasir Arafat's historic return to Gaza and he said, "It is not important. It is just politics. We are struggling for freedom everywhere, not just in Gaza." I started to ask him about the peace process and he interrupted me. "I am not talking about Palestinians. We are only disabled people fighting for freedom." Before he said good-bye, Radwan thanked me for coming to meet him in Mokassad Hospital in Jerusalem in 1988, and he thanked me for the wheelchair. He has a new one now. The old one is in use today at a rehab facility on the West Bank in the town of Rammallah.

"Those little wheels were so very bad in Nusirat camp, so I changed them. It is better now, John," Radwan told me. "There is a lot of sand in Gaza. Do you remember all of the sand?"

I told him I remembered.

Khomeini's
Revenge

*A*n estimated 1 million people died in the Persian Gulf War, which was not the Gulf War that everyone watched on TV in the 1990s. The Iran-Iraq war that nearly spanned the entire decade of the eighties was the longest sustained military conflict of the twentieth century between two sovereign powers. Its battles, and casualties, were all conducted and disposed of well out of sight of any media. Tucked away in the cold war's last years, the battles between Iran and Iraq seemed irrelevant and out of place in the world. But it is the regional conflicts like the Iran-Iraq war that would prefigure the world of the next century, while the cold war faded into an abrupt obscurity.

For much of the world, the twentieth century ended a few years early anyway. In Eastern Europe, Russia, Africa, and the Middle East, the towering themes and intractable conflicts that had produced a pair of world wars, a generation of cold war allies and enemies, stadiums full of spies, villains, heroes, and a numbing onslaught of technology evaporated in the 1980s. Not only did the twentieth century leave early, it had arrived fourteen years late with World War One, "the war to end all wars." Seven decades later, the best the world could manage was a shorter military attention span. The preferred wars were quick and contained and over places like Panama, Grenada, and the Falkland Islands. The protracted horrors of Eritrea, Ethiopia, Afghanistan, Iran, and Iraq were largely unseen.

The first Persian Gulf War, and a Godlike leader's failure to win it, brought a century of dreams to a close in Iran. Persia had begun the twentieth century attempting to take its place as a constitutional government, free of colonial and western economic domination. Ayatollah Khomeini was the leader who would finally make good on that promise. Khomeini swept to power in a staggering political movement that marshaled Iran's religion, Shi'a Islam, its oil, and the most powerful military in the Middle East to end its self-loathing, forge the first truly Iranian national destiny, and piss off the entire world in the process.

If the Iran-Iraq war didn't get much TV coverage in the West, the American government's obsession with Khomeini more than made up for it. The Ayatollah was a far more comprehensible enemy to people in the United States than the Soviet Union's Andropov, Chernenko, and Gorbachev were, and much better known. To the people of Iran, Khomeini wasn't much for fireside chats, but he told them which days would live in infamy, and that the only thing Shiites had to fear was fear itself.

The eight-year war with Iraq was started by Saddam Hussein, but it became a focus for Khomeini's Islamic revolution. At the end, ground to a stalemate, with a half million dead, Iran's military had become a pitiful war machine struggling to trade hostages for American spare parts. Its oil revenue was declining, and Khomeini had publicly surrendered. In a speech on July 18, 1988, after promising to fight to the last drop of his own blood, Khomeini told his people he would agree to a cease-fire. "Taking this decision was more deadly than taking poison," Khomeini said in a statement read on Tehran radio. "I submitted myself to God's will and drank this drink for His satisfaction."

Having surrendered to Saddam Hussein, Khomeini's legacy had become clouded, even if his hold on the people of Iran was as strong as ever. In the end the Ayatollah was the head oracle of an Iranian bureaucracy wrapped in hesitation and backbiting and run by lesser Ayatollahs. Khomeini's edicts were received like tremors rather than policy in the West. Who had the upper hand? The State Department, the CIA, and the media pundits all asked. Was it the radicals or the moderates, the pragmatists or the zealots? The Iranian people also wanted to know, and they presumed Washington could tell them.

Along with its other contributions to world culture, Iran is a nation of conspiracy theorists capable of unbridled paranoia over the most outlandish scenarios. In a sunny living room in the southern city of Ahwaz, an Iranian white collar worker told me in all sincerity, "We Iranians were fooled in the beginning, but now we believe that Khomeini was a CIA plot to destroy Iran" (the CIA had actually helped install the Pahlavi family in power, inaugurating the "shah of shah's" back in 1956). "Look around you," he said. "It worked." He was not interested in or persuaded by my suggestion that the U.S. was as surprised by Khomeini as the fifty-two hostages at the U.S. Embassy in Tehran had been. "That was their plan all along," he replied without a blink. "They wanted us to think that."

He told me what he enjoyed most now was to watch Western TV shows, which he could pick up across the gulf on Bahrain TV. His favorite show was "The Equalizer." For the ten months that followed Iran's surrender to Saddam Hussein, the people of Iran drifted, simply waiting for Ayatollah Khomeini to die. On June 3, 1989, he did.

The media had been waiting as well. It had been a lean year for news in the Middle East. Most members of the press corps had not seen their names on a front page in months. There were long faces in a bar in Amman, Jordan, in the autumn of 1989, when a group of Middle East reporters was in town for one of King Hussein's periodic and timid little experiments in democracy. Normally this kind of thing made the front page. But mock-controlled elections for a mock-controlled parliament was not going to make the news that night. Democracy's main event was in Berlin. A hard day of Jordanian election coverage would be tossed into the rubbish. I encountered Alan Cowell of *The New York Times* sitting with Middle East correspondent Caryle Murphy of *The Washington Post,* who was just beginning an assignment in the region.

"You might as well order a beer." Cowell shrugged as he greeted me. "The Berlin Wall is coming down, right now, tonight." He raised his glass and handed me a piece of wire copy with the words: "Bulletin— Berlin wall falls."

"It's the End of Days." Cowell's toast referred to the Islamic day of judgment, at which point Caryle Murphy looked at both of us and wondered aloud, "Maybe I made a mistake coming to the Middle East." Two years later Murphy received the Pulitzer Prize for her reporting in Kuwait during the Iraqi invasion.

In 1989, Khomeini's death seemed to be about the sole guaranteed front-page story left in the Middle East. The Soviet Union and Eastern Europe were crumbling. Democracy was coming to China. For weeks the students and workers were massing toward a showdown in Beijing's Tiananmen Square. Khomeini's final taunt to the infidel journalists who had been writing about him for a decade was to go and die on the day before the Tiananmen Square massacre. The routine wire story of Khomeini's death made the front pages, but the funeral and the waves of features and think pieces were all going to have to struggle to make it to page two.

June 5 was an emotional day in Tehran. The Ayatollah's funeral would bring an entire nation into the streets. There were to be a couple of ceremonies, the first a religious service to be held at Khomeini's North Tehran home. The second would be the burial at the Beheshed al Zahra cemetery outside the capital. The day of mourning began very early. By 6 A.M. the streets were jammed with vehicles. The buses were overflowing. Bicycles and motor scooters typically carried four or five people. Down every street, whole families walked together in a somber, disorganized parade. Tehran is a sprawling, noisy city of more than 14 million people. On the day of the Ayatollah Khomeini's funeral, with more than a third of its citizens in the streets, Tehran was quiet.

The mood was broken as groups of reporters were spotted by people massing along the route to the Ayatollah's house. I rolled past a crowd of people and they began shouting, "Death to America!" in a kind of stupored frenzy; a familiar ritual of anti-American eyes seeking American camera lenses. When they discovered that I was American, the crowd began to smile as they yelled. Between chants, some people assured me that they loved the American people. "Why does America hate Iran?" someone shouted from the crowd.

I considered a detailed response, noting the colonial history of Iran and the demoralization of the United States in the post-war era. The phrase "Death to America" had at least one virtue on a hot day in the middle of a crowd of Farsi-speaking Shiites: we all knew what we were talking about. Instead of a history lesson, I replied that it was possible, just possible, that Americans took some offense at being told to die.

This proposition seemed dubious to one man who looked at me as though I had just endorsed the Warren Commission Report at one of Oliver Stone's dinner parties. "The American people know we are speaking of the government. They understand." I suggested that possibly most Americans had missed this detail. "Then they are brainwashed." "By whom?" I asked. He delivered his answer without a pause. "The Brookings Institute and the rest of the thinking tanks." As a precaution I suggested that he modify his chant to say "Death to the American government." He shook his head. "Too long. Who would say this? It won't fit on signs."

A man who said his name was Oskar stepped forward and asked where in America I was from. Most of the regular down-home Americans so beloved of these chanting Iranians would have had trouble locating the nation of Iran on a map of the world, let alone identifying one of its major cities. I named the last city I had lived in back in the States—Washington—to which he replied without a pause, "D.C. or state?"

Oskar then grabbed the handles on my wheelchair and began to push me in front of the crowd, all the while shouting, "Death to America," along with everyone else. I protested the pushing while I mused over the irony of the message "Death to your country, now sit still while I help you move along here." It was a venerable message in this part of the world. Certainly the Iranians were used to sitting quietly while colonial masters decided their nation's future. Oskar was going to push me. That's all there was to it.

I had an attack of performance anxiety. I was in Iran to report on the death of the Ayatollah. Detained by the chanters and arguing with Oskar over who was going to push my chair, I had gotten separated from the rest of the press corps. The walking media was somewhere up ahead of me. The news, I assumed, couldn't possibly be where I was. It must be up where the rest of the reporters were. I had stopped to get one little comment from an Iranian citizen about the death of their leader and had gotten sucked into a discussion about conspiracy theories, and an argument with an Iranian Jerry Lewis named Oskar.

In what looked to be a large school parking lot at the edge of an endless crowd of mourners, three helicopters were parked. Oskar rolled me up to a red-faced Iranian revolutionary guardsman who was trying to fend off the angry mob of television crews, all insisting on an aerial view of the funeral. The big networks all had large, grinning Iranian thugs and fixers to get their way. NPR and I had only Oskar, and we were a bickering comedy act in broken English.

"Please, don't push."

"Mr. John, it's okay. It is no trouble for me."

"I know it's no trouble, but please, it is better for me that you do not push."

"Mr. John, it is no problem, thank you. I will be your legs."

"I can push."

"No, I will push, it is no problem for me."

"I can push."

Woodward and Bernstein we were not, and it looked like it could take more than Watergate's burglars to get me a helicopter ride that morning. The crowd of international media hovered around the red-faced Iranian officer, screaming and cajoling in equal measure. I would try to get in line or get my name on the official list to ride on one of the choppers. The list was scribbled on a scrap of paper and passed from officer to officer, who added names and crossed others out as everyone argued over who should take the first helicopter and why their deadline was the most important. Who was on the official list, and why, was a complete mystery.

The journalists seized on various ways of interceding and gaining the upper hand. In an effort to appease everyone, which was also an apt metaphor for Iranian politics, the officers ended up masterfully playing the American reporters off against the Brits, the Japanese, the Russians, and the French. They also played the television people off against everyone else. For all of the irritation he was causing, the Iranian guardsman commander was having no fun. Despite sowing derision and mutual suspicion among all present, from the look on his face he seemed to be trying to please. He was not just scalping tickets for helicopter rides to view Shiite madness, he was attempting to allow the West to view the last rites of the Ayatollah. He said things like, "All those who wish to see the holy remains of the blessed Imam Khomeini, will you please stand in a straight line. We want to cooperate with you, the ladies and gentlemen of the international press." You could see that he believed Khomeini had definite plans for his funeral weekend. Whatever those plans were, this officer did not want to get anything wrong.

Eventually Oskar stepped forward and addressed the Iranian officer on my behalf with an emotional speech. In a somber, passionate oration delivered entirely in Farsi and incomprehensible to me, he apparently evoked the Islamic revolution, the spirit of the dead Imam Khomeini, and the officer's mother. Perhaps Oskar simply offered to mow the officer's lawn every other Thursday. Whatever Oskar said, the officer suddenly motioned for me to get on one of the choppers. I rolled excitedly across the tarmac and hoisted myself triumphantly aboard as a British cameraman shouted, "Hey, why send him? He's radio."

As we lifted off, there was Oskar with my chair, rolling into a crowd of mourners estimated at 2 million, all wearing the same black outfits. My wheelchair was black. I had known Oskar for all of ten minutes. The first words I heard him utter were "Death to America." Now he had my wheelchair and I was hanging from a helicopter over a sea of Iranian mourners who had hung on Khomeini's every word while he was alive.

From the helicopter we could see a nation bidding its leader goodbye. The hills and fields and streets around north Tehran were packed with people. The helicopter banked and circled over a mottled surface of humans, all facing the place where Khomeini's body lay in a box of green glass. The glass glinted with each occasional ray of sunlight that broke through the clouds. It was early morning and the city was blanketed in its usual spotty fog. From above, the dignified mob had assembled in a quiet chaos that stretched as far as the eye could see. The heads of the women veiled in solid black were distinct from the uncovered heads of the men. Segregated by sex, the crowds of women standing together looked like vast puddles of black in a sea of bowed male heads. With its buildings jutting up into the morning air, the whole city of Tehran was marbled in a coating of black and gray, delivering the impression that an enormous swarm of motionless bees had descended over the capital in the night. The din from the helicopter drowned all of the sound from below. On cue, the mourners followed the lead of the sheik directing the service. From above, the synchronous bowing and prayer rippled in waves to the horizon.

In the middle of it all were the remains of the man who had led Iran away from an alliance with the United States and Israel to become the mortal enemy of both, and into angry isolation from much of the world. If there was a way back, Khomeini would not be leading these people. The prayer and ceremony of the funeral prolonged the moment and delayed having to think about what came next. The helicopter circled the coffin twice and made several long, steeply banked turns around the vast crowd. There was time for me to reflect on the moment of Khomeini's passing.

He took power in 1978 and had called on Iranians to rewrite their history and to invent a future where none had been before. At no time in sixteen centuries of Islamic history had the government of a major Muslim nation been completely in the hands of the clergy, though Islam is the only religion that explicitly claims to offer a blueprint for national politics. It was just one measure of the boldness and brutality with which Khomeini would confront Iran's place in time and space. He had taken power when the price of oil was at an all-time high, and when the political strength and will of the United States, which had controlled Iran's destiny for much of this century, was at an all-time low. It was a perfect moment for Iran. But under Khomeini, it was a moment squandered in lives and oil and Iranian riyals.

Iran's history on the world's stage predates Islam and Christianity. While the early Jews struggled, the Persians flourished. The Persian Empire even befriended the exiled people of Israel in a story retold in the Old Testament book of Ezra. Such ironies abound in Iran's history. The layers in its historical bedrock are distinct. There is very little that overlaps from one to the other. A new regime or movement ascending to

power in Iran repudiates and obliterates the previous regimes and out-
looks. Khomeini was no exception. Everywhere in Iran there are stun-
ning monuments and public works projects that attest to Iran's heroic
triumphs and are named for whatever historical event, religious or secu-
lar, seems convenient to those in power. The names change with the
political seasons and the successive regimes doing the naming. Reza
Square becomes Martyr's Square. The Interior Ministry becomes the Institute for Religious Guidance. The U.S. Embassy becomes "The Center
for the Study of the U.S. Espionage Den's Documents."

For more than a decade since the taking of the American hostages in
Tehran, Iran and Khomeini dared to confront a land where popular history was crystal clear, with all the annoying impurities and contradic-
tions filtered out: the United States. We were the good guys, we were
number one, we played by the rules, end of story. They were ungrateful,
uncivilized, beyond the pale, fanatical Muslim zealots gone mad with oil
money. So the question for me in the helicopter gazing down at the
millions of mourners was, who was this Oskar who had my wheelchair
somewhere below? Was he a devout, struggling Iranian anxious to enter
the future in a post-Khomeini era, or an ungrateful, fanatical, Muslim
zealot gone mad? An even better question was: which person was more
likely to return it?

Rolling the wheelchair in front of him Oskar emerged, smiling, from
the crowd as my helicopter landed. He waved off the armed security
guards who were keeping the crowds of mourners away from the reporters and rolled right up to me. I felt ashamed of having been so
nervous about my chair. Beaming with pride, Oskar looked as though he
would have faced one of Saddam's chemical weapons attacks to return it
to me. I thanked him and hopped back into the chair. Oskar shook my
hand, then turned around, making a kind of overly dramatic farewell
salute, and shouted, "Death to America, Mr. John. Nice to meet you."
The armed guards then herded him back into the teeming mass of
mourners, where he disappeared.

The place where the Ayatollah was to be buried was a large, dusty
field around which trucks had piled metal shipping containers into a
barrier to keep the place from being overrun with the millions of self-
flagellating Shiite mourners who were gathering in the noonday sun.
There was no confusion about this flight. About sixty reporters flew in
what seemed to be a very old American Chinook troop transport helicopter that might last have been serviced about the time the Shah was
overthrown, nearly a decade earlier. The Chinook lurched into the air

with all the grace of a cat climbing up a wet shower curtain. I took the wheelchair this time

As we flew to Beheshed al Zahra cemetery, we could see the roads around it clogged with every sort of vehicle as an even larger crowd than the one which had gathered for the morning prayer was now converging on the cemetery. In the distance, the dust kicked up by the feet of five million mourners walking toward Khomeini's final resting spot was visible as a yellow cloud slowly rising on a windless horizon.

The pilot attempted to get us close to the crowd of mourners, but the only safe place to set the chopper down was in a cauliflower field about 1,000 yards away from the plateau on which the cemetery stood. There were deep ridges in the field and large boulder-sized clumps of dirt everywhere. As the chopper landed, I noted the terrain with some alarm. There would be no rolling across this field. The large cargo door of the Chinook creaked open and the crowd of reporters carrying cameras, notebooks, and Ray Bans rushed out and off toward the dusty crowd of mourners. I moved my chair and backpack full of equipment slowly down toward the door. The Iranian helicopter crew saw me in the empty cargo compartment and asked why the other reporters had left me behind. It seemed like a silly question. I understood completely that they would all run away. I would not ask them for help, and they would not offer. That was the agreement, but the Iranian pilot looked shocked and concerned that I was alone, struggling to get out of the helicopter into a field I clearly couldn't roll through, while my colleagues had run away without so much as a good-bye. "They are in a hurry," I said.

Most of the crowd had not even arrived yet. Thousands of people were moving slowly across the field where we were. As I settled down into the dirt, and the pilot was considering how he was going to take off again with me sitting right next to the Chinook, a family of Iranian mourners bounded over toward the helicopter. Without a word of explanation, two of them picked me up. One person took my chair, another my equipment, and we all headed off toward the cemetery. The relieved pilots shouted good-bye and took off as soon as we were clear of the rotors.

"We will take you to Imam Khomeini, Mr. John," they shouted as we ran headlong through the field. The two men carrying me were named Saddeq and Darius, and I asked them if they were sad that Khomeini was dead. "We are not sad because Khomeini destroyed Iran. We are happy." In broken English we talked about the new president, Ali Akbar Hashemi Rafsanjani, whom that morning Tehran radio had taken to calling Ayatollah instead of Hojatolislami, a lesser designation. "It seems he has a promotion now," Darius said.

When we reached the crowd, it was possible to roll again on flat ground. I got back in my chair and rolled toward the center of the mourners, who became more passionate and emotional the closer we got to the burial site. Darius, Saddeq, and their brothers stayed with me, striding along with luminous smiles on their faces as we slowly made our way. The dense crowd moved according to its own whims, sweeping everyone into its current. There was no possibility of cutting across the flow of people. Low to the ground, I negotiated my way through the crowd as a fish might swim through thick black seaweed. A line of people would approach, pause, look startled, then part for me to roll through. The same thing would happen with the next wave. The women who saw me would pull their black shador veils more tightly around their faces, while the men just looked confused. I could see some of the other reporters off in another part of the crowd. As they were recognized as journalists, particularly if they had cameras, a crowd would gather around and begin to chant the familiar "Death to America, Death to Israel."

Darius and Saddeq quickly decided that I was not making fast enough progress toward Imam Khomeini's final resting place, and so they began to shout at people to move out of my way. Through a crowd of millions, they took it upon themselves to confront, on my behalf, the people whose pictures were just beginning to appear on Western television newscasts as the Shiite zealots who wanted to die along with their beloved Imam.

I stopped to interview some of the mourners. One woman said that she felt that Iran was alone in the world now that Khomeini was dead. She said that the war with Iraq was horrible for Iran and had killed many people she knew. "But," she said, "it was God's will." Most people I spoke with, though, believed that things would be better for Iran now that Khomeini was gone, something Darius explained to me by saying, "Khomeini was better as Imam than as President. The people know he is still Imam Khomeini here at Beheshed al Zahra." Darius pointed at the ground under his feet.

The crowd was a solid mass of people as we approached the two-tiered container walls around the burial site. Saddeq was no longer able to shout people out of my path, and from all sides they were beginning to stumble into me like falling dominos. When Darius spotted an ambulance with its red crescent painted on the side slowly making its way through the crowd, he began to point and gesticulate dramatically. I thought he was asking for directions to a clear route into the grave area. Instead, Saddeq and Darius had commandeered the ambulance. They hurried over to me, smiling broadly, and told me to hop in the back.

The sun was at its peak, beating down on several million people dressed in black, most of whom were busy working themselves into an emotional frenzy. The heat had already produced a number of truly exhausted people who I had seen being carried through the crowd. I did not need an ambulance. I came from the place Khomeini had routinely called the Great Satan, I was an infidel. I wasn't about to drive off in an ambulance meant for the fatigued and faithful among a crowd of five million Shiite mourners.

There was no arguing with Darius. He motioned for me to get in, as did Saddeq and the driver, and when I hesitated once more, the crowd around the ambulance began to insist along with them. The people were all pointing for me to go to see Imam Khomeini, and beckoning toward the ambulance. I climbed in.

From the inside of the ambulance we burrowed through the crowd, which opened before us and closed around us as we moved forward. The black of the mourning garments, the wailing of the people as we approached the grave, and the intense sun all composed the place into a lost world churning with uprooted souls on their way to somewhere else. The dust swirled and settled like parched dew until we were indistinguishable ghosts. We inched our way toward a post-apocalyptic Calvary to watch a helicopter deliver a dead god to millions of mourners who, whatever they thought of Khomeini politically, would forever measure their lives by how well they had said good-bye to him on this day.

A group of men carrying someone who appeared to have passed out from the heat came toward us. The man was semiconscious and continued to wail as he was carried. His back was drenched in sweat and blood from self-inflicted whipping. The men attempted to place him into the ambulance, but Darius told them to go away. I said it appeared that this man needed an ambulance far more than I, and that we should make room for him. "There is nothing wrong with this man," Darius said to me, as if bringing him aboard the ambulance was the silliest suggestion I could possibly make. "He is just one of the religious." He was one of the extremely devout mourners who professed their piety by reenacting, on their own bodies, the martyrdom of Husayn, maternal grandson of Muhammed, and prophet of Shi'a Islam, who died at the hands of the treacherous general Yazid at Karbala, Iraq, in the year A.D. 680. Darius and Saddeq insisted that the man not get into the ambulance, pointed to my wheelchair hanging on the tailgate, and the two mourners with him nodded and carried the wailing man back into the crowd.

More than a dozen mourners would die or be injured from such overly enthusiastic expressions of piety. Hundreds would pile into the grave along with Khomeini's body, insisting that they be buried along with him. Most of the people at the cemetery expressed a quieter reverence for the Ayatollah. They stood in the heat and watched, finding their own way to say good-bye.

"Why did you come here?" I asked Darius. "You said you were happy that Khomeini is gone."

"Yes, but there is only one Imam Khomeini," he replied. "I will miss him. All Iran will miss him."

It occurred to me that not only Iran would miss the Ayatollah. He was America's perfect bad guy, an end of the century Tojo, uncompromising and extreme. His hostage crisis was Pearl Harbor for the post-war generation. He set aside national holidays to burn American flags: "Death to America" days, he called them. He issued a commemorative stamp in English showing the taking of the American hostages, "The Takeover of the U.S. Spy Den." The stamps provoked high-level meetings at the White House, and an official U.S. policy that any mail carrying the stamps was to be refused by the U.S. Postal Service. For this reason, the stamps were not used much by Iranians, but they were a very popular item for Western reporters, who could be seen buying sheets of them at the Tehran hotels on their way to the airport.

Khomeini had bagged one American president, Jimmy Carter, and had made a run at Ronald Reagan during the Iran-Contra scandal. Khomeini seemed to me to be very much like Reagan. They both were simple, uncompromising, and capable of saying almost anything. Khomeini could call for the death of Salman Rushdie, Ronald Reagan could publicly compare nuclear war to the Book of Revelations and joke about beginning "the bombing in five minutes." Iranians thought of Khomeini as a better Messiah than a president, and for that reason he could do no real wrong. Most Americans would probably agree that Ronald Reagan did better being a movie-star father figure than he did with the mechanics of leading the United States from the White House. Like Khomeini, even Reagan's critics claimed to miss him when he was gone.

Khomeini's funeral was the people of Iran's slow return to consciousness from a national dream. Since 1989, many other nations have similarly awakened. Eastern Europe, Russia, South Africa, and the United States, perhaps last of all on the world stage, have begun to emerge from grip of the twentieth century's supposedly ironclad truths to discover that they were made out of so much gossamer thread. Swept away in the first breezes of the millennium, they have been replaced by a horizon with few recognizable landmarks.

My last image of the Beheshed al Zahra cemetery was of sitting in the crowd of mourners, watching as a helicopter made several attempts to land over the outstretched arms of thousands of wailing people. I could not see the grave, and when the helicopter dropped out of sight I could see only hundreds of dusty hands around me, all grasping at the cloudless, straw-colored sky.

Back at the hotel, many hours later, I learned what much of the world had already been told: that after making several passes over the grave, the helicopter crew carrying Khomeini's body dropped the Imam ". . . into the hands of the people," in the metaphoric words of an Iranian television commentator. I filed my stories back to NPR in Washington, where the editors were completely preoccupied with the aftermath of the Tiananmen Square massacre in Beijing. There was plenty of time for a long dinner at the hotel café.

I talked about the events of the day with an English-speaking waiter, who was most interested in hearing about what I thought of the Iranians I had met: Oskar, Darius, Saddeq, and the millions of mourners at the cemetery. I suggested that there was a chance I could have been trampled in the crowd, or attacked by grieving people who might object to an American on sacred ground, or have lost my wheelchair to Oskar during my morning helicopter ride.

The waiter was adamant that there wasn't the slightest possibility that anything like that would have happened to me under any circumstances. Especially the part about losing the wheelchair. He insisted something to the effect that if you can't trust an Iranian you have known for ten minutes on the day of Imam Khomeini's funeral with your wheelchair, then who can you trust? Who, indeed? I had to agree that he had a point.

"Mr. John, there was no problem," the waiter said. "Iran is a religious country. It is not like in New York."

Public Transit

*N*ew York was not like Iran.

It was a shock to return to the United States in 1990, where it routinely took an act of God to hail a taxi. There was nothing religious about New York City, even on Christmas Eve. I had taken a cab from midtown to Riverside Church on the west side of Manhattan only to find that my information about a Christmas Eve service there was mistaken. The church was padlocked, which I only discovered after getting out of the cab into the 40-mile-an-hour, 20-degree weather. I tried all of the doors of the church and found myself alone at close to midnight, without a taxi, on December 24 at 122nd Street and Riverside Drive.

I was wearing a wool sports jacket and a heavy scarf, but no outer jacket. There were no cars on the street. Being wrong about the service and having come all the way uptown was more than a little frustrating. I suspected that I was not in the best psychological condition to watch the usual half-dozen or so New York cabs pass me by and pretend not to see me hailing them. I knew the most important thing was to try and not look like a panhandler. This was always hard. Many times in New York I had hailed a cab only to have the driver hand me a dollar. Once I was so shocked I looked at the cabbie and said, as though I were correcting his spelling, "No, I give you the money."

"You want a ride?" he said. "Really?"

The worst were the taxis that stopped but had some idea that the wheelchair was going to put itself into the trunk. After you hopped into the backseat, these drivers would look at you as though you were trying to pull a fast one, tricking them into having to get out of their cabs and load something in the trunk that you had been cleverly hiding. Some cabbies would say that I should have brought someone with me to put the chair in, or that it was too heavy for them to lift. My favorite excuse was also the most frequent, "Look, buddy, I can't lift that chair, I have a bad back."

"I never heard of anyone who became paralyzed from lifting wheelchairs," I said. My favorite reply never helped. If the drivers would actually load the chair, you could hear them grumbling and throwing it around to get it to fit, and smashing the trunk lid down on it. When we arrived at our destination, the driver would throw the chair at me like it was a chunk of nuclear waste and hop back behind the wheel. The only thing to do in these situations was to smile, try not to get into a fight, and hope the anger would subside quickly so you could make it wherever you were going without having a meltdown.

There were some drivers who wouldn't load the chair at all. For these people, at one time I carried a Swiss army knife. The rule was, if I had to get back out of a cab because a driver wouldn't load my chair, then I would give the driver a reason to get out of his cab shortly after I was gone. I would use the small blade of the knife to puncture a rear tire before the cab drove away, then hail another one. A few blocks ahead, when the first driver had discovered his difficulties, he was generally looking in his trunk for the tire jack when I passed by, waving.

The trouble with this idea was that other people often did not have the same righteous attitude that I did about tire puncturing in Manhattan traffic, and using knives to get freelance revenge in New York City under any circumstances. Most of my friends put me in the same league with subway vigilante Bernhard Goetz and concluded that I needed serious help. So I had stopped using the Swiss army knife and was without it that Christmas Eve on 122nd and Riverside Drive.

The first cab drove toward me and slowed down; the driver stared, then quickly drove by. A second cab approached. I motioned emphatically. I smiled and tried to look as credible as I could. Out in this December wind I was just another invisible particle of New York misery. The driver of a second cab shook his head as he passed with the lame, catch-all apologetic look New York cabbies use to say, "No way, Mac. Sorry, no way I can take you."

I had one advantage. At least I was white. Black males in New York

City have to watch at least as many cabs go by as someone in a wheel-chair does before getting a ride. Black male friends of mine say they consciously have to rely on their ritzy trench coats or conservative "Real Job" suits to counter skin color in catching a cab. If I could look more white than crippled, I might not freeze to death on Christmas Eve. I was a psychotic, twentieth-century hit man named Tiny Tim, imagining all sorts of gory ways of knocking off a cabbie named Scrooge. The wind was blowing furiously off the Hudson, right up over Riverside Drive.

A third cab drove by. I wondered if I could force a cab to stop by blocking the road. I wished I had a baseball bat. For a period of a few minutes, there was no traffic. I turned and began to roll down Riverside. After a block I turned around, and there was one more empty cab in the right lane coming toward me. I raised my hand. I was sitting directly under a streetlight. The cabbie clearly saw me, abruptly veered left into the turn lane, and sat there, signaling at the red light.

I rolled over to his cab and knocked on the window. "Can you take a fare?" The driver was pretending I had just landed there from space, but I was freezing and needed a ride, so I tried not to look disgusted. He nodded with all of the enthusiasm of someone with an abscessed tooth. I opened the door and hopped onto the backseat. I folded the chair and asked him to open the trunk of his cab.

"Why you want me to do that?" he said.

"Put the chair in the trunk, please." I was half-sitting in the cab, my legs still outside. The door was open and the wheelchair folded next to the cab. "No way, man." he said. "I'm not going to do that. It's too damn cold." I was supposed to understand that I would now simply thank him for his trouble, get back in my wheelchair, and wait for another cab.

"Just put the chair in the trunk right now. It's Christmas Eve, pal, why don't you just pretend to be Santa for five fucking minutes." His smile vanished. I had crossed a line by being angry. But he also looked re-lieved, as though now he could refuse me in good conscience. It was all on his face. "You're crazy, man. I don't have to do nothing for you." I looked at him once more and said, "If you make me get back into this chair you are going to be very sorry." It was a moment of visceral anger. There was no turning back now. "Go away, man. It's too cold."

I got back into the chair. I placed my backpack with my wallet in it on the back of my chair for safekeeping. I grabbed his door, and with all of my strength pushed it back on its hinges until I heard a loud snap. It was now jammed open. I rolled over to his passenger window, and with two insane jabs of my right fist I shattered it. I rolled around to the front of the cab, and with my fist in my white handball glove took out first one, then the other, headlight. The light I was bathed in from the front of the cab vanished. The face of the driver could now be seen clearly, illuminated from the dashboard's glow.

I could hear myself screaming at him in a voice that sounded far away. I knew the voice, but the person it belonged to was an intruder in this place. He had nothing to do with this particular cabbie and his stupid, callous, insensitivity; rather, he was the overlord to all such incidents that had come before. Whenever the gauntlet was dropped, it was this interior soul, with that screaming voice and those hands, who felt no pain and who surfed down a wave of hatred to settle the score. This soul had done the arithmetic, and chosen the weapons. I would have to live with the consequences.

I rolled over to the driver's side and grabbed the window next to his face. I could see that he was absolutely terrified. It made me want to torture him. I hungered for his fear; I wanted to feel his presumptions of power and physical superiority in my hands as he sank up to his neck in my rage, my fists closed around his throat. I attacked his half-open window. It cracked, and as I hauled my arm back to finish it, I saw large drops of blood on the driver's face. I looked at him closely. He was paralyzed with fear and spattered with blood. There was blood on his window, as well. A voice inside me screamed, "I didn't touch you, motherfucker. You're not bleeding, Don't say that I made you bleed. You fucking bastard. Don't you dare bleed!"

I rolled back from the cab. It was my own blood shooting from my thumb. It gushed over the white leather of my gloves: I had busted an artery at the base of my thumb, but I couldn't see it because it was inside the glove. Whatever had sliced my thumb had gone neatly through the leather first, and as I rolled down the street I could hear the cabbie saying behind me, "You're crazy, man, you're fucking crazy." I rolled underneath a streetlamp to get a closer look. It was my left hand, and it had several lacerations in addition to the one at the base of my thumb. It must have been the headlight glass. The blood continued to gush. Wind blew it off my fingers in festive red droplets, which landed stiffly on the frozen pavement under the streetlamp. Merry Christmas.

Up the street, a police squad car had stopped next to the cab, which still had its right rear door jammed open. I coasted farther down the street to see if I could roll the rest of the way home. With each push of my hand on the rim of my chair, blood squirted out of my glove. I could feel it filled with blood inside. The cops pulled up behind me. "Would you like us to arrest that cabbie? Did he attack you?" All I could think of was the indignity of being attacked by him. I thought about screaming, "That piece of human garbage attacked me? No way. Maybe it was me who attacked him as a public service. Did you donut eaters ever think of that? I could have killed the bastard. I *was* trying to kill him, in fact. I insist that you arrest me for attempted murder right now, or I will sue the NYPD under the Americans with Disabilities Act." I thought better of this speech. Intense pain had returned my mind to practical matters. Spending the night in jail for assaulting a cabbie after bragging about it while bleeding to death seemed like a poor way to cap off an already less than stellar Christmas Eve.

"Everything's fine, officer. I'll just get another taxi." I continued to roll one-handed and dripping down Riverside Drive. The cops went back to talk to the cabbie, who was screaming now. I began to worry that he was going to have me arrested, but the cops drove back again. Once more the officer asked if I wanted to file a complaint against the cabbie. As more blood dripped off my barely white glove, the officers suggested that I go to the hospital. They had figured out what had happened. As I started to explain, they told me to get in the squad car. "Let's just say it was an unfortunate accident," one officer said. "I think you gave that driver something to think about tonight. I don't think he'll ever stop for someone in a wheelchair again. If we can get you to the emergency room in time, maybe you won't lose your thumb."

I got in the backseat while the cops put the chair in the trunk. Seven blocks away was the emergency room of St. Luke's Hospital. Christmas Eve services at St. Luke's included treatment of a young woman's mild drug overdose. An elderly man and his worried-looking wife were in a corner of the treatment room. His own scared face looked out from beneath a green plastic oxygen mask. A number of men stood around watching CNN on the waiting-room TV. A woman had been brought in with fairly suspicious looking bruises on her face and arms. One arm was broken and being set in a cast. She sat quietly while two men talked about football in loud voices. The forlorn Christmas decorations added to the hopelessness of this little band of unfortunates in the emergency room.

When I arrived, everything stopped. Police officers were always an object of curiosity, signaling the arrival of a shooting victim or something more spectacular. For a Christmas Eve, the gushing artery at the base of my thumb was spectacular enough. The men sitting around the emergency room shook their heads. The overdose patient with the sunken cocaine eyes staggered over to inspect the evening's best carnage. "Where did you get that wheelchair?" She looked around as though she was familiar with all of the wheelchairs in this emergency room from previous visits. "It's my own." I replied. "That's a good idea," she said. "Why didn't I think of that?"

I got nine stitches from a doctor who suggested politely that whatever my complaint with the taxi driver, I was one person on the planet who could ill afford to lose a thumb. The deep laceration was just a few millimeters from the nerve and was just as close to the tendon. Severing either one would have added my thumb to an already ample chorus of numbness and paralysis. The thought of losing the use of my thumb was one thing, but what was really disturbing was the thought of its isolation on my hand, numb in the wrong zone. Trapped on a functional hand, a numb and paralyzed thumb would have no way of communicating with my numb and paralyzed feet. It would be not only paralyzed, it would be in exile: an invader behind enemy lines, stuck across the checkpoint on my chest.

Today there is a one-inch scar that traces a half circle just to the left of my knuckle. The gloves were a total loss, but they no doubt saved my thumb. Nothing could save my pride, but pride is not always salvageable in New York City. I have taken thousands of cabs, and in each case the business of loading and unloading delivers some small verdict on human nature. Often it is a verdict I am in no mood to hear, as was the case on that Christmas Eve. At other times the experience is eerie and sublime. At the very least, there is the possibility that I will make a connection with a person, not just stare at the back of an anonymous head.

In my life, cabbies distinguish themselves by being either very rude and unhelpful or sympathetic and righteous. Mahmoud Abu Holima was one of the latter. It was his freckles I remembered, along with his schoolboy nose and reddish-blond hair that made his Islamic tirades more memorable. He was not swarthy like other Middle Eastern cabbies. He had a squeaky, raspy voice. He drove like a power tool carving Styrofoam. He used his horn a lot. He made constant references to the idiots he said were all around him.

He was like a lot of other New York cabbies. But out of a sea of midtown yellow, Mahmoud Abu Holima was the one who stopped one afternoon in 1990, and by stopping for me he wanted to make it clear to everyone that he was not stopping for anyone else, especially the people in expensive-looking suits waiting on the same street corner I was. His decision to pick me up was part of some protest Mahmoud delivered to America every day he drove the streets of Manhattan.

His cab seemed to have little to do with transporting people from place to place. It was more like an Islamic institute on wheels. A voice in Arabic blared from his cassette player. His front seat was piled with books in Arabic and more cassettes. Some of the books were dog-eared Korans. There were many uniformly bound blue and green books open, marked and stacked in cross-referenced chaos, the arcane and passionate academic studies of a Muslim cabbie studying hard to get ahead and lose his day job, interrupting his studies in mid-sentence to pick up a man in a wheelchair.

I took two rides with him. The first time I was going somewhere uptown on Third Avenue. Four cabs had passed me by. He stopped. He put the chair in the trunk, and to make more space there, brought stacks of Arabic books from the trunk into the front seat. He wore a large, knit, dirty-white skullcap and was in constant motion. He seemed lost in the ideas he had been reading about before I got in. At traffic lights he would read. As he drove, he continually turned away from the windshield to make eye contact with me. His voice careened from a conversation to a lecture, like his driving. He ignored what was going on around him on the street. He told me he thought my wheelchair was unusually light. He said he knew many boys with no legs who could use such a chair. There were no good wheelchairs in Afghanistan.

"Afghanistan, you know about the war in Afghanistan?" he asked.

I said I knew about it. He said he wasn't talking about the Soviet invasion of Afghanistan and the American efforts to see that the Soviets were defeated. He said that the war was really a religious war. "It is the war for Islam." On a lark, in my broken rudimentary Arabic, I asked him where he was from. He turned around, abruptly, and asked, "Where did you learn Arabic?" I told him that I had learned it from living in the Middle East. I apologized for speaking so poorly. He laughed and said that my accent was good, but that non-Muslims in America can't speak Arabic unless they are spies. "Only the Zionists really know how to speak," he said, his voice spitting with hatred.

I thanked him for picking me up. He removed my chair from his trunk, and as I hopped back into it I explained to him that it was difficult sometimes to get a cab in New York. He said that being in America was like being in a war where there are only weapons, no people. "In Islam," he said, "the people are the weapons."

"Why are you here?" I asked him.

"I have kids, family." He smiled once, and the freckles wrinkled on his nose and face, making him look like Tom Sawyer in a Muslim prayer cap. The scowl returned as he drove away. He turned up the cassette. The Arabic voice was still audible a block away.

The second time I saw him I remembered him and he remembered me. He had no cassettes this time. There were no books in the car, and there was plenty of room in the trunk for my chair this time. Where were all of the books? He said he had finished studying. I asked him about peace in Afghanistan and the fact that Iran and Iraq were no longer at war. He said something about Saddam Hussein I didn't catch, and then he laughed. He seemed less nervous but still had the good-natured intensity I remembered from before. "Are you from Iran?" I asked him, and this time he answered. He told me he was from Egypt. He asked me if I knew about the war in Egypt, and I told him I didn't.

Before he let me off he said that he wanted me to know that America would lose the war against Islam. He said that we won't know when we have lost. "Americans never say anything that's important." He looked out the window. His face did not express hatred as much as disappointment. He shook his head. "It is quiet now."

He ran a red light and parked squarely in the middle of an intersection, stopping traffic to let me out. Cars honked and people yelled as I got into the wheelchair. He scowled at them and laughed. I laughed too. I think I said to him, "Salaam," the Arabic word for peace and good-bye. He said something that sounded like *"Mish Salaam fi Amerika,"* no peace in America. Then he said the word "Sa'at." In Arabic it means difficult. He got into his cab, smiled, and drove away. On February 26, 1993, cabbie, student of Islam, and family man Mahmoud Abu Holima, along with several others, planted the bomb that blew up the World Trade Center. Today he is serving a life sentence in a New York prison.

If you use a wheelchair and you want to avoid cabs in New York City, you can pay ten thousand dollars a year in parking to have your own car, or you can try your luck at public transit. There are para-transit wheelchair vans which are bookable far in advance. Then there is the subway, which has only twenty elevator sites out of hundreds of stations. And there are the buses.

The buses in New York have wheelchair lifts, and if the driver is carrying a key to operate the lift, and the lift has been serviced recently, and the bus is not too crowded, and the driver notices you at the stop, then you have a chance of getting a ride. Because the fare box is at the front of the bus and the lift is at the back, you can ask the driver to put your bus token into the box, but he will refuse. "I'm not allowed to touch your money," is what they usually say, and so they hand you instead a self-addressed stamped envelope for you to mail a check for a dollar and twenty-five cents to the Transit Authority. The bus lifts are better than nothing, except that when the city buys new buses, the new wheelchair lifts don't work properly, so there is a period of months when a bus drives up and the driver shrugs and says that his bus is one of the new ones. Only in New York would the new buses be the ones you can count on not to work.

Attempting to use public transit involves taking the risk of finding no bus lift, no elevator, or that either one will stop working while you are in the middle of using it. The transit system in New York sometimes seems like an elaborate trap for people in wheelchairs, lured like mice to cheese with promises of accessible transportation. For years, in New York's Herald Square there were signs indicating an accessible subway station with an elevator. The space for the elevator was a large cube covered with plywood that looked as though it hadn't been disturbed for years. Wheelchair signs had arrived before the elevators, but that didn't keep the Transit Authority from putting the signs up even when there was no way to use the train at this stop. While they waited for the long-delayed elevator, the Transit Authority covered the little wheelchair symbols on the Herald Square subway station to prevent confusion. To-day the elevator works, but the signs for it are still covered. The Transit Authority apparently wants it to be a surprise.

When I returned to New York City from the Middle East in 1990, I lived in Brooklyn, just two blocks from the Carroll Street subway stop on the F train. It was not accessible, and as there appeared to be no plans to make it so, I didn't think much about the station. When I wanted to go into Manhattan I would take a taxi, or I would roll up Court Street to the walkway entrance to the Brooklyn Bridge and fly into the city on a ribbon of oak planks suspended from the bridge's webs of cable that appeared from my wheelchair to be woven into the sky itself. Looking down, I could see the East River through my wheelchair's spokes. Look-ing up, I saw the clouds through the spokes of the bridge. The bridge was made for me and me for the bridge. It was always an uncommon moment of physical integrity with the city that ended when I came to rest at the traffic light on Chambers Street, next to City Hall.

It was while rolling across the bridge one day that I remembered my promise to Donna, my physical therapist, and how I would one day ride the rapid transit trains in Chicago. Pumping my arms up the incline of the bridge toward Manhattan and then coasting down the other side in 1990, I imagined that I would be able physically to accomplish every-thing I had theorized about the subway in Chicago in those first days of being a paraplegic back in 1976. In the Middle East I had climbed many stairways and hauled myself and the chair across many filthy floors on my way to interviews, apartments, and news conferences. I had also lost my fear of humiliation from living and working there. I was even intrigued with the idea of taking the train during the peak of rush hour when the greatest number of people of all kinds would be underground with me.

I would do it just the way I had told Donna back in the rehab hospital. But this time I would wire myself with a microphone and a miniature cassette machine to record everything that happened along the way. Testing my old theory might make a good commentary for an upcoming NPR radio program about inaccessibility. Between the Carroll Street station and City Hall there were stairs leading in and out of the stations as well as to transfer from one line to another inside the larger stations. To get to Brooklyn Bridge/City Hall, I would make two transfers, from the F to the A, then from the A to the 5, a total of nearly 150 stairs.

I rolled up to the Brooklyn Carroll Street stop on the F train carrying a rope, a backpack, and wired for sound. Like most of the other people on the train that morning I was on my way to work. Taking the subway was how most people crossed the East River, but it would have been hard to come up with a less practical way, short of swimming, for a paraplegic to cover the same distance. Fortunately I had the entire morning to kill. I was confident that I had the strength for it, and unless I ended up on the tracks, I felt sure that I could get out of any predicament I found myself in, but I was prepared for things to be more complicated. As usual, trouble would make the story more interesting.

The Carroll Street subway station has two staircases. One leads to the token booth, where the fare is paid by the turnstiles at the track entrance, the other one goes directly down to the tracks. Near the entrance is a newsstand. As I rolled to the top of the stairs, the man behind the counter watched me closely and the people standing around the newsstand stopped talking. I quickly climbed out of my chair and down onto the top step.

I folded my chair and tied the length of rope around it, attaching the end to my wrist. I moved down to the second step and began to lower the folded chair down the steps to the bottom. It took just a moment. Then, one at a time, I descended the first flight of stairs with my backpack and seat cushion in my lap until I reached a foul-smelling landing below street level. I was on my way. I looked up. The people at the newsstand who had been peering sheepishly down at me looked away. All around me, crowds of commuters with briefcases and headphones walked by, stepping around me without breaking stride. If I had worried about anything associated with this venture it was that I would just be in the way, but just as on that day under curfew in Gaza, I was invisible.

I slid across the floor to the next flight of stairs, and the commuters arriving at the station now came upon me suddenly from around a corner. Still, they expressed no surprise and neatly moved over to form an orderly lane on the side of the landing opposite me as I lowered my chair once again to the bottom of the stairs where the token booth was.

With an elastic cord around my legs to keep them together and more easily moved (an innovation I hadn't thought of back in rehab), I continued down the stairs, two steps at a time, reaching the chair at the bottom of the steps. I stood it up, unfolded it, and did a two-armed, from-the-floor lift back onto the seat. My head rose out of the sea of commuter legs, and I took my place in the subway token line.

"You know, you get half-price," the tinny voice through the bullet-proof glass told me, as though this were compensation for the slight inconvenience of having no ramp or elevator. There next to his piles of tokens the operator had a stack of official half-price certificates for disabled users. He seemed thrilled to have a chance to use them. "No, thanks, the tokens are fine." I bought two, rolled through the rickety gate next to the turnstiles and to the head of the next set of stairs. I could hear the trains rumbling below.

I got down on the floor again, and began lowering the chair. I realized that getting the chair back up again was not going to be as simple as this lowering maneuver. Most of my old theory about riding the trains in Chicago had pertained to getting up to the tracks, because the Chicago trains are elevated. Down was going well, as I expected, but up might be more difficult.

Around me walked the stream of oblivious commuters. Underneath their feet, the paper cups and straws and various other bits of refuse they dropped were too soiled by black subway filth to be recognizable as having any connection at all to their world above. Down on the subway floor they seemed evil, straws that could only have hung from diseased lips, plastic spoons that could never have carried anything edible. Horrid puddles of liquid were swirled with chemical colors, sinister black mirrors in which the bottoms of briefcases sailed safely overhead like rectangular airships. I was freshly showered, with clean white gloves and black jeans, but in the reflection of one of these puddles I too looked as foul and discarded as the soda straws and crack vials. I looked up at the people walking by, stepping around me, or watching me in their peripheral vision. By virtue of the fact that my body and clothes were in contact with places they feared to touch, they saw and feared me much as they might fear sudden assault by a mugger. I was just like the refuse, irretrievable, present only as a creature dwelling on the rusty edge of a dark drain. By stepping around me as I slid, two steps at a time down toward the tracks, they created a quarantined space, just for me, where even the air seemed depraved.

I rolled to the platform to wait for the train with the other commuters. I could make eye contact again. Some of the faces betrayed that they had seen me on the stairs by showing relief that I had not been stuck, or worse, living there. The details they were too afraid to glean back there by pausing to investigate, they were happy to take now as a happy ending which got them off the hook. They had been curious as long as they didn't have to act on what they learned. As long as they didn't have to act, they could stare.

I had a speech all prepared for the moment anyone asked if I needed help. I felt a twinge of satisfaction over having made it to the tracks without having to give it. My old theory, concocted while on painkillers in an intensive care unit in Pennsylvania, had predicted that I would make it. I was happy to do it all by myself. Yet I hadn't counted on being completely ignored. New York was such a far cry from the streets of Jerusalem, where Israelis would come right up to ask you how much you wanted for your wheelchair, and Arabs would insist on carrying you up a flight of stairs whether you wanted to go or not.

I took the F train to the Jay Street-Borough Hall station. The train ride was exhilarating. I had a dumb smile on my face as I realized that the last subway ride I had taken was in February 1976, when I went from Garfield on the Dan Ryan train in Chicago to Irving Park on the north side to visit a friend. The Chicago trains had a green ambient light from the reflection off the industrial paint on all the interior surfaces. The New York trains were full of yellows and oranges. But the motion and sound of the train was familiar. The experience was completely new and just as completely nostalgic.

The Jay Street station was a warren of tunnels and passageways with steps in all of them. To get to the A train track for the ride into Manhattan I had to descend a flight of stairs to the sub-platform; then, depending on which direction I was going, ascend another stairway to the tracks. Because it was a junction for three subway lines, there was a mix of people rushing through the station in all directions, rather than the clockwork march of white office-garbed commuters from Brooklyn Heights and Carroll Gardens on their way to midtown.

I rolled to the stairs and descended into a corridor crowded with people coming and going. "Are you all right?" A black lady stopped next to my chair. She was pushing a stroller with two seats, one occupied by a little girl, the other empty, presumably for the little boy with her, who was standing next to a larger boy. They all beamed at me, waiting for further orders from Mom.

"I'm going down to the A train," I said. "I think I'll be all right, if I don't get lost."

"You sure you want to go down there?" She sounded as if she was warning me about something. "I know all the elevators from having these kids," she said. "They ain't no elevator on the A train, young man." Her kids looked down at me as if to say, "What can you say to that?" I told her that I knew there was no elevator, and that I was just seeing how many stairs there were between Carroll Street and City Hall. "I can tell you, they's lots of stairs." As she said good-bye, her oldest boy looked down at me as if he understood exactly what I was doing, and why. "Elevators smell nasty," he said.

Once on the A train I discovered at the next stop that I had chosen the wrong side of the platform and was going away from Manhattan. If my physical therapist, Donna, could look in on me at this point in my trip, she might be a bit more doubtful about my theory than I was. By taking the wrong train I had probably doubled the number of stairs I would have to climb.

I wondered if I could find a station not too far out where the platform was between the tracks, so that all I had to do was roll to the other side and catch the inbound train. The subway maps gave no indication of this, and the commuters I attempted to query on the subject simply ignored me or seemed not to understand what I was asking. Another black lady with a large shopping bag and a brown polka-dotted dress sitting in a seat across the car volunteered that Franklin Avenue was the station I wanted. "No stairs there," she said.

At this point, every white person I had encountered had ignored me or pretended that I didn't exist, while every black person who came upon me had offered to help without being asked. I looked at the tape recorder in my jacket to see if it was running. It was awfully noisy in the subway, but if any voices at all were recorded, this radio program was going to be more about race than it was about wheelchair accessibility. It was the first moment that I suspected the two were deeply related in ways I have had many occasions to think about since.

At Franklin Avenue I crossed the tracks and changed direction, feeling for the first time that I was a part of the vast wave of migration in and out of a Manhattan that produced the subway, all the famous bridges, and a major broadcast industry in traffic reporting complete with net-work rivals and local personalities who have added words like rubbernecking to the language. I rolled across the platform like any other citizen and onto the train with ease. As we pulled away from the station, I thought how much it would truly change my life if there was a way around the stairs, and I could actually board the subway anywhere without having to be Sir Edmund Hillary.

The incoming trains were more crowded in the last minutes of the morning rush, and back at the Jay Street station there was a roar of people rushing to catch that lucky train that might make them not late after all. As I was sliding my folded chair toward the steps down to the platform, a young black man with a backward baseball cap walked right up to me out of the crowds. "I can carry the chair, man," he said. "Just tell me where you want me to set it back up." I looked at him. He was thin and energetic, and his suggestion was completely sensible. I didn't feel like giving him my speech about how I didn't need any help. "Take it to the Manhattan-bound A train," I said. "I'll be right behind you."

One train went by in the time it took to get up the flight of stairs, but going up was still much easier than I had imagined. My legs dragged along cooperatively just as my theory had predicted. At trackside, the boy with my chair had unfolded it and was sitting in it, trying to balance on two wheels. A friend of his, he explained, could do wheelies ever since he had been shot in the back during a gang shooting. "Your chair has those big-ass wheels," he said, commenting on the large-diameter bicycle wheels I used, as if to explain why he was having some trouble keeping his balance. "I never seen those kinda wheels," he said as I hopped back into the chair.

As the train approached, he asked me for some cash. I thought that I must be some kind of idiot to go through all this and end up spending more to get into Manhattan than anyone else on the subway that day. The smallest bill I had was a five. I handed it over to him and boarded the train, laughing to myself at the absolute absurdity of it all. When I looked up, I could see commuters looking up from their newspapers. They cautiously regarded my laughing, as though I had just come from a rubber room at Bellevue Hospital. I let out a loud, demented shriek, opening my eyes as wide as I could. The heads bobbed quickly back behind the newsprint.

On the last flight of stairs leading onto City Hall Plaza at Centre Street and Chambers, the commuters in suits poured into the passageway from six trains. There was not a lot of space, and people began to trip over me. One gray-suited man in headphones carrying a gym bag nearly fell down, but he caught himself and swore as he scrambled up to street level, stepping on one of my hands in the process. A tall black man in a suit holding his own gym bag picked up my chair and started to carry it up the stairs. In a dignified voice he said, "I know you're okay, right?" I nodded.

Behind him a Puerto Rican mother with two identically dressed daughters in fluffy flowered skirts with full slips holding corsages offered to take my backpack and cushion up to the top so that I could haul myself without worrying about keeping track of the loose things. At the top, as I unfolded the wheelchair, the mother told me that she was on her way to get married at the Manhattan municipal building. Her two daughters were bridesmaids. She said she was going to put on her wedding dress, which she had in her gym bag, in the ladies' room before the ceremony. I wished her good luck and hopped back up into the chair as the commuters streamed by. It was a familiar place, the same spot I always rolled to so effortlessly off the Brooklyn Bridge.

I turned to roll away and noticed that the two little girls had come back. In unison they said, "We will pray for Jesus to bring back your legs, mister." "Thank you," I said. As though I had just given them each a shiny new quarter, they ran back to their mother, who was waiting for them with her hand outstretched to take them across busy Centre Street. It was not the sort of thing I ever cared to hear people say, but after the ordeal of the subway, and the icy silence of what had seemed like every white person I met, I didn't mind at all. For once, I looked forward to riding home in a cab.

Since 1976 I had imagined the trip on the subway. I knew it was possible, while my physical therapist back in Michigan had known it would be utterly impractical as a form of transportation. We were both right, but neither of us could have imagined the America I found down there. The New York subway required only a token to ride, but on each person's face was the ticket to where they were all really going, the places they thought they never had to leave, the people they thought they never had to notice, or stop and apologize to for stepping on them. Without knowing it, I had left that America behind long ago. I discovered it alive and well on the F train.

Sealed Rooms

*T*here was never a moment during the two years I spent in the Middle East when I wasn't convinced that everyone was going to make it to ground zero while I was trapped in the men's room, or stuck in sand, at the bottom of stairs, or in an elevator. When I returned to the region at the end of 1990 to cover the war with Iraq, all of those same fears returned. But the Gulf War put this same competitive dementia and fear of failure into much of the world press corps. In the days before the United Nations deadline for Iraq to withdraw from Kuwait, my most familiar anxiety was also afflicting most of my colleagues.

During wartime, journalists become possessed with the overriding paranoia that they are missing the story; this was nowhere more true than in the Middle East in January 1991. In the hotel coffee shops and press briefing rooms, from Dhahran, Saudi Arabia, to Baghdad, Amman, and the lobby of the Tel Aviv Hilton, reporters sat around watching each other leaving and arriving, all the time wondering if they were talking to the wrong people, if they were going to be the last to find out, or be looking the wrong way when whatever was supposed to happen, happened.

One of the great myths about war is that there is a ground zero, a center stage, where the terrible forces unleashed by it can be witnessed, recounted, and replayed like the launching of a rocket. War is a human

activity far too large to be contained in the experience of a single reporter in a single place and time in any meaningful way. When war
comes, it happens to everyone. Everything is in its path. Yet this is the
allure of war reporting, the chance of acquiring some personal mother
lode of truth to beam back to the living rooms of a waiting nation. The
fear that comes from reporting on a war is as much a fear of missing
this mother lode as it is of being injured or killed in battle, and it sets
reporters apart from the people who have to fight wars. Soldiers have
their own agonies to think about as a battle approaches. Missing the war
is not generally one of them.

Because simply removing Saddam from Kuwait was too prosaic a reason to mobilize the entire free world, George Bush inaugurated the
New World Order and openly declared that the Gulf War was an opportunity for America to put something called "the Vietnam syndrome" to
rest once and for all. "This will not be another Vietnam." At the very
least, the American reporters who were in a frenzy to be there at the
moment of destiny in Kuwait, Saudi Arabia, and Baghdad were counting
on another Vietnam. The war was an opportunity for the "Live at Five"
generation of journalists to show their Vietnam-era elders that they had
no monopoly on journalism's oak-leaf clusters.

The Vietnam story had also started out as something of a generational
marker for the journalists raised on World War Two in the era of Edward R. Murrow and the younger men and women of the fifties and
sixties. The reporters remembered today for their coverage of Vietnam
did more than just show up. They may have begun by telling the story
of the heroic rescue of a regime in Saigon from the forces of global
communism, but they ended up telling the American people a different
story, about the fall of regimes in Laos and Cambodia, and the slow,
methodical assault on the people of Vietnam as a way of bringing down
the regime in Hanoi. To tell that story, those same reporters would take
on the combat generals in Saigon, the military planners in the Pentagon,
and the regime in the White House.

There was little challenging of military assumptions in Kuwait and
Iraq. The Gulf War was more like Vietnam than even the Vietnam War.
It was alleged to be surgical. It produced overwhelming devastation. It
rendered the enemy invisible except through the gun sights. It was followed by chaos and slaughter in Kurdistan and southern Iraq on the
order of, if not the scale of, Cambodia's genocide after the U.S. with-
drawal from Indochina. The people of Iraq lived through an incendiary
horror while American politicians, generals, and reporters speculated
about the mind of Saddam, about tactics, strategy, and technology. They

obsessed about their careers. The only ones who really knew what was going to happen during the second Persian Gulf War were Norman, Colin, Saddam, George, and possibly the Mossad. The rest of us would just have to wait and pay attention.

Unlike my first trip to the region two years before, when I had no idea what to expect, in late 1990 I thought I knew how to make things work for me in the Middle East. Though I had grave reservations about the morality of the war, I was determined to cover it on the same terms as any other reporter. To have any chance of challenging the premise of Desert Storm, I would have to find my way to its mythical center, and whatever it took to get there I would do. The possibility of proving to all the world it could be done from a wheelchair was most tantalizing of all. I was not moved by the idea of walking the corridors of military history to witness unimaginable brutality, heroism, and the terror of wagering everything to get the story. I was moved by deeper forces that were known only to me, and they had little to do with the war and the people who would die because of it. I wanted to go to Baghdad for my own reasons. It was a question of editorial balance, I argued to my editors, having learned long ago not to mention wheelchairs to them. We had so many people stationed on the Saudi side of the war, I told them. NPR listeners would expect us, above all, to be broadcasting from Baghdad.

"We can't guarantee your safety in Iraq, John," said an editor. I had gone to a lot of completely insane places for NPR and had never heard about this safety guarantee before. The foreign desk was also concerned that other news agencies were leaving Iraq. The White House had said that reporters in Baghdad were in "grave danger."

"Since when has NPR guaranteed my safety or anyone else's?" I queried the foreign desk. "We do the story and take our chances. If I get in trouble," I told NPR, "I don't expect you to launch a cruise missile to save me."

"Would you like to go to Saudi Arabia?" an editor asked.

"Baghdad," I said, knowing that at this late date the possibility of obtaining passage to Baghdad was going to be expensive, extremely hard to arrange, and unless I had an Iraqi visa, impossible.

"We'll start you out in Israel," the senior foreign desk editor, Cadi Simon, suggested. "Then we'll see about Baghdad." Cadi had held her breath hundreds of times, worrying about me on deadline. She had been the calm voice on the Washington end of many calls that originated in chaotic, violent places where no one expected me to arrive, let alone file from. She would always scold me for making her worry, and then, over the phone, I would hear her turn to the producers waiting with her to learn if there would be a story that night, and dismiss them. Her voice beaming with pride and intensity, Cadi would say, "Of course there will be a story," hiding her doubts and mine. "John will be filing in ten minutes."

"Good luck," she said to me, and then shutting the door to her office she confided, "I feel better knowing you will be there." Cadi was herself an Israeli who had become a U.S. citizen. Her mother was still in Israel. She was sparse with praise, but when she delivered it, you could count on it making more than just your day. As a taskmaster, Cadi was someone who could make you mad enough to throw a phone across a room, but she was also the kind of editor you would die for without a second thought.

Israel looked to be far from the center of Desert Storm in the hours leading up to the United Nations deadline, but I much preferred Tel Aviv to Saudi Arabia. It was a short drive to Jordan, where passage could be booked to Baghdad overland from the northwest. After the war started, there would be only one way to get to Baghdad from Dhahran, Saudi Arabia, and that was straight through the front lines. Israel seemed to be a better place to start from.

Relatively fresh from my experience in the New York subway and having had a sobering experience of accessibility, American-style, in my few months home, my assumption was that in the middle of an all-out war the Americans were going to be the last people in the world to care about my physical problems covering Desert Storm. I knew people in Israel who would help me. I also had good friends in Jordan and Egypt. My best friends in the press corps were in Baghdad. I would take my chances with them rather than stand in line with the hordes of newly deputized Middle East experts who had descended on Saudi Arabia hoping for the official Pentagon-eye view of the coming battle. The war they would analyze for so many earthshaking global implications would quietly produce thousands of paraplegics, quadriplegics, and amputees. Nobody was going to waste their time on a disabled reporter.

Israel approached the war with an eerie unreality. Saddam's bellicose rhetoric threatening to set Israel on fire was laughable, but it made its point. Shortly after arriving, I went to see a young Israeli boy I knew to get his impressions of the impending war. In the two years since I had first met him, Avi Koolik's little-boy voice had acquired the raspy honks and squeaks of early adolescence. In the Israel he knew, "Peace is never coming, and war is never coming," he had told me. Now everything seemed to be changing, and when he thought about what might happen to him if the war came to Israel, he sounded like a young man nervous about going to a school dance. "I'm very afraid," he said. "This is only my first war, you know."

War was a historical reality for every generation of Israelis, but the possibility of a chemical attack hit close to an old nightmare for twentieth-century Jews. The gas mask demonstration videos that played on Israeli TV leading up to the war were profoundly unsettling. Their matter-of-fact tone only made the unstated Holocaust imagery that much more vivid. For weeks before the first air raids, newly arrived Soviet immigrants stood in line at Israel's Ben-Gurion Airport to receive government-supplied gas masks and so-called "countermeasures" that came in a little box covered with Hebrew lettering.

Iraq had access to cold–war era nerve gas and World War One vintage chemical agents, including mustard gas, and the Hebrew instructions indicated what to do in case of either. The mask would work for mustard gas, while the hypodermic antidote injected into the blood would be the response in case of nerve gas. The masks had labels and instructions but the gas, if it came, would have neither. Uncertainty quieted voices and softened faces into a calm, almost desperate attentiveness in the echo-filled hall at Ben-Gurion Airport. They recalled the grim, gray huddles of men, women, and children in the photo record of the Polish ghetto facing Hitler in the thirties.

Even as gas masks were being handed out, the likelihood of Iraq being able to deliver a chemical warhead over the 600 miles between Baghdad and Tel Aviv seemed, by all reasoning, to be extremely small. There was no evidence that Saddam had the ability to keep fragile chemical agents intact over the rough ride and extreme temperatures of a missile trajectory. There was also no evidence that he could detonate a chemical warhead in the air and spread the poison over a wide area. Chemical weapons launched into the dirt kill plants and livestock. Only a precise detonation over a populated area delivers the lethality advertised in chemical warfare.

But it was hardly reasoning that was driving events. In Israel, simply the prospect of poison gas and massive death was enough to transform the prosaic twentieth-century Israeli air raid shelters into concrete gas chambers. Everyone was required to have a sealed room in their home. Weeks of elaborate instructions on how to seal up ordinary rooms had caused a run on duct tape and plastic sheeting.

On the first night of the war, along with everyone else in Israel except the government officials who could tune in all three U.S. networks, the press corps watched CNN. John Holliman, Bernard Shaw, and Peter Arnett crawled around in a hotel room in Baghdad while the producers in Atlanta kept re-running pictures taken by an ABC News cameraman of the first bombs falling over Baghdad. Israel listened in, and one Israeli, Likud party luminary Benjamin Netanyahu, even got to reminisce tearfully about past wars with Bernard Shaw over a phone line broadcast round the world.

Israeli TV was broadcasting CNN pictures with simultaneous translation and commentary into Hebrew. As CNN transmitted, Israelis noted the air raids on Baghdad and the ascendancy of former Israeli journalist Wolf Blitzer, filing constantly from the Pentagon. He had been the Washington correspondent for *The Jerusalem Post.* The Israeli TV commentators remarked on how well Blitzer was doing on CNN. Israelis speculated on the future of his beard. The consensus was that once he was a big star, he would have to shave. Blitzer didn't lose the beard. It was just one of the predictions that never came true at the beginning of the war with Iraq.

That first night of the war the broadcast reporters in Tel Aviv just waited to go on, and most of them had a long time to wait. Israel was way down on everyone's list in the package, or spin down. There was remarkable uniformity network to network. ABC was the first to report the beginning of the air war, but when the live video links from Baghdad were cut by the Iraqi government, only CNN was left with a live voice signal, and therefore the capability to go live from every major theater of the war. For everyone else, the opening shot or opening audio was CNN: three television guys trying to do radio from a hotel room, interrupting each other and hanging microphones out the window. For someone who had spent a decade working for National Public Radio, this was a particular irony.

The second lead was from the forward command in Dhahran, Saudi Arabia. Next, to Riyadh for the really big generals to repeat what had just been said, then to the Pentagon for spokesman Pete Williams to repeat what had just been repeated, dramatically break in for a reaction from the White House, and finally back to the live TV general in the studio to explain what had just been said twice, and to try to imagine what hadn't been said, and to pretend that anybody actually knew what was going on. Next, to the Arab analyst to explain either that Saddam was insane, or that his cruel and dubious strategy of national suicide was actually brilliant. Finally a quick pop from the White House, a recap from Dhahran, a commercial break, and, "When we come back, reaction in Israel."

But there was no reaction on that first night. There was nothing to report except the "atmosphere of tense calm" and the "wait and see attitude" of the Israeli government. Israeli officials were not used to being a Middle East sideshow after forty years of invasions, wars, secret antiterrorist missions, and preemptive strikes, so this was an unusual situation. With no national emergency, and the war safely to the east by about 600 miles, the Israeli spokesmen indulged in a favorite pastime: spinning. Since there was nothing particular to spin on the war, they would offer the theory that Israel might have inside information on the massive destruction going on in Baghdad. Israeli officials would say, "We are monitoring the situation very closely." Roughly translated, this means: "I just got off the phone with Colin Powell and Dick Cheney."

One rumor was that the Israelis knew from moment to moment where Saddam Hussein was. One of the juicier stories in Tel Aviv was that one of Saddam's wives or mistresses was actually an Israeli agent. At one briefing, a lot of time was spent talking about whether Israeli Intelligence would reveal to the Americans where Saddam was hiding, or would they take him out themselves. Without giving away either their inside knowledge or their ignorance, the Israeli military sources would simply say, "We are monitoring the situation very closely."

Very little of this officially embellished fantasy made it into print or on the air. There was little appetite among editors for wild speculation and the "wait and see attitude" from Jerusalem with bombs falling in Baghdad live, on camera, and in prime time, with Peter Arnett's steady voice narrating. The reports from the air war were too good to be true. It was a systematic, high-tech blitzkrieg on live television that seemed unstoppable, and hardly something Saddam Hussein could stand for long. As the damage estimates from the first waves of the bombing reached the White House, there was elation. Wolf Blitzer reported from the Pentagon that some U.S. officials were talking about an Iraqi surrender within days. After the first night of the air war, an Israeli foreign ministry official, holding his gas mask, remarked that perhaps the vast phone banks set up for the media in Tel Aviv and Jerusalem would soon be closed down. "We are monitoring the situation very closely," he said. "This thing is not going to take very long."

At 2 A.M., about twenty-four hours after the first bombs began falling in Baghdad, the war seemed closer to Washington than to Israel. I had gone back to Jerusalem, where the city and my hotel were quiet in the pre-dawn hours. I was sprawled on a couch in the lobby of the Hilton Hotel, along with my gas mask, tape recorder, and a small pile of miscellaneous junk piled on my wheelchair like a table. I was going over some notes. It had been a long day of waiting, watching, and forgetting to eat. I had just ordered a tuna fish salad, the one food available twenty-four hours a day in Israeli hotels. I had taken three bites.

When the Gulf War found Israel in the early hours of January 18, 1991, the nation was awakened by an unthinkable nightmare that announced its arrival in familiar, moaning, air raid sirens that were no drill. All of the precautionary play money in the weeks leading up to the war was suddenly redeemed. When the SCUDs began to fall, a terrified Jewish nation ran to escape from poison gas.

I vaulted from the lobby couch into my chair, nearly knocking it over and spilling my notes and equipment all over the lobby. I grabbed a microphone, tape recorder, and a small shortwave radio and headed out the front door of the hotel to record the sound of the air raid sirens. There had been six SCUD missiles fired from Iraq at Tel Aviv and Haifa, but on the radio there was only the announcement that sirens were sounding all over the country, and that people were supposed to now do what they had been rehearsing for the past few weeks: "Go into your sealed room and await further instructions." This was also the message from the frantic hotel staff, who tried to convince me and the one other person outside to come in and go to the shelters and sealed rooms. I told him to shut up, worried that his voice would ruin the recording I was making to send back to Washington. "Mister, you must come, I will help you." His voice and his face, terrified over what he thought might happen to me after he left, were a part of the moment. The news was the sound of the siren.

When the recording was finished, I returned to the hotel to call Washington and found that the switchboard was closed because the staff of the hotel had all gone into the shelters. On the way back down to the lobby, I discovered that all but one elevator was turned off, another security measure, but this one made me nervous since an absence of elevators would require some truly fancy gymnastics to get from the eleventh floor, where my room was, to the lobby.

The lobby was empty. The hotel was completely deserted. Radio messages continued to urge everyone into sealed rooms. I went to the press filing room in the basement and found table after table of completely functional phones. I called Washington and sent the sound of the air raid siren over the phone, editing around the voice of the hotel employee who pleaded with me to come inside. I did some live reporting of the very preliminary details available from the friends and government officials around the country I was able to call.

The radio began to report that missiles had landed in Israel without specifying where. The other NPR reporter in Israel, Linda Gradstein, was already in her sealed room with her gas mask on. There was some speculation on the radio and on the wire reports from back in the U.S. quoting unnamed sources in Israel that there was gas involved in this initial attack. I was on the line with half a dozen NPR reporters and anchors, and the din and confusion made it hard to know when to speak. Around me, I could see that I was alone in a room full of phones in a hotel that was completely empty. I could hear the discussion in Washington focus on the reports of a chemical attack in Israel. "What have you heard, John?" I was asked. At this point we knew nothing. I began to feel like the canary in the coal mine. I looked at the box containing my gas mask. I smelled the air. I told NPR that I thought I would try to find a sealed room and that I would call them back once I found one.

I returned to the eleventh floor and looked at the signs in the hall indicating where to go. The possibility that a substance could cause death the moment you became aware of its presence in your breath made me dizzy. The dizziness made me suspicious of the air. The suspicion made me afraid. The fear made me dizzier. I rolled toward the designated room. The door was narrower than the other doors in the hall, but it looked as though I could still just get my wheelchair through it. I opened it and discovered that there was an inner door. The outer door had a loose seal of plastic and rubber, which formed a passive barrier to the outside. The inner door was significantly modified, with plastic sheeting poking out from underneath and over the top.

I tried the door handle. It turned but was locked. I heard muffled voices from inside. A voice I could make out was asking me if the outer door was closed. I closed it and said yes. There was a click, and the inner door slowly opened. It was seriously encumbered with the plastic sheeting and duct tape that lined it all the way around. When the door was fully open, a wall of plastic sheeting was still between me and the people inside. In the plastic there was a slit a person could step through, after which the plastic could be folded back and resealed with tape. The plastic wall was attached directly to the doorway on all sides.

Inside was a group of people wearing gas masks. They were hard to place. Tourists, Israelis, immigrants, I could not tell. Their eyes were all that could be seen through the large, round lenses in the masks. Faces and heads were buried; the elongated filters over the mouths and chins gave everyone an unearthly look of uniformity, like a colony of bugs. There was a radio in the room. Three married couples were huddled together. A family with three children were all back in the corner. The children's faces were averted from the door. That they were all wearing their gas masks made my predicament seem that much more terrifying.

A tall, thin, hotel employee, obviously an Israeli, was standing near the door. He and I inspected the doorway. I was unable to step through the plastic, so I would have to roll into the room. But moving the wheelchair over the threshold would tear down the elaborate plastic seal, violating its integrity. Each second the inner door was open, the anxiety of the people inside the room visibly increased. It was an inaccessible room. I was flooded with all of the reactions I had ever had in that situation. Anger, embarrassment, and the good-natured ingenuity to make the situation work despite the physical limitations. On the other side of the plastic, wearing gas masks, a group of people huddled inside a Jewish nightmare recreated by Saddam Hussein.

The tall man at the door spoke to me awkwardly. "It is too small," he said. He looked back at the group in the corner. They had terror in their eyes. One man shouted in a voice muffled by his gas mask, "There are old people and children in here, for God's sake. Close the door." The longer the door stayed open, the more frightened the people behind the plastic became. The children started to cry. I reached down to the door frame and fingered the plastic sheet with the intention of pulling it away from the door so as to open a space, slip through, and then reseal the plastic.

As I did, the older woman and man sitting closest to the door gave me a look that I will not forget in my lifetime. Their eyes widened. The woman grabbed the shoulder of her husband and they both acquired a look of fatal, breathless horror as they gazed at the prospect of the plastic seal being broken. The mother in the back of the room grabbed her children and held them close. I could hear through the filters on their masks a cry that caught in their throats and a tinny, quavering sob that emerged from their masks like a bad soundtrack from an old movie.

At the height of a twister, and holding her little dog, Toto, Dorothy Gale walked alone around the back of her house in Kansas to the wooden doors of the basement shelter. There was no wicked witch on the screen during, what was for me, the most terrifying scene in *The Wizard of Oz*. Dorothy kicked the doors with her heel, but they would not open. "Why didn't they let Dorothy in?" I asked my parents. They had no answer. "It was just too late," they would say. "They couldn't open the doors. The twister was right there," my mother said. "See it?" I saw it. Dorothy was on her own. So was I.

There is no more disquieting fear than the realization of being on your own, separated from everyone, cut off by fixed circumstances everyone can see, no matter what side of the dividing line they are on. The tall man at the door looked at me, and then back at the people in the room. His face seemed to say that he wanted to let me in, but now that the missiles had come, it was too late to break the seal.

I was trying to enter their flimsy sanctuary, but the expressions on the faces in that little room stopped me cold. On opposite sides of the plastic seal, my presence posed the question: who would be sacrificed, the lone man in the wheelchair or the family with children and two married couples? I did not begrudge this calculation. The line was drawn. The terror on their faces made me hurt inside. I could not deny their terror, I could not understand it. I could not protect myself. After three years of working in the Middle East, I understood that I could not enter this place. It resonated through my identity as a man from the Christian West, and a man in a wheelchair. It rang as an impenetrable certainty, fully real but only partially understood. I do not know why I turned and rolled away and didn't demand to be allowed into their sealed room. I only understand that if the same situation presented itself in the future I would have to do it again.

I raised my hand and smiled. I started to leave. The tall man looked apologetic. The couples' faces broke into relief and they gestured in a kind of good-bye that quickly became a motion for the inner door to be resealed. The mother in the back of the room looked like she had started to say something, but I did not wait to hear it. "I'm sorry," the tall man said as he closed the door. In the dark space between the outer and inner door of the sealed shelter, I felt as the people who climbed on the trains to go off to the Nazi death camps might have felt, a combination of heroic resignation, deep fear, and an even deeper loathing. I knew I had to go, as they apparently knew. Why do we know such things? Because I occupied some unspoken rung on an unstated ladder of humanity's chilling hierarchies, I felt deeply ashamed. I had betrayed all that I believed in, as did each of the people on the trains. Yet they also gave their lives for something they believed was the quiet dignity of a people who shared faith, pain, and a common history. There is no one who can begrudge them that even if their epitaph consists of piles and piles of shoes and boxes of human hair in sober memorials to the death camps.

Recalled today as a minor footnote of destruction in a small war, the SCUD attacks against Israel on that first night reduced people to random slabs of meat on opposite sides of plastic sheets, staring, terrified, from behind gas masks. Saddam's little pranks forced us all to do six-column moral arithmetic in our heads to win back our lives. War makes people turn somersaults like chimps on a game show; dragged through its brutal necessities, we prayed to escape with our souls intact.

I opened the outer door, returned to the elevator lobby, and went back to the phone bank on the basement level. I had my phone book with the numbers of all the people I knew in Israel. I presumed they would all be at home. I called Washington. The story from Israel was now leading the newscasts around the world. Linda Gradstein was back on-line to NPR from her own sealed room and had been filing news from the Israeli radio reports. I decided to call everyone I knew and try to get the lowdown from various cities.

With Washington in one hand and every other major city in Israel on-line down the table, I filed stories and did live updates for more than two hours. There were a number of missiles. Based on information from people at various points around Tel Aviv and Haifa, which I plotted on a map in front of me, it seemed as though between three and six missiles had landed. (The official count revealed weeks later was six.) There were casualties, although the extent and the nature of the casualties was unclear. The government was trying to withhold as much information as possible so as not to supply the Iraqi missile launchers with information on the accuracy of the SCUDs.

When the all clear signal was called, the rest of the hotel emerged from the sealed rooms and the other reporters gradually filtered into the press room to find me with four phones up to my ears. It was not clear if there had been no gas in this attack or if gas was attempted and something had malfunctioned. Authorities were not ruling anything out in the first hours after the attack.

I wanted to see where the missiles had landed, but I had no transportation. The reporters just coming out of the sealed rooms still had to file their stories, and getting an international phone line at that point was nearly impossible. Phone traffic between the U.S. and Israel in the hours after the first attack jumped from about three thousand calls per hour to three-quarters of a million. My friend Lou Salome, a reporter for the Cox newspaper chain, had a car. As he came up to me, he could see that I had an open phone line to the States. I patched him through to his desk in Atlanta, and after a quick conversation and some dictation, he and I went off to see the missile damage for ourselves. Lou and I would have a head start. We threw our gas masks into the backseat of the car and drove toward Tel Aviv.

According to my map, there was missile damage in at least two neighborhoods, Ramat Gan, east of the city, and a south-side neighborhood where recently arrived Russian and Georgian immigrants were living alongside Jews from Morocco and Yemen who had settled there long ago. The drive to Tel Aviv with Lou was a relief from the tension in the early, solitary moments of the air raid. The road was deserted; we passed no one along the way. The reports of chemical weapons were disturbing, but if they were true, we presumed that we would have heard about monstrous casualties by then. We drove as fast as we could, both of us feeling very much ahead of the pack and invulnerable until the final turn on the road into Tel Aviv.

On our left, a quarter-mile from the road, was a building lit up with flames. An industrial plant for producing textiles had clearly been hit by something. We had arrived before any emergency vehicles and decided to investigate before proceeding into the city. We reckoned our way to the plant along unmarked, unlit roads. The complex had sustained a direct hit in one of its main buildings, and power to the entire surrounding area was out. The fire had engulfed much of the structure.

As we turned a corner around the back of the building, we suddenly found ourselves behind an Israeli military vehicle packed with fully armed soldiers, each one wearing the white, hermetically sealed suit of chemical weapons specialists. The soldiers stared back at us through their bubble-suit helmets and smiled. Lou and I looked at each other and immediately reached out to roll up our car windows. It was an instant of feeling absolutely checkmated. I said to Lou, "I guess we're dead." Then after a long overdue breath, "I guess we're not dead." There were no chemical weapons here. We kept our windows open and drove with the soldiers to the center of the complex, where the flames were heaviest. As we looked at the crater the SCUD had left in the factory, some of the soldiers were standing around with their helmets off.

It was a different scene in Tel Aviv, where by daybreak it was clear that this first attack had only been with conventional warheads. It had killed no one, but the psychological implications of an attack from the air 600 miles from Israel had struck deeply. In south Tel Aviv, a group of neighbors stood around an athletic field where a warhead had poked through three layers of concrete to make an ugly crater where boys had played soccer the week before.

"It was a dud," one of the neighbors called out, noting that the warhead had not exploded, but had simply burrowed into the wreckage where police and military experts were trying to determine if it could be safely removed. The Russian Jews pointed knowingly and insisted that it could not explode if it was a Russian SCUD. "It is shit, this weapon, and all weapons of Russia," said one man from Minsk. An Iranian Jewish family recalled how Saddam had shot missiles at Tehran during the first Persian Gulf War. "He must be trying to find us," they said. I asked another family where they were from, and a man looked around at the crowd and announced, "We are from Baghdad, Saddam is sending us a message." The crowd began to cheer and shake the hands of these Jews from Iraq. I tried to imagine the reception an American from Tokyo would have received in such a crowd the day after Pearl Harbor.

The second attack came the next night at about the same time. This time Tel Aviv did not fare as well. A missile plowed into an apartment complex in Ramat Gan, nearly leveling a four-story building. I arrived on the scene to see the soft concrete walls of a block of apartments sheared away, exposing the undisturbed furniture and living spaces, like a dollhouse opened for play. A newly arrived Russian immigrant woman stood sobbing on the street in a satin nightgown and slippers, wrapped in sable furs that looked as if they had come from one of Gloria Swanson's closets. An Israeli man and woman sat in the living room of one of the exposed apartments, looking down on the police and fire rescue workers as though they were watching street life from their newly constructed balcony. The old man's pastel blue bathrobe had clumps of gray concrete mud on it, which his wife was wiping away with a wad of tissue paper.

I rolled toward the center of the jam of emergency vehicles and fire trucks, where a police officer saw me and insisted that I leave the area. "It is too dangerous for you here," he said.

"I'm working," I told him, pointing at the microphone and tape recorder in my lap.

"We are working too." He was unmoved. "Go back now."

He was not saying this to any of the other reporters who were walking toward the most seriously damaged apartment. I ignored him, rolled forward, and discovered thick fire hoses on the street, swollen from pumping pressurized water. The officer came up to me, shouting.

"I thought I told you to get out!" He began to pull my chair from behind.

"Leave me alone," I said, gripping my wheels to stop him from moving me while with my other hand I tried to keep my recording equipment from falling off my lap. I moved forward and toward the fire hoses blocking my path.

"See, you can't go," the officer said as I tipped up on two wheels and hopped over the first swollen fire hose, then two more, and into the middle of where debris from the apartments was being removed. The crowd of neighbors watched this maneuver and cheered when I made the jump. I looked up, and the couple in the blown-up apartment waiting to be rescued were smiling and pointing at me and the police officer. The rescue workers were smiling as well. Only the police officer was still angry. He came up to me and began shouting, "I said get out of here. You can't be here. Now go."

"Why?" I asked. "I'm here already."

His face was red and blotchy with rage. "You are in a wheelchair!" He shouted this directly into my face. In his eyes was a frustration born more of the circumstances of the evening than anything about me. He had watched apartments fall down and missiles falling from the sky. He could do nothing about any of that. The one thing he thought he could control on that evening, in the middle of destruction and fire hoses, was me.

"It's okay," a voice said. "Let him move." I looked up, and there was big, bald Moshe, who had carried me up the stairs to the Temple Mount observation post in Jerusalem three years before. I hadn't seen him in more than a year. "You come back for more, Crazy?" He laughed, and with a few words, his frustrated junior officer, who had just been preparing to throw me back over the fire trucks into the crowd, walked away. "Saddam is making a big Intifada here," Moshe said. I told him I had to agree. "Can you see everything good now?" he asked, hinting that he wasn't going to be carrying me up any stairs on this morning. I nodded and he said good-bye, wished me good luck, and walked back into the twisted wreckage.

Over time, as the count of missiles and separate attacks rose, the flaming junk Saddam was sending over the horizon ceased to have the intensely symbolic value that it had had in the first hours of the war. The SCUDs' effect on Israelis and Palestinians became something of a signature, producing different reactions depending on where a person lived or what he believed.

The most popular night spot in curfewed Tel Aviv was a place named for a popular movie: The Baghdad Café. It was mobbed with young people sipping beer and waiting for the sirens as midnight approached. The Palestinians on the West Bank, who had watched the missiles screaming overhead at six times the speed of sound on their way to Tel Aviv and Haifa, cheered for Saddam. As subsequent missiles began to fall short and land in Palestinian villages, the cheering stopped. Men would stand around nervously and insist, for the record, that Saddam was standing up to Israel, while wives and mothers would speak of the terror for their children and the insanity of being under occupation from one side and bombed by another.

"Saddam is stupid," one wailing, angry mother told me in the West Bank village of Deir Ballut where a missile fell 20 miles northeast of Tel Aviv. "Shamir is stupid. This war is stupid. Is your President George Bush stupid? Go home and ask him." She had nothing more to say.

The most agitated Israelis were the leftists. The most serious were the conservative Likud leaders like Deputy Foreign Minister Benjamin (Bibi) Netanyahu, who prided himself on being cool under fire even as he and others in the government had to explain why Israel had agreed to a Bush administration demand not to respond militarily to the Iraqi SCUDs. Netanyahu was on American television live during one attack, and the army officers I was with at the time took bets to see if Bibi would put his mask on or tough it out maskless on camera. Most of the officers bet that Bibi would not put on his mask. "He will put it on, but he will be the last one," one officer who claimed to be from the opposition Labor party told me. He won twenty bucks when, after looking around to see if everyone else in the studio was wearing a mask, Netanyahu put his on and continued the interview.

The Israelis who seemed most at peace during the missile attacks were the Orthodox followers of the Lubavitcher Rabbi Menachem Schneerson, who died three years after the war. Before the war and seven thousand miles away, from his headquarters in Brooklyn, New York, Rabbi Schneerson had flatly declared that no serious harm would come to Israel from Saddam Hussein. As each missile landed and caused destruction but no deaths, the smiling pale-skinned Lubavitchers would deliver an elaborate Talmudic "We told you so" to anyone who would listen. "We believe in the rebbe and we are absolutely sure that nothing can hurt us now," one man told me at Ben-Gurion Airport as he welcomed a drove of people arriving in Israel to witness in person Rabbi Schneerson's millennial remote-control accuracy about the Iraqi SCUDs.

In contrast, the older, leathery, suntanned Zionists who walked the North Tel Aviv streets named after the legends of Israel's modern history were morose and fatalistic about the missile attacks. "We have lived here for so long and have no peace when these flaming bombs can come down from the sky," they said. "Everything we have made here is for nothing." Peace movement activists and world-famous writers A. B. Yehoshuah and Amos Oz held a news conference at the Tel Aviv Hilton in which they called for war against Iraq, declared all talk of sanctions to be Nazi-era appeasement, and said that the world should recognize the potential for a new Holocaust against the Jews. Israel, the writers said, should defend itself and not take orders from a United States demanding restraint. In response to a reporter's question, Oz, perhaps Israel's most celebrated peacenik, said flatly that a tactical nuclear strike in Iraq would be preferable to the annihilation of Jews by poison gas. Long after Saddam's surrender, it was reported that in the early hours of the war the Israeli nuclear arsenal was on full alert and aimed at Iraq in the event of the chemical attack that never came.

By the fourteenth missile attack from Iraq, the inaccuracy of the missiles was apparent, and many of them were falling out of the sky like patched-together spare parts. Israel was overrun with American reporters doing feel-good stories about the brave Israelis. The press room in Tel Aviv had the sentimental atmosphere of the phone bank at a PBS fundraiser. I decided to leave Israel on the day a reporter from the *Boca Raton Jewish Weekly* arrived from South Florida with two photographers in tow and asked me if I knew any "injured missile people" for a feature she wanted to do.

Israel was once again a sideshow. Whatever the effect of the SCUDS in Israel, the bombing campaign over Iraq would be thousands of times greater. The coming land war would be the test of Saddam Hussein's decision to invade Kuwait, and the culmination of George Bush's decision to confront him. I told Cadi that I was intent on getting to Baghdad, no matter what, and that I was going to go ahead and get an Iraqi visa. In words I would live to regret, I told her that I was not going to miss the war just because NPR couldn't make up its mind. There was still time to make it to Baghdad.

Looking back on those weeks in 1991, it is the obsessive pursuit of the Baghdad story that seems so shallow and pointless while so many of the subtler details, that seemed irrelevant at the time, are today full of meaning. There was the wasted time spent pursuing an Iraqi visa in the PLO offices of Bassam abu Sherif in Tunis, trying to get Yasir Arafat to intercede on my behalf through his direct line to Baghdad.

But there was also the evening in the apartment of an Arab family in Casablanca watching General Schwarzkopf deliver a briefing on CNN. With a pointer, he described the features in a fuzzy gun-camera picture of a bridge on which an Iraqi truck was driving. Schwarzkopf made some very matter-of-fact points about the significance of the bridge and how selectively the high-tech "smart" weapons chose their targets. As I sat in the living room, I noticed that all of the people watching were focused intently on the moving truck, their heads moving from left to right as the bridge came closer into view, indicating that an impact was imminent.

I noticed that General Schwarzkopf had a little smile on his face, while there in the living room with me the Arab family was riveted in suspense. There was a white flash on the screen and the bridge took a direct hit at a point that looked to be about 100 feet behind the moving truck. The truck seemed to speed up after the blast. I could see what was going to happen next. Schwarzkopf was working the crowd of reporters in Riyadh. The Moroccan family sitting with me sighed deeply with relief that the driver was unharmed, while on CNN Schwarzkopf put his pointer on the picture of the now-speeding truck and turned to the reporters in the briefing room. "He's the luckiest man in Iraq today." The roomful of reporters burst out laughing.

"Why are they laughing?" All of the people in the living room turned to me in shock. They wanted the only American present to explain the joke to them. "The driver was almost killed," they said. "What is funny here?"

I had no explanation. Morocco was a part of the allied coalition against Iraq, the other Arab nations in the coalition being Syria, Egypt, and Saudi Arabia. The souls of the reporters may have been with Norman Schwarzkopf and his smart bombs in the briefing room, but the heart of those Moroccans and, I suspect, every Arab who watched those pictures, was with the driver of that Iraqi truck. They did not consider him to be a very lucky man.

After a week of phone calls and meetings trying to arrange passage into Iraq, the PLO's advice was to take a letter from Arafat to Amman and use it to obtain a visa to Baghdad at the Iraqi Embassy there. The letter, in Arabic, claimed, among other things, that I had been wounded in the Vietnam War, a detail entirely fabricated by Arafat's people. They were too discreet to ask me directly, so they explained my wheelchair themselves, in a way, they told me later, that was sure to impress the Iraqis.

My last night in Morocco was spent trying to do a story about the reaction to the Allied ground offensive that was expected to begin any day. The war had become an eerie stalemate with the Allied air campaign unabated, and Iraq's ability to launch missiles deteriorating, but there was no sign of surrender. Much of the broadcast reporting on the reaction in the Arab world had been about the ritual protesters in Egypt and Jordan who, day after day, claimed their undying allegiance to Saddam Hussein, on cue and in time for the evening news in America. Yet outside Cairo and Amman, the war had produced a deep sadness in the Arab world, not unlike the fatalistic reactions of some Israelis, nostalgic for a peace they had never known.

I found a group of young men at a restaurant in Casablanca and we sat around talking about the war. There was the same blustering speech-making until I pulled out two copies of the Koran, in English and Arabic, and asked each of them to think of a verse from the Muslim holy book that applied to the eve of what Saddam had called "the mother of all battles." The speeches stopped and everyone pointed to one thin young man who had been quiet up until then. He took my Arabic Koran in his hands and as the other boys gathered around him he turned precisely to a verse about two thirds of the way through it. Then he stood and in the beautiful singing Arabic of the mosque, he read the verse in a boy soprano voice that quieted the restaurant and caused the people in the street walking by at dusk to stop and listen.

I understood nothing he had read except that everyone listening bowed and said *al Hamdu-lillah* (God is willing) when he had finished, and a woman in the street wiped a tear from her eye as she walked away. The patrons of the restaurant quickly paid their bills and left the place empty but for me and my two Korans. I looked at the place where he had been reading, in the sura (or chapter) called Luqman. These were the words in English:

"Lo! Allah! With him is knowledge of the hour. He sendeth down the rain, and knoweth that which is in the wombs. No soul knoweth what it will earn tomorrow, and no soul knoweth in what land it will die."

I thought of the Allied and Iraqi soldiers spread out along the Saudi border waiting for their orders, wondering when and where they would take them. I had heard considerable analysis of Desert Storm from decorated generals and other high-ranking officials during the Persian Gulf War, but nothing as true as those words sung by a young boy on a February night at a café in Morocco.

I arrived in Amman and went immediately to the Iraqi Embassy's locked front entrance. The long line of reporters waiting outside communicated with the embassy staff through a little window that swung open and slammed shut at the whim of the Iraqi functionaries inside. I knew that the Iraqis, once they saw my wheelchair, would allow me to come inside, where it would be easier to see the ambassador and present him personally with my PLO letters of introduction. The line of journalists from all over the world had been waiting every day since January 15 in front of the embassy door, never seeing beyond the door. They watched the Iraqi staff lift me over their heads and inside.

By the middle of February, the Iraqi Embassy in Amman had become a nasty, desperate place where visas were dangled in front of women in return for "evenings alone." The embassy staff did a brisk trade in smuggled goods, particularly cases of Scotch whiskey, which were understood to be part of the price of official admission into Baghdad. Each shuttle from the Rashid hotel in Baghdad brought a laundry list of items for the reporters and diplomats there. Another list carried by the drivers who worked for the Iraqi Information Ministry contained items for the Iraqi officials that, it was understood, would be supplied by the new people going in.

I gave the embassy officials my letter from Yasir Arafat. The PLO was right about the Iraqi interest in Vietnam. For once, I did not deny being a veteran when they asked me about how I got "wounded." I felt cheap and slimy when an official claimed that more Americans would die in the coming land war with Iraq than died in Vietnam. "You should warn the people in America," he said. "They will listen to a veteran like you who sacrificed so much." It made me sick to listen to him and sicker not to tell him the truth, but all I wanted was the visa. The embassy staff took my papers and passport and told me to return the next evening to pick up my visa.

I went to the hotel in Amman bursting with energy and optimism and ran into (at eye level) Nora Bustany, my four-foot eleven-inch friend from *The Washington Post* who was also waiting to get an Iraqi visa. I told her about my experience at the embassy. She said she thought my plan for getting a visa was as good as any she had heard of, but she was cautious about the Iraqis' intentions.

"They will do what they want, and they just don't care about the media anymore." She told me that she had just found out that the Iraqis had approved a visa for *The Washington Post,* but she didn't seem happy about it. "I won't be going," she said. "They know I am Lebanese and can speak easily with the people. They said anyone but Nora can go." She seemed deeply disappointed that something she believed made her better at her job could be the reason she was not going to be permitted to do it.

I went to my room and there was a call from Cadi in Washington. "I have bad news, John," she said, sounding upset. Before she could tell me, I blurted out that I thought I would be getting a visa the next day and could be in Baghdad the day after that. There was a long pause on the phone.

"We can't send you, John," she said. "Your instructions are that if NPR gets a visa tomorrow, you're not to use it." She proceeded to tell me that another reporter in Amman would use the visa instead. I would be staying behind.

There had been a meeting about whether it was safe to send me into Iraq and that they had decided not to find out. The story she told was rambling and the word wheelchair was not mentioned even once, as though no one could bring themselves to mention the name of a relative who had just died. NPR management, Cadi said, had called the heads of ABC News, CNN, and the BBC, all of whom had operations in Baghdad.

"Since when do we need their permission to do our stories?" I shouted at her. I could feel what was coming. "Listen, John," she said. "We asked them, that if we sent you in, would they be willing to tell their staff people to help you if you needed it, and they said no." I said nothing. "They said they were too busy and besides, they think it's too dangerous for you to go."

"Cadi, what did you expect them to say? Don't you think they would have said the same thing if we'd asked them about any of the other outlandish places you have sent me?"

Cadi's voice was determined; she was doing what editors all over the world were doing in the final hours before the ground offensive began. The safety of the reporters in Iraq and Saudi Arabia was a crucial issue for everyone in the media, but for Cadi and me it brought to a head issues that had never before been discussed. Her voice was tinged with a kind of shame and sadness, as though it fell to her to carry out what she thought was someone else's dirty work. "John," she said as if to drive some point home and be done with a horribly awkward moment, "the elevators at the Rashid Hotel don't work. The bombs took them out."

I realized then how much I had wanted to do something and how impossible it was going to be to do it now. I considered defying NPR and going into Iraq anyway, but my vengeful feelings only revealed how selfish my reasons for wanting to go had been to begin with. I was humiliated that NPR would have such a meeting and that it would be the only time they ever thought about the effort required for me to do what I had been doing for so long. NPR had never asked about the elevators before, when I had been carried up or had climbed up stairs, or had slogged through the mud in Romania with bullets flying everywhere, or had been stuck in the sand in Gaza with gasoline bombs blazing. But it all seemed so silly now. All along, I had wanted their unhesitating confidence. In a moment I realized that it was probably unobtainable. I was sobbing now. I said to Cadi, "Do you think for a minute that I didn't realize the elevators were out at the Rashid? It has always been my job to deal with those things. Why did you change the rules?"

There was a pause. "Sometimes I hate this job, John," she said.

"So do I, Cadi." I hung up.

The next day there was no visa at the Iraqi Embassy for me or anyone from NPR. It was to be the last trip into Iraq from Amman before the ground war started. There had been no serious consideration of a visa for me. The slimy business of pretending to be a Vietnam veteran on the PLO letter was all for nothing. On the night the ground war began, Jordanian TV broadcast the movie *Coming Home* with Jon Voight playing a Vietnam veteran in a wheelchair. What the Jordanians were thinking by choosing that movie I couldn't fathom. It seemed to speak directly to me, a failed symbol, sitting in a hotel, while outside, hundreds of miles away, a war was real.

I had wanted to go to Baghdad for the wrong reasons, but NPR had refused to let me go for what I thought were equally wrong reasons. Now there was nothing left to do but wait and see how it all turned out. I felt liberated for the first time in my life from this need to prove something. I could get on with the business of doing my job. The cease-fire between the armed forces of Iraq led by Saddam Hussein and the allied coalition led by General Norman Schwarzkopf, General Colin Powell, and President George Bush took effect on February 28, 1991, exactly fifteen years to the day I had tumbled down a hill in Pennsylvania, never to walk again.

Four weeks later I rolled down a crowded road filled with Kurdish refugees hauling their possessions and what was left of their lives out of northern Iraq. On either side of the road was the human waste of a people laid low by disease and death. The refugee tableau stretched to the horizon in Kurdistan, and of all the images of the Gulf War this would become an emblem of the century's end, as the Kurds were soon overtaken in the world's attention by the unimagined refugee horrors to come in Sudan, Somalia, Bosnia, and Rwanda. Today that line always seems to be stretching over the horizon.

As I rolled down the road back into Iraq, the terrain became more difficult until it finally ended in the squeeze of space between vehicles fighting for the narrow ledge hugging the cliff along the Iraqi border. There was a man with a donkey there. He offered to give me a ride. We negotiated a price. I gave my wheelchair to a taxicab driver and told him to meet me at the border post in a few days. I climbed onto the donkey without a thought of Baghdad or wheelchairs or elevators. From the shoulders of the beast I could see the crowd of refugees better, and all the people living under plastic sheets and sticks for shelter. I could see the mass graves and the yellow-gray flesh of their bodies off to the side of the road. I thought to myself how recently it seemed that I had imagined I might miss the war I had been sent to cover. I looked around and felt ashamed as I took my first steps on the donkey's legs. I had missed nothing.

25

Charles Peter Slagle

The town of Newark, New York, is compact and square, the blockish model of a northeast American village. Arched over by trees and iron streetlights, the concrete and stone sidewalks are jostled by old tree roots into difficult undulations. Once they were flat, but today they are full of obstacles. I roll over them with care to avoid the places where the stones are detached by as much as a few inches. I would roll in the street, but there is too much traffic in the city. All of Newark's churches and schools, its five- and dime-store, and the old public library are within the city limits. The Newark State School for the Mentally Ill, where my uncle was sent to live out his life in his eighth year, was built just outside the city limits.

On the road from Newark to Phelps, where Uncle Charles Peter Slagle now lives in a smaller facility for severely retarded adults, the Newark State School can still be seen on the left. The campus of brick buildings is set away from the road, down a hill across a rolling lawn. My uncle lived most of his life here. For most of my life I never knew he was here, or if he even existed. All I had been told was that he was a total vegetable, that he could not recognize anyone. I do not know him, nor is there any expectation that he will know me, or that I will know him any better after I see him. We will not have a nice chat. We will not go for a nice walk. He will not tell me to pick some things up for him at the drugstore. We will not talk about old times. He will not say hello when I arrive and he will not say good-bye when I leave.

The perverse irony about my uncle's condition, PKU, is that since the 1960s it has become completely treatable even though little more is known about the disease other than what was first observed about it back in the 1930s. The treatment came long after it could have been of any use to my uncle. Once detected, PKU ceases to be harmful when an infant's diet is modified to avoid proteins that are toxic in PKU babies. But medical science cannot say for sure whether untreated PKU babies ever have a functioning mind, before the effects of the disease in their blood turns them all into "idiots" or "imbeciles". The question has never really been studied. What is obvious about the untreated victims of PKU is that they were almost uniformly miserable throughout their early lives, as though they were experiencing a numbing persistent discomfort.

The early medical literature is replete with PKU case histories. In 1961 a report on the early symptoms of phenylketonuria looked at three dozen Canadian children. A girl, Lori B., had a normal birth. Her parents noted a peculiar odor and difficulty with food in her first two weeks of life. She was described as unhappy by her mother after three months. By nine months Lori's mother presumed she was retarded. At seventeen months Lori was spastic and having seizures; at twenty-two months she was diagnosed with PKU.

Baby William was admitted to a hospital at ten weeks. The report says: "His mother did not think he was retarded, though this was evident in the hospital." Other children were irritable until their diets were modified, and then became, according to their parents, "placid," "good" babies. The details in each of the cases suggest the struggles, failures, and successes of parents and the cries of their children. But it is all buried beneath the medical data.

An older study of children from all over North America from the late fifties attempts to chart the developmental history of untreated PKU babies. These children would most closely mirror the experience of my uncle. In neat columns of numbers, the cases of 106 children are laid out according to when they demonstrated certain behaviors deemed clinically indicative of development. There is a column for "Sat Unsupported," another for "Walked Alone," a third for "Talked(words)." The study found that PKU babies typically sit by themselves after about a year, walk by themselves after two and a half years, and talk in some form some time between the third and fourth years of life. More than half of the group were capable of some walking. Virtually all could sit unsupported, although when this happened it was quite frequently delayed well beyond the sixth month, when normal babies are said generally to begin to sit by themselves. Only 8 percent of the severe PKU babies were ever said to have talked.

When I asked my grandmother if Peter knew any words, she said "moon". "We used to sit every night at the window and I'd look out and point to the moon and he'd smile and say 'moo.' " "Moo" was the closest Peter ever came to saying a word. Doris Slagle has never doubted that her son understood what he was pointing at. She spent virtually every waking moment of his first six years working with Peter. She worked with him on the blanket to get him to crawl, or sit up, or walk. "He liked to sing the songs 'Always' and 'Whispering.' At one time he could sing 'Red River Valley' with me. I don't know if he can do that today," she said. "It wasn't singing really, but he liked to do it. I'm sure of it."

Regarding the significance of talking, the PKU study of 106 children notes that, "This repeating of words spoken to the child by parents is perhaps more akin to a conditioned trick such as playing patty-cake, or waving 'bye-bye' . . ." Such abilities had no significance, the study concluded. Doris Slagle reports that her son Peter could wave good-bye. He preferred playing "this little piggy," according to mother and sister, to playing the game "patty-cake."

Whatever the medical details, Charles Peter Slagle is alive, is still my uncle, my mother's brother, my grandparents' only son, and I am his nephew. Nothing can change this, even though to visit him is to jump across an enormous chasm in time and to confront the set of values that sent him to the Newark State School in the first place. To the state and medical professionals charged with his care, and to the people in his family who gave him up so long ago, Charles Peter Slagle has other names. He is a "total vegetable," "an idiot," a PMR (for profoundly mentally retarded), an MRDD adult (mentally retarded developmentally disabled), a ward of the State of New York, connected to the state bureaucracy that pays his bills and buys his socks and pays minimum wage to the people who feed him day in and day out. I long to believe that there was no other way, that my uncle had to be sent away, his circumstances so unique, compelling, and clear-cut that my family can be absolved of his banishment, a life sentence for a nonexistent crime.

From the words of his mother and sisters I have pieced together the details of Charlie's life. They constitute so little of the life he ended up living, and Charlie's connection to me now isn't in them. As I roll in my wheelchair toward the place where he lives, I understand that my uncle and I share the experience of being different. Our lives are lived in the crawl space between our strangeness and other people's reactions and fears. The instinctive human fear of those who are different has defined both of our lives. The forces that put my uncle away would also place me in a category from which there is no escape. Inside me is the engine that thrashes about never stopping, always mindful that someday those same forces could decide my fate, claim that I am really helpless, that my life is not worth living, give me a label, and send me away to a place for all those like me. Much as the Holocaust haunts the soul of every Jew, I can see my uncle's exile as both some cold, logical inhuman consequence of history and as an utterly arbitrary exercise in evil with me a possible target.

My connection to my uncle also stems from a mystery only my long-dead grandfather can resolve. Why did he reject his son so completely and accept me, his grandson, without question? The experiences of mental retardation and paraplegia are quite different. My grandfather had nineteen years to know me before I became a paraplegic, whereas his son was retarded almost from birth. Yet I can't help thinking that somehow my grandfather's unhesitating acceptance of me is related, even implied by the equally definitive rejection of his son. It is something I cannot ever know. But it haunts me nonetheless.

Among all the memories of my grandfather John Slagle there is one dim, confusing image of a time he and I spent together a long time ago when I was a little boy, and he was still quite new at being a grandfather. It was some time around the 1960 Kennedy-Nixon campaign when he and I went for a drive. He said he had some work to do. Even as a little boy, I knew that Grandpa worked for the Jackson & Perkins Rose Gardens, a mail-order flower company, of long-standing and some national repute in Newark. He was a middle-level executive but I thought he was a captain of industry, his fame visible to me in every rose petal and in the advertisements for J & P roses on the back of the TV magazine in our Sunday paper. His job was the reason we had spectacular rose-bushes years ago in our backyard in Binghamton, New York. To me, roses were a sign of the mark I believed he had made in the world. I was fascinated by them with their thorns, their amazing, fragrant flowers, and even more amazing to a little boy, the silvery Japanese beetles that ate the leaves and had to be picked off one by one as part of my backyard chores.

Grandpa and I parked outside a brick building I had never seen before, and he walked a long distance across the lawn to the building even though there were plenty of places to park right there in the lot near the door. This was not the Rose Gardens, this was not where Grandfather worked. He left me in the old gray Plymouth for a long time on that street in Newark. When grandfather returned, he told me not to tell anyone what had happened, and because nothing had happened, I said nothing.

There was no particular reason to remember that day, and it was only the feeling of boredom that lingered in my mind. Grandfather had given me nothing to do to amuse myself in the car while I waited for him. He had just said good-bye and had walked slowly away. Grown-up things took a long time. Whatever grandfather had to do, I thought, it must have been a very grown-up thing. It is why I did not forget the image, and why it came back to me as a lightning bolt on the day I rolled from Newark to Phelps in my wheelchair to see my uncle.

I stopped in the hot sun, while the bugs and crickets buzzed in the roadside brush, and I looked across a lawn to a campus of brick buildings. I recognized the place. My wheelchair was near the same spot where Grandfather's old Plymouth had parked so long ago. Like the sudden matching of lines on two separate pages placed together and held up to the light, these two pictures matched in my memory. Here I had waited while grandfather did his work that afternoon. I couldn't tell which building he'd gone into, but the hill, the lawn, and the place by the road were the same.

The place had been developed into something of an industrial park in the years since 1960. The sign on the lawn contained the names of businesses and at the bottom the letters NDC. They stood for Newark Developmental Center, the politically correct name for the old town asylum, the Newark State School for the Mentally Ill, the nuthouse. NDC was an acronym devoid of meaning. You had to know where to look, to discover where to look away. I had been here before. I knew where to look.

In my short life I had traveled from Pennsylvania to Mount Saint Helens, Jerusalem to Tehran to Africa. My every breath was about pushing some limit I imagined I was chained to, always breaking free and triumphantly holding the broken end of that chain as I plunged headlong to the next place, only to start pushing all over again. I had covered so much distance in those years. I looked at the brick buildings where my uncle had spent more than twice the number of years I had lived in my wheelchair. His world must have consisted of the distance from his bedroom to the washroom on the floor of his ward, except on those days when he might have been taken outside with some of the other patients. His world was the end of that familiar chain in my life, the rusty metal ring in the concrete wall I was running from.

What my grandfather might have done that afternoon long ago, while I waited outside in the car, if he had even seen his son inside the building, is unknown. My uncle would have been in his mid-twenties then. Did my grandfather have a special relationship with his son that no one knew about? Did he go there on his own, to interrupt the exile he had decreed for his son? I estimated the distance from the road where my grandfather had parked the Plymouth to the door of the building he went into thirty-three years before at about 200 yards, shorter than I remembered. It was probably the closest I had ever been to my uncle.

I sat there staring at the grass, trying to pry open the old memories as if they were fossils. I struggled to remember my grandfather's face when he said that he would be right back, and the way he had looked when he had returned. I tried to recall if he had been smiling or crying. Perhaps he had spent happy, private moments with his son that day, or perhaps in shame he had taken steps to further disown him. There was nothing in my mind to make a picture, and no one alive today to confirm it even if I could. As hard as I tried, all I could remember was Grandpa leaving, Grandpa coming back, and the childhood boredom of waiting. Perhaps this was the feeling that my uncle often had. For years after he was sent away as a little boy he had waited for his parents, possibly wondering why he was there in such a strange place; and then after enough time had passed, perhaps he no longer waited, no longer wondered, finally convinced that the strange place where he lived was now home. My uncle would certainly not be expecting me to visit. I continued rolling down the two-lane highway toward Phelps.

Uncle Peter was sent away in September of 1943, a few years after he took his first steps. Doctors and specialists had lots of theories about why the little boy, whose mental retardation was now confirmed and presumed to be irreversible, should be removed from the house. Over time those theories and suggestions from doctors became a substitute for the clarity my grandparents never had with their unusual son, who could not speak and never got any better. For much of 1942 and 1943 Doris and John resisted the doctor's insistence that the boy would not improve, and the accumulating opinions that he be removed from their house. It was John Slagle who finally had enough. With his wife's consent they planned to send Peter away. The decisive argument had to do with the effect doctors said Peter's condition might have on others in the family. My mother was told that if her brother stayed in the house it could affect her own intelligence. There was nothing contagious about Peter's condition; PKU was not something he had gotten from the water or a dirty doorknob, that much was clear even back in the forties. But the idea of contagion was so central to the notion of disease that it could not easily be set aside.

Peter's condition was always presumed to be contagious, independent of any biological truth. It was an element of fate that would entwine itself around the family if left to itself. Peter's condition reflected on the Slagle name in some way that profoundly disturbed his father, that caused him to park far from the door and walk the distance to the building where his son lived. Putting Peter away was a socially acceptable form of moral quarantine. John Slagle could not make his son better, but for the good of his family he could be convinced that an institution was the best place for him.

My grandmother can remember everything she packed in several suitcases for her son. "We even took his little wooden rocking chair," she said, recalling how he loved to rock back and forth, something he could do far better than he could walk. She smiled as she spoke of how in his moments of shrieking and hitting himself he would often find that little chair and in a dim flash of memory plop down in it, remembering once again how to rock. Grandmother particularly remembers a nurse named Miss McCaffrey. It was Nurse McCaffrey who would be most closely responsible for Peter's well-being. She was tall and severe in a white nurse's uniform, unmemorable in every way except that it was to this woman that Doris Slagle gave her son away. It would be Nurse McCaffrey she and her husband would call to receive any news of Peter.

Nurse McCaffrey took Peter's hand and walked him to the center of the room where she let go of him. In the office of the doctors, they watched while Peter did his worst, hit himself repeatedly, made his loudest noises, had a seizure. The doctors noted his reactions. Someone suggested that Peter immediately be fitted with a helmet to protect his head from his self-abusive punches. Doris Slagle wanted to comfort her son, as she had always done since he had been born. She wanted to hold him while he screamed and shook and had one of his fits, but her husband held her back. "The doctors needed to see everything, I guess," she said.

My mother can also recall the trip to the state school with her brother. Peter sat in the backseat and bit himself a couple of times before falling asleep. When they arrived, everyone carried a suitcase except John Slagle, who alternately carried and walked with his son, holding his hand. In the suitcases were clothes and toys. My mother can recall that Peter's favorite toy, Jocko the monkey, was in one of the bags. She remembers hexagonal tiles on the floor, dark wooden doors that were huge and had a funny smell. My mother also remembers Nurse McCaffrey.

While her parents spoke with the doctors, my mother, Nancy, sat in a big overstuffed chair that smelled old and metallic like everything else in the hospital. There was an echo in the halls. There were other children in an adjacent room sitting on blankets and in cribs. My mother speaks in whispered horror of the faces of the children. "The ones with the small heads, you know," she said. "The microcephalics and the ones who kept bobbing up and down and opening and closing their fingers over and over again." She remembered the honking voices and thinking that the people at the school were all like her brother and that he might be happier among them, as an injured bird returns to soar with its own flock. But the eerie smell of the state hospital made it hard to feel good about leaving her brother behind.

From the upper floors of the patient wards, eleven-year-old Nancy recalls the pale, blank faces staring down at her as she walked to and from her parent's car. For much of her life she has had nightmares about those faces. In the worst of those nightmares the face of her brother appeared in one of the windows, looking down, looking for his older sister. "I always thought he must have wondered what had happened to us," my mother says, speaking of her nightmares. Her brother's absence had a life of its own, parallel and just out of sight. On each of her birthdays and during every subsequent milestone in her life— graduation, marriage, and the birth of me, her first child—Nancy Slagle thought of what her brother might be doing at the same moment. In her mind, she sketched his face into every family portrait. Because she did not really know what had happened to her brother in all those years, she thought the worst. In her face is the shapeless guilt of a child who had held the lantern as her parents had buried a body long ago. The light and shadows from that moment formed the same old questions in her eyes. "If it had been me, I wonder if I would have been sent away," she mused out loud.

The papers were signed. Charles Peter Slagle became a ward of the State of New York. Until they retired in the sixties, Doris and John would pay the state a monthly stipend, about sixty dollars, for food and clothes but from that moment on their influence over their son's life would be miminal. From now on it would be lived here. Nurse McCaffrey came over to the boy in the little toy rocking chair and gathered up his things for the orderlies to carry up to his room. She called him Charles and took him by the hand. The boy my grandfather called Petey would now be called by his first name, the name on the commitment papers. Peter became Charlie forever.

While his parents and sister watched, Nurse McCaffrey took Charlie by the hand and led him down the hall to the elevator and pressed the button for the floor where he would live for the next thirty years. My grandmother can remember watching him walk all the way to the end of the hall, reveling in each step he took, proud of each step she had taught him to take, secretly wanting him to turn around and run back into her arms. Before the elevator door closed, she thought that if her son had turned around and waved or even acknowledged his mother down the hall she would have defied her husband, called the whole thing off, put him back in the car, and driven home. But he did not turn around, the elevator doors closed, and they drove away without their son. Doris sobbed the whole way home. "He just didn't even know me. I think that is what always hurt the worst."

It was up to Charlie to save himself by doing something he could never do: turn around and wave to his mom and dad. Charlie Slagle's mental retardation made it very difficult to be sure about what he knew or didn't know about anything, including recognizing his parents. Doris Slagle's seven-year-old boy could have been fascinated by being in an elevator for the first time. Perhaps, after the doors had closed he had waved, or had looked around to find his family; perhaps he did nothing unusual. Peter may not have been able to clearly recognize his mother on the day he was sent away. But more than fifty years later, having spent most of his life in an institution, it is absolutely clear that Charlie Slagle doesn't know her.

At first, there were weekly visits to the hospital and a few overnight trips home for Charlie. All contact stopped after 1945, when the Slagles' third child was born. Sometime around the day that Susan was born, my grandfather and my mother took Charlie to an abandoned field that afternoon for lunch. Grandpa spent the trip back to the state school talking to his daughter about how Charlie didn't know any of them any-more, about how he was much happier where he was, living with peo-ple just like him. My mother said nothing. It was the last time she would see her brother at his new home for decades.

Charlie came home for the very last time Christmas 1943. John Slagle brought him home from the state school on Christmas Eve to a house-hold full of anticipation. Mother and older daughter were anxious to see if Charlie remembered his old house and how to do things like open the refrigerator. "He remembered applesauce," my mother recalled. She had told all of her friends that her brother was coming home for Christmas. There were four stockings hanging over the fireplace that Christmas, John, Doris, Nancy, and Peter.

These moments seem so golden to me, observing it all from the distance of a subsequent generation, probing memories for the remains of something so long gone. It could always have been like that at Christmas in the Slagle household. Kids screaming. Charlie honking. My mother playing the role of chatterbox, spouting her theories of what Charlie might or might not have been thinking, John and Doris the proud parents accepting the situation, good and bad. The grandchildren, me among them, could have worn out the adults by asking them why Uncle Charlie made that noise, or wore that helmet, or sat in that wheelchair.

My life would certainly have been different if Charlie had stayed home, or if we had known him while we were growing up. We would always have noticed the width of doorways. The houses we lived in would probably have been wheelchair-accessible. My brothers and I would have quarreled over who was going to push Uncle Charlie when we visited him. We would never have called people "retards" at school. We might have charged a full fifty cents to the neighbor kids to come over and see him when he visited. Charlie was more amazing than one-armed Grandpa Hockenberry. When bicyclists started wearing fiberglass helmets for protection, we would have noted that they were just like the one Uncle Charlie wore. If he had been a part of our lives I would not be rolling down a road on a hot summer day in 1993 to meet him for the first time.

That Christmas Eve in 1943, there was a terrible argument and early the next morning John Slagle took his son back to the state school. Nancy was told that her brother had become sick and had to see a doctor. This is what she told the many friends and neighbors who knew that Charlie was going to be home for Christmas. He had come down with pneumonia, she said. This is what she assumed until she found out more than forty years later what had really happened.

Charlie was not sick that Christmas; he had an accident in his bed that night and woke up honking and thrashing about. Charlie was not toilet trained, a skill beyond most people with untreated PKU retardation. He was quite a mess by the time his parents found him. While cleaning him up, my grandfather made the decision to take Charlie back to the state school for good. He was driven back on Christmas morning, delivered abruptly to the nurses, never to see his parents outside the institution again.

Christmas dinner was grim that evening. In the middle of it my grandfather burst into tears and sobbed uncontrollably in front of his wife and daughters. Doris and her husband went into their room, and my mother listened to her father sob from the other side of the closed bedroom door. Her memory of that Christmas is sitting alone at the dining-room table, staring at the turkey. From that moment on, mention of Charlie was increasingly rare. Gradually, within a matter of months, he was not mentioned at all. By the time Susan was a toddler it was clear that Charlie was not ever to be mentioned. Grandfather was going to act as though he did not have a son. Everyone was required to play along. It was an edict that remained in force until after John Slagle died, forty years later.

As a toddler, Susan played in her brother's room and slept in his little maple bed for years without knowing that he was alive and just a short walk away at the Newark State School. My grandfather had sworn his wife and daughter to secrecy about Charlie. Susan was not to know where her brother was. Their motive was to protect her from knowing that she had a brother in the nuthouse.

My aunt Susan and I share this total blank page when it comes to Charlie. We each knew vaguely of his existence, but nothing more. In Susan's case, she knew about her brother because of the family portrait in the back of the upstairs hallway with Charlie's face in it. There was a brother, but "he was lost," they said. They did not say he was dead, and so Susan imagined that he lived somewhere she couldn't get to. That place in her mind was a firehouse she had driven by one time. She thought of him upstairs, behind a closed, curtained window. Other than that image, there was nothing. I saw the same family picture as a little boy, and for me Charlie's face floated in an ether of adult seriousness. He was the ghost of grave looks and head shakes and sentences that trailed off. No one had ever told me he was dead. There was just not enough detail for him to be alive in my mind.

Susan discovered her brother's actual whereabouts when she was fourteen years old and I was just four. In 1960 she found a routine letter from the state school to the Slagle house buried underneath some papers. There had been lots of letters over the years, all carefully hidden away. But this routine medical report on Charlie's condition confirmed to his sister that he was one of her neighbors, and that he had been for practically all her life.

Susan demanded to know why she had never been told. Each member of her family responded that it was for her own good. They didn't want her to be hurt, they said. They wanted to protect her from knowing what they knew. Susan's discovery was a scandal in the Slagle household. She was told by her mother that she might know about her brother, but it was made clear to her that she was not to see him. "I understood that they were the ones who would be hurt if I went to see him," she said. "Especially Daddy."

Grandfather could not reverse what he had set in motion in the forties. To John Slagle, sending his son away was something he had done for his daughters, and he bore the pain for them. For them to want to know and visit their brother would have meant that he and his wife had borne all that pain for nothing. As I rolled toward Phelps to see Charlie for the first time, I could feel the physical sensation of defiance in my own numb body. John Slagle's edict was an old one, something my grandmother, mother, and aunt dared not defy until after his death.

My aunt Susan said that all she had wanted was to see her brother, to see what he looked like, to see him as a person rather than as this dark corner in the family no one could speak about. This was forbidden. To see Charlie was an act of rebellion that obliterated him as a brother, son, or uncle. In exile he could only be a symbol, never a human being. It is the symbol that has defeated the humanity in Charlie's life, and in the lives of so many people in America who were perceived as different or "in the way" as we marched across the continent and down through history. Healing and reclaiming the humanity from each one of those individual defeats is perhaps the most difficult mission before us as a nation. It is the real American Revolution.

My mother tried to see her brother Charlie once in the late sixties but was too afraid to go through with it and turned around on the way to the hospital. She made the trip again in 1981 after her father died. She sat in her brother's room as a nurse went to collect him from a recreation area. She looked around the room and saw nothing familiar. Everything she and her mother remembered packing for Charlie nearly forty years earlier was gone. The room was empty except for a small bed and a pair of slippers.

She could hear him coming down the hall before she saw him. There was the sound of clumsy steps as he was being led by the hand. "Well, Charlie," the nurse said, "look here, you have a visitor." She was the first relative to visit since his parents had last seen him in the 1960s. It was the first time his sister had seen him since 1945. It was the first time she had ever heard him called Charlie. He was wearing a helmet, but she could see that her brother's face was now that of a man's.

"He crossed his feet and put them underneath him and sat down in a strange little ball, like a fetal position, and he looked at me a little bit. There was no 'What took you so long?' kind of thing. I mean, there was no recognition of me whatsoever," my mother said. It was the nurse at the state school who recognized my mother. She said she went to the same Presbyterian Church as the Slagles and would often see the family standing together in a pew. On Sunday she would see Charlie's parents, and during the week she took care of their son. I wondered if she ever talked to Charlie about his parents while she fed him or gave him a bath. "I saw your mother in church today, Charlie," she might have told him.

"You used to sing in choir once in a while, I remember," the nurse said to my mother. "I would see you when you would come home from college." My mother asked about Charlie's health and learned that he had a few problems but was basically fine. She asked to look at his chart. There was a place on it to list his visitors over the years. The page was blank. She put her name on the page and left. She has never returned.

My aunt met her brother for the first time in 1988, and she has been to see him each year since. My grandmother went to see her son in 1989, and once more in 1991. She remarked to her daughter that he was quite small, and that he seemed to resemble her late husband's side of the family. Charlie was not the little boy Doris Slagle remembered who had walked clumsily into the elevator holding a toy and the hand of Nurse McCaffrey. The doors had closed in 1946. When they opened more than forty years later, the little boy was gone and his mother had become an old woman. When he had gone into the institution, Charles Peter Slagle was profoundly retarded, but he was not a stranger to his parents, much as they might have thought so. By 1989 he had truly become both.

On the last flat road before the turn to Charlie's group home the pavement opened up on a strip of car dealerships and farm equipment companies. Across the street there were cornfields stretching to the horizon. It was a left turn. Just back from the road on a circular drive was a large but residential-looking prefabricated house with some picnic benches and playground equipment on the lawn. I rolled up the driveway and saw the front door of Uncle Charlie's house. It was beautifully ramped and welcoming to someone who had rolled a wheelchair for eleven miles in the sun that day, and for seventeen years before that. I rang the doorbell and a nurse pushed a button and buzzed me through the front door.

"I'm here to see Charlie Slagle," I said. "Are you a relative?" she asked. "Yes," I said. "Welcome," she said to me as I rolled inside. I was nervous. It had been a long time since I had visited one of these hospitals. In the years since I'd left rehab I had really not seen that many wheelchairs. I was usually the sole crip in my group. I was the hotshot paraplegic, the role model, the brave reporter, the pitiable victim. "They," the rest of the world, were out there being normal, staring at me, getting inspiration from me, ignoring me, asking if I needed help with the door, or if I was lost. Here no one was going to do any of that. In this place, I was the normal one. It felt very strange.

In the hallway walking toward the nurse was an older woman whose face was divided into two distinct halves. One side was unremarkable, but the other side was filled with dark purple blisters that bulged, obscured, and obliterated her left eye and much of her nose. She had an extreme case of rosacea, a chronic skin eruption associated with what also appeared to be severe mental retardation. The purple skin hung off her like the aftermath of an explosion. She stared straight ahead and moved her fingers in the air in front of her face as though she was sewing or conducting an orchestra. The side of her head I could recognize as a face was smiling. The smile reached the center axis of her face and vanished into the shapeless, purple, disfigured left side. The nurse caught me staring. "Come this way," she said. "I think Charlie is eating dinner right now."

I rolled into a large dining area where a number of people were sitting with bibs on. Some were being fed, others were feeding themselves. They looked up at the rare dinner-time visitor. One man's eyes registered a kind of befuddled amazement and he looked to the nurse for an explanation. "This is Charlie's nephew, everyone," she said. "And he's brought a guitar."

In the center of the room, sitting at a long table by himself, was a little man in a wheelchair with a bib on being fed a mixture of green mush and brown mush. I rolled up to him. His head was moving around as he ate. His eyes were darting aimlessly around the room. "Look who's come to see you, Charlie." The nurse spoke first. It occurred to me that though he had been an uncle for more than thirty-five years he had never before heard the words I now uttered. "Hi, Uncle Charlie. I'm John. Your sister Nancy is my mother." His head stopped moving. He looked straight at me. His hair was blond. He looked very much like my grandfather, and just as my aunt had told me, he looked very much like my mother.

We sat there for a time as I stared at him. He was staring at me. The people in the room were all staring at the two of us. I had told myself that I wouldn't care if he acknowledged me or not. He did not have to prove anything to me. He could be a total vegetable, he did not have to look at me even once, or know that I was there, and I would still accept him. This would be my repudiation of all that had happened to him. I was not going to care that he couldn't return my affection. I was going to be someone who would make no conditions. He was Charlie Slagle. He was alive. It was up to me to accept that on his terms.

As I saw the resemblance to my dead grandfather, my resolve crumbled and I searched his face greedily for a sign of recognition. I touched him and spoke. "Uncle Charlie, I've heard so much about you. I saw pictures your mother has of you as a baby. I feel like I have missed you, Charlie." A stream of words, stupid and heartfelt, poured out of my mouth. He was moving his head while I spoke and occasionally, as he began to look away, his eyes held mine for a moment. "Moo. Do you remember the moon, Charlie? How your mother would point at the moon at night, and you would point too, and you would say moo? Charlie, do you remember the moon?" His head resumed moving back and forth.

I sat with him, searching for some magic word, trying out all the little songs and any of the things my mother, my grandmother, or my aunt had told me. I was twirling the tumblers to crack the safe and see his face burst with recognition. I would reveal for all time the Charlie inside. "He was in there all the time," I would be able to say. "He was trapped, but I brought him out. He was unable to find us, but I found him." It was the old myth, that the real Charlie was inside. I was going to find the little boy who would have grown up to play baseball with his father; the boy John Slagle would have made things for. I wanted to tell Charlie that I had his cutting board back at my house, the cutting board his father had made for me. I felt as I sat there that it was really his cutting board. I looked into his eyes, and I wanted to tell him that I had slept in his little maple bed as a boy, that I had played in his room with some of his toys. I really wanted to thank him and have him look at me and just acknowledge me with an eyebrow, a movement of the head, a twinkling of the eye, a half smile, a little noise to show a sign that he had heard me.

When the words and songs and suggestions all emptied out of me, there was just silence. Charlie and me. Although he would not recognize it in the same way, I must have looked like everyone else who had ever visited him from his family. I was another one of those people who showed up every few years to rattle his cage, or tap on his glass tank to get a rise out of him and then run away to tell someone about it like a dog stealing a shoe. In the end, there was no metaphor for Charlie. The most important thing was simply to be there near him and allow who he really was to sink in. If I really wanted to know him, I had to sit quietly and listen to the details of his life, something people so rarely do. Just as people looked for the shortcuts for knowing about my life in a wheelchair, I was looking for the same thing to understand my uncle Charlie. I was staring now. I was human, just like him.

Charlie picked up one of his hands, made a little fist, and with a slow windup smashed himself in the face, landing a blow squarely against his jaw. "Now, Charlie," the nurse feeding him said. "What is the rule about doing that, Charlie?" She looked at me. "He has a history of self-abuse, but he's been better about it lately." She turned back to Charlie and her voice got louder. "Haven't you, Charlie. Haven't you been better about hitting yourself?"

I took out my guitar and played a few songs; everyone in the dining room seemed to enjoy listening. Charlie finished his dinner and watched me. I spoke with the chief nurse, who told me a few things about Charlie's health problems, when he lost his teeth, how closely they watched his diet. She said he hadn't been wanting to eat over the past few years, and so it was difficult keeping his weight up. It was small talk. She could tell that my mind was racing. "You shouldn't worry about your uncle. He is happy here. This is all he knows. Few people at this home get many visitors. It is fine this way." After all the years apart there was no other way for it to be.

I went outside with Charlie and took a few pictures of him. He watched me and wondered who I was, or perhaps he simply detected a disturbance in his daily routine. A stiff breeze came up from across one of the adjoining cornfields. We went back inside and sat in a large room with a television and some stuffed chairs. He sat in a chair in the corner of the room and curled his legs up and put his arms over his head. Occasionally he would try to hit himself and I would gently take his hand and say no. He would open his eyes and look straight at me as if to say, "Why not?" Then his eyes would flutter as though he'd forgotten what he was thinking, and he would raise his hand once more.

We sat like this for many hours as the sun began to set through the window. It made his blond hair look golden. I looked at him and thought of all the things that had happened in his life and mine. I thought of all the reasons put forward to explain why he was sent away, the reasons why I didn't know him and why I never really would. I saw much more than a little mentally retarded man with blond hair and the features of my mother and grandfather in his face.

I looked into his eyes, and it made me angry that he was here in this place and that he had never known the places my brothers and sister and I had grown up in. I had been told by my grandmother, my mother, and my aunt that Charlie wouldn't know me and could never acknowledge his family. But we could all still acknowledge him. Because Charlie didn't recognize his family, he was to be put away and forgotten? To be loved, Charlie had to pass the one test he was sure to fail. To be loved and accepted by his family, Charlie had to be aware enough to show that he knew them. Charlie could never do this. In failing that test, Charlie became a stranger to me. In the quiet evening light, with me sitting there next to him strumming the guitar, Charlie had nothing more to prove. So why did I still have so much to prove?

I thought back to how my hands had felt as I had grabbed the saddle of the donkey and pulled myself up for the ride into Iraqi Kurdistan. I remembered the marathon races in Chicago. I remembered staring up at the bed slats in Martha's room, wondering what I was doing there. I wondered the same things while rolling through the crowds in Iran after Khomeini died. I remember the hot shrapnel under my tires on the road in Tel Aviv when the missiles fell, the people in the gas masks in the sealed room, how I agreed that they would stay and I would fend for myself in the wheelchair. I thought of the eyes of every cabbie who had refused me a ride, every person who had handed me change or asked me if I was lost. I was a slave to every one of those tests. Every line drawn for me to cross, I would cross. Every lowered expectation I would raise. In a life of breaking chains and surmounting obstacles I had only bound myself more tightly to the idea of fighting for my freedom.

Fighting for freedom is America's national ritual, and it is where, I think, things often go so very wrong for America. After more than two centuries of telling Europe and the other doubters that we have not yet begun to fight, we don't know how to stop. Our history consists of flinging ourselves at all of the obstacles and railing against the doubters. There have been two centuries of resentment, of watching to see if they were making fun of us, watching to see if they would hold the door for us or would ask us for help. We have spent two centuries trying to prove something that people long ago lost interest in, and now we are lonely as the world's only superpower. We defeated them all many times over, showed them unequivocally that we did not need their help, and today we stand around arguing with ourselves. There have been two centuries of dealing with our disabilities as a nation and ignoring those things which we couldn't face. Today, fighting for freedom is done among ourselves, inside our own borders, something the U.S. Constitution claims no American should ever have to do to be free.

Someone outside draws a line in the sand and questions whether we are a superpower and America crosses it like a rat going for the cheese. Khomeini did it, so did Saddam Hussein. But if Americans ask for freedom, access, to be included in their own country, they are shouted down or ignored. We know best how to fight to be recognized as a world power, but we haven't given much thought to what we would actually do in a free society. The faces of the people trampled, left behind, or sacrificed to make us a superpower are all still here. They haven't stopped staring, and try as they might, they can't get America's attention like Saddam or the Ayatollah can. What is different about them is not that they are black, or red, or yellow, or poor, or disabled. What is different about them is that they have not been included. It is why they are staring. In the beginning, people in America are told that freedom belongs to them; then they discover that they must fight for it.

What we call civil rights in America is people jumping through hoops for their freedom, then having their scores tallied like figure skaters in the Olympics. Uppity niggers score low, so do illegal immigrants and welfare mothers and crips who ask too loudly why there is no ramp into the theater. "We fought for it, so it's only fair that you should have to." It is America's real declaration of independence that poisons and isolates blacks, Jews, Asians, and whites from each other. It is less about race today than it is about this brutal free-for-all of who gets what, who deserves more, who's being fair, who's taking advantage.

We started our national history trying to escape the divisions and hatreds of the lands we all came from and we have ended up creating our own. In the game of freedom fighting, I have scored very high in my life, but now I find I can't stop playing. Just as America can't stop insisting that it's still number one, I sit in my wheelchair and dare someone to say the wrong thing. Inside, the soul that would be free churns in a turmoil of bondage, anger, and servitude, like the violence on America's urban streets.

Charlie doesn't argue. Charlie doesn't want to fight. I sit with him and he teaches me something about freedom. None of the historical details I had learned about my uncle prepared me to meet him. For nineteen years I was a young white man of comfort and suburban privilege in America. The winners and losers in America's battles were, like Uncle Charlie, out there somewhere. People like me only stared at them. The truths about their experiences and the truths they represented were in code. One might know historical details about the tragedy of the American Indian, the African-American experience, the struggles of everyone from Asians to industrial workers, but being white and free in America is to be more like a spectator. It is rarely from experience that a white person learns history; more likely it is from reading the program notes.

It is for this reason that I have come to find myself grateful to have been a crip for the past nineteen years: I may miss walking, running, or tree climbing from time to time, but I do not miss being a spectator. The forces that tore the vertebrae from my ribs and the spinal nerves from the protected flesh in my back also parted a curtain for me. Looking at Uncle Charlie sitting there in his chair I can see for the first time who he is, separate from the forces that kept him from me, from his family, and locked up here in this place. The impulses that put my uncle Charlie away know no race or religion, and they are alive for me now as though history has awakened from its own dream. Uncle Charlie is the last plank of a bridge that as a white man in America I believe I could only have crossed in a wheelchair. It has been a long time coming.

Though this is a nation of suspicious enclaves and ignorant spectators, I have come to believe that the experiences of struggle that define the peoples of America, and ultimately this world, can be shared. We are taught to believe that knowing what others have been through is impossible in our rainbow coalition of American enclaves (members only need apply). With hate and suspicion, each group claims that no one outside its enclave can know their experience, and that the indecipherable walls around each group grow higher. The T-shirt says: "It's a Black Thing." The codes of experience are like closely guarded family secrets where the key to the code has been thrown away. As a white person I understand the feeling of not knowing the code, as a person in a wheelchair I know the experience of selfishly guarding the code and punishing those outsiders who don't know it.

It is not as though a spinal-cord injury is some ridiculous antidote to ignorance. It is to understand that if a car accident on a sunny Pennsylvania day and the arbitrary exercise of gravity on my bones has brought me closer to America's walled-in ethnic, racial, and economic enclaves, how indecipherable can they be, really? In Genesis, upon observing the Tower of Babel the Lord said of the world he had made, "Behold, the people is one, and they have all one language; and this is the beginning of what they will do; and nothing that they propose to do will now be impossible for them." I suppose that would include climbing on donkeys in Kurdistan.

If he had been born at another time, Charlie's PKU would have been treatable. If I had gotten in a different car than Margaret Zinn's beige Chevrolet in 1976, I would still be able to walk. These are the suppositions that presume to blame fate or time for the lives we end up living. In Charlie's case nothing can change the fact that he is my uncle, that he looks like me, that I am connected to him, and always have been. As

Peter, the name his parents called him by, he was imprisoned in shame and rejection; as Charlie, and by living his own life, in his own way, my uncle is free.

I stayed with him until it was nearly time for bed. I spoke with the other workers at the group home and said that I would visit again soon. I put my name on Charlie's visitors' list. I went over to him one more time to say good-bye. I took his hand. "Uncle Charlie, it's been very nice visiting you." I looked into his eyes as I spoke. "Good-bye, Uncle Charlie." His face twisted into a scowl, his eyes darted up to the ceiling, and he turned away. I rolled out through the big, wide-ramped front door and sat waiting in the driveway for a moment, watching Charlie through the window, sitting in his wheelchair. I caught him looking out the window for an instant. I reared up on two wheels and pushed with my arms.

My grandfather went to his grave, according to my grandmother, having spent every day of the last thirty-four years of his life thinking about his son Petey's exile up there at the state school. His wife and daughters have done the same. I rolled out of the driveway and down toward a waiting taxi. I wished it were a gray Plymouth waiting with my grandfather inside. I would tell him that I was sorry I took so long, but I just wanted him to know that everything was fine. "Petey is okay," I would say to him. "You know, Grandpa, they call him Charlie now."

I drove away.

Somalia

*I*n October 1992 there was nothing but death and chaos in all of the coverage of the disastrous famine in Somalia. On my way to Mogadishu for ABC News, I laid over in London to refit my wheelchair for what promised to be very rugged conditions. In the hotel room that night, I fell asleep after an evening of wrenches and axle plates, re-greasing bearings, and tightening spokes. I had a walking dream.

I was wandering around alone in a field of dead people. The people who remained alive gestured toward me, but I could not speak with them. They motioned in desperation, but I could not understand what they wanted. I walked past them for miles, it seemed, until my legs began to get sluggish and it became nearly impossible to me to walk. I tried to ask them what they needed. One man whose head was atop a scrawny tree trunk was saying something that I couldn't understand. Then he turned his head and I could see that each thin branch of the tree had a head on it and that they were all looking at me and talking. I knew why they had died, but I couldn't tell them. Soon I was so tired and sluggish that I couldn't take another step. The heads on the trees finally said something I could understand.

"You can't walk," they said, as though they were accusing me of something.

I knew that, I thought. I realized that I had misplaced my wheelchair somewhere, and wondered how I was going to find it. Then I woke up.

On the eve of leaving London for Somalia, I called Rick, my college roommate before the accident in Pennsylvania, for the first time in two years. I had thought of him as I looked out the window of the plane on the flight to London. The plane had cast a shadow on the thick clouds below. Far below the clouds was the Atlantic Ocean, in the shadows which concealed all evidence of our crossing. Horizons curved away in all directions. I was a random spot on an infinite globe. Through the window of the plane I peered around behind me, looking for the sun. It was hard to move in the plane seat, and I was reminded of another cramped seat next to a window. For an instant I was looking out, trying to find Ricky. His hand and voice had been there once before, right behind my ears.

I reached Rick at home. There was no particular reason to call him, but a single chilling thought of not returning had come and passed. There wasn't much in the way of authority in Somalia in October 1992, two months before the media feeding frenzy and the starvation stampede to the beaches of Mogadishu. We made small talk at first. "I'm in London. I leave for Somalia tomorrow." We were both quiet guards, barring entry to the places we had closed away years ago. We were also cold from being locked outside. Over the years, while we each guarded our own door, we grew to wish that the other one would force the latch and demand entry. We both knew that in such a case we had decided, quietly, secretly, and independently that we would stand aside and let the other in.

"Somalia, it sounds pretty insane over there." He was listening for other words from me. They came in a rush, things I had half-thought from all of the awkward moments encountered, and had then filed quickly away.

"Rick, I'm sorry that I never wanted you to push my chair. I didn't mean any harm in it. I just wanted you to know that I have been all right all these years."

He paused, and I could hear the tremble in his breathing. "I just wanted to say that I really appreciated what you did."

"But I didn't do anything," he said, his voice very soft now.

"Ricky," I said, "I've missed you all these years." I looked back to the moment on the hill when everything inside the car was warm with my own blood, and outside the car Ricky was scared and so alone, frightened and cold.

"I wanted to thank you for saving my life back there in Pennsylvania. I know that you did, and for the past few years I wondered if anyone had ever thanked you. I don't think anyone ever did."

A low moan came from the phone. Something holding us together and keeping us apart gave way and we both just hung there in space together. It was the first time we had spoken of the accident since February 1976.

"I didn't save you," he said. "I didn't think you were going to make it. You told me that you couldn't walk. I was watching the fire. You kept making jokes. I wanted to get you out of there. I couldn't. That girl driving was hurt so bad. At least I could talk to you." Ricky was sobbing through the phone now. "It's been so long." He whispered as he said it. "I didn't save you. We just didn't die."

"You aren't to blame," I blurted out to him. "Never once have I ever thought so." In tears, over the phone we began to exhume all of the ghosts untouched from that day. The reasons we were hitching. The reasons we got in that car with those girls. The reasons I held all of the guitars and Ricky held all of the clothes and sleeping bags. "Ricky, I know you were hurt bad from the accident and nobody ever noticed." His voice came back to me from 1976. "It's okay, man. It's going to be okay." I could hear him next to my ear through the crack in the window.

There was a pause on the phone. A heart had started beating again. My best friend and I had been so far apart for so long. Our lives had changed so much in that time. The ripples out from the accident had crested now, and we sat blinking on beaches, holding telephones. An ocean was between us. I said into the phone, "Did we make it, Ricky? Is everything okay?" Rick was always the leader, always the scared smart one while I was always reckless.

"Why do you go to these places?" he demanded to know. I had no answer for him. "I put out one fire long ago that was about to kill you." Ricky's voice had a sudden edge. "I don't know if this other one can ever be put out."

We landed in Baidoa, aboard a U.S. Army C-130 transport. The moonscape of Somalia was accessible only by military plane. Once we departed from the transport we were alone, a solitary crew roaming from one end of Somalia to the other with armed escorts every moment. At the airport an Australian official from CARE, in a gaucho hat, urged us to get back on the plane and return to Kenya. He said that it was impossible to guarantee our safety. We would have to leave. There was shooting in town. Our armed escorts were paid and were waiting for us to get on board. The man from CARE said, "You're on your own." We thanked him and had started to drive away when a Somali carrying a sidearm and an assault rifle stopped us. He wore wraparound sunglasses and a green silk shirt from Venice Beach, California, and had his own entourage of armed escorts.

We followed him. He was the security chief for the Baidoa airport. He took us past dozens of roofless buildings covered with rifle and artillery shot. What used to be an official building was now a windowless ruin with only three of its walls intact. Outside what had been a front entrance, two bullet-scarred statues of monkeys watched as we drove slowly by. They looked unspeakably evil, like outposts of a place beyond the ends of the earth.

Even at this end of the earth you needed a press pass. We drove into a parking lot full of debris and were told to enter what looked to be an abandoned and vacant building. A crowd of well-armed boys greeted us. After a moment, three older men appeared. Their age and the fact that they weren't wearing Nike or Club Med T-shirts set them apart. Their cotton shirts with buttons and collars gave them a certain dignity, apparent despite the overpowering smell of human waste. Inside the building was a table and some rusted, rickety chairs downsized from the ruins of an elementary school classroom. The building might have been a school at one time, or perhaps the school supplies had been brought here from the looting of a nearby school. On the table was a single box of paper clips. Squares of paper sat on the table, clipped together with sheets of carbon paper.

One of the older men collected our passports and began to fill out the sheets of paper with our names, nationalities, and passport numbers. While he wrote, the young boys in the room pointed at the wheelchair and chewed the intoxicating herb we saw everywhere in Somalia, *chat* or *qat*. They pointed at the tires and spokes with their rifle barrels and conversed intently about something. We were invited to pay ten dollars for each permit. Our security guards angrily disputed the permit charge, and they waved their weapons at the security boss with the silk shirt and the sunglasses. All smiles vanished.

Everyone in the room was aware that we were carrying thousands of dollars in cash and thousands more in equipment. Five bullets, and they could divide all of our money peacefully. Instead they were prepared to open fire in a closed cramped room over, at most, fifty bucks. We paid the fees. The smiles returned. We were officially welcomed to Somalia and the Baidoa district. As we left, one of the elder men spoke with Khaled, a young Somali man serving as our translator. After a moment Khaled climbed into our jeep and we drove off.

"He was talking about you," Khaled said to me. "He was liking your cart." My "cart" was strapped to the top of the Jeep with two elastic cords. "He said he hoped it would not be stolen. We need these carts in Somalia." I looked back through the window at the parking lot and building. The crowd that had just welcomed us was gone, vanished into

the ruins. The roofless, sun-bleached stone and brick looked undisturbed, as before. It was hard to believe that we had just been there. In
my pocket the scribbled papers we had just paid for had no meaning
beyond that parking lot. But my chair had value. If we lost our cash and
equipment we might be able to purchase our lives by giving up the
chair. In a Jeep full of heavily armed security boys hanging out the windows and off the roof, I felt completely naked.

We were an apparition driving through a nation of ghosts. A thin boy
attempted to lead his staggering family down the road. Along the side
of the road were the bones of some who hadn't made it. A skeleton
undisturbed next to a bush mimicked the last motions of a human being
now long gone. A man had once been draped over these bones. At first
it seemed that he had knelt down. There were indentations in the soil
below his knee joints. There were none below his elbows, which perhaps had held his head and shoulders up above the earth for a time.
They were lighter than his legs and hips. His emaciated arms had barely
depressed the soil. The white skull rested near the bones of his hands.
A brown garment fluttered in the wind. In October 1992 the weight of
Somali bones could not hold down even this piece of burlap. A walking
stick lay where it had fallen.

The phenomenon of starvation that had descended on Somalia mani-
fested itself in vast, cruel landscapes of human misery punctuated by
crueler pockets which, without explanation, the plague of hunger had
missed. It was not only the boys with the weapons who had food. All
around the country there were heavily defended enclaves of the well-
fed. Whole villages watched as other displaced and starving people
walked by on their way to the feeding centers that dotted the countryside. Why one group was alive and the other near death were two opposite and profoundly unequal mysteries. Skeleton people, the Somalis
called their own unlucky countrymen, walking by on their way to die.

The well-fed people paid attention to the television camera. The starving people did not. In one prosperous village it was the wheelchair that
attracted a crowd. We stopped to shoot some pictures. I would be the
decoy. The village would follow me, so Alex the cameraman would be
free to shoot pictures. I rolled up and down the center of town and the
crowd followed. Our armed security escorts stayed close to me. They
were city boys from Mogadishu. It was easy for a crowd of villagers to
get in their way. The villagers were not in my way.

Our high-strung security detail came with two vehicles. Three hundred bucks a day got you two Toyotas, two drivers, a roof-mounted .50-
caliber machine gun, five guys with AK-47 assault rifles, and a twelve-

year-old carrying an M-60 grenade launcher and wearing a T-shirt that said "I'm the Boss." We called him Boss. The job of Boss and his older companions was to protect us. They took the job seriously. It was the only employment available in Somalia in October 1992.

The most popular T-shirt in Somalia was "I'm the Boss" in various colors. The one Boss wore was black with yellow letters. Strapped loosely around his kid frame, a canvas belt needed an extra hole punched in it to keep it from falling down. The belt held grenades, and he carried at least ten in the individual pockets, which bulged around his hips like a floating life ring for a child just learning to swim. In his hands he carried the launcher, a sawed-off short-barrel affair that broke in the middle, Schwarzenegger-style, for loading one cartridge at a time. It looked and felt light and portable, as though it was made for twelve-year-olds who needed to stop armored vehicles or other twelve-year-olds with grenade launchers. One was more likely to meet the latter than the former in Mogadishu in October 1992.

I rolled through the crowd in the village. The only words that were reliably understood were Arabic numbers, which were of no use at all, but since they were the only words all of us knew, we would call out numbers one through ten, laughing and squealing. *Wahad, tneen, talatta, arba; wahad, tneen, talatta, arba.* Alex worked to get pictures of the huts and empty shops clustered together. Literally hundreds of people raced along next to my chair. The youngest boys quarreled over who would push me. For a while I let them push. We ran faster and faster. Occasionally they would push my chair over the feet of a slower moving older woman. After a couple of these collisions I stopped the chair and insisted as best I could in my bad Arabic, which they understood about as poorly as I could speak it, that I would push the chair.

Here communication broke down. The crowd pressed in close. People inspected the chair and commented on the man in it. It seemed that the entire village was surrounding me. Some boys tried to push from behind once again. I looked back around at them with as severe an expression as I could muster. I expected to continue having this wordless argument over pushing my chair while Alex finished taking his pictures. I could not see him or the rest of our team. They stared at me and I stared at them.

Our Mogadishu security detail was impatient to get back on the road. They considered these villagers to be ignorant bumpkins unworthy of respect. While we were interested in making some sort of contact with them, our security detail barely tolerated them. One tall man who normally sat next to the .50-caliber machine gun on the roof of one of our

Land Cruisers began to shout at the boys behind me. He did not like it that the boys were still trying to push my chair. In a few moments two of our security people were firing their AK-47's into the air to disperse the crowd around me. Again the smiles vanished. Children scattered, screaming. We finished up quickly and were on our way before something truly awful could happen.

The two Toyota Land Cruisers were piled high with equipment and weapons, and just behind the back seat was a 55-gallon drum filled with gasoline. This was our fuel supply. On average, it lasted three or four days. In the beginning the big drum full of inflammable liquid wasn't noticeable, but over time, as the gasoline in the drum made its way into the Toyota's tank (usually the boys would siphon it in while standing around smoking and laughing), you could hear sloshing in the tank as we drove over the wretched bumps and pits and completely roadless stretches around the Somali countryside.

As we got closer to Mogadishu, little boys would stand by the road and do an elaborate dance, waving a piece of colored fabric to get vehicles to stop. Some of the boys had been repairing holes in the road and held out their hands for payment. Other boys had dug their own holes in the road, which they would refill to suggest that they had been doing the same thing. Others relied exclusively on their dancing and performance to bring in money. There was someone begging every 100 yards on the last 10 miles into Mogadishu.

The city was a crowded ruin. On the right side of the road, as it turned toward the center of the city, a white wall ran for more than a mile. Inside the wall had been the U.S. Embassy compound. Its buildings were still there. The facility had been completed just a few months before it was closed down. Its relative newness shone through smudges of graffiti, charred wreckage, and walls shattered long ago by artillery and grenades.

It was a flash both forward and backward in time to see the debris. On a coastal promontory, the U.S. Embassy stood facing the Red Sea. The compound was overgrown with weeds that waved obscenely as the wind blew through the blackened holes blasted through walls and floors. One place had been hammered with the heaviest of weapons, its armor melted into slag before it cooled. It looked like metal and glass ice cream. The local Somali warlords said that two people had entered a secret chamber in the ambassador's residence to steal, and the door had shut behind them. For two days, the story went, gunmen fired at the vault. When it was finally breached, the two men inside were long dead. There was no evidence of this now. Only neglect. Not even squatters gathered here. In a few months, the U.S. Marines would enter this compound as part of the Operation Restore Hope deployment. For now it was abandoned. The men that stayed here holding off the uninterested with a few AK-47's did not even take shelter in the spacious residence, which was one of the few unguarded places in Mogadishu with a basically intact roof. They stayed in the rocky field. Their fire flickered at night in the foreground while the unlit embassy building on the hill poked a blunt, black hole in Mogadishu's brilliant night sky.

There were no ramps at the embassy, and I rolled over pieces of shrapnel and long-spent ordinance to get inside the residence. On the lawn of the secure inner compound the last chopper had taken off the first week in January 1991 under cover of marine fire and the world's preoccupation with the impending war with Iraq. In that helicopter, the U.S. ambassador and the Soviet ambassador were evacuated with their tennis rackets in hand. A generation of cold-war sideshow in Ethiopia and Somalia came to an end in that helicopter ride. Each nation held the distinction of having at one time been both U.S. and Soviet allies. Now a quite different horror show would begin.

Downstairs, on the back side toward the sea, stood the remains of two spectacular bedrooms. On the wall of one, scrawled in a hand that clearly did not know English, were the words "Please can you sind helb us." There were scant signs that anyone but low-grade militia had ever paused here. The only evidence of a warlord's presence was the enormous hole punched through one of the interior walls with a heavy cannon shot that could only have come from the better armed, and therefore most important, of the clan functionaries.

On the porch off one of the main-floor bedrooms was a birthday card that was never sent. In big, round, girlish letters it talked about loneliness and the rising tension around the time it must have been written, in late 1990, just before the fall of the government. The card concluded with a deeply sad postscript: "I hope to see you in my palace by the sea. Love, Kathleen." The card's bright fuchsia trim was the only color left on this smudged ruin of an ambassador's residence.

On the floor inside the bedroom was another small dot of color, a game card from an old edition of the popular board game Trivial Pursuit. One of the questions on the card was about Elvis and Graceland. The geography question asked what the longest river in America was. Of all the billions of dollars spent here in Somalia, of everything U.S. policy in Africa had armed, built, supported, and ultimately abandoned, this card and tons of useless military hardware were all that remained.

"We are a nation of monuments now." A gentle Somali man from the northern port town of Berbera spoke while sitting on the burned-out wing of a fighter half-buried in the sand. "This is the best museum from the cold war. It is also the best junkyard. The junk is doing fine, as you can see. What has been ruined is my country." The Somalis understood best of all that in the grand cold-war scheme of things, their nation was a trivial pursuit. The final insult to more than a generation of weapons shipments and proxies and payoffs to dictators in the Horn of Africa by Moscow and Washington was that when the scenario of global conflict actually ensued, when Iraq invaded Kuwait, when the regional trip wire was tripped, Somalia didn't figure in anyone's military plans. Somalia's bases and ports and airstrips rusted in the sun while the Allies flew their smart bomb missions from aircraft carriers just over the horizon in the Red Sea and the Persian Gulf. Meanwhile, the people of Somalia began to starve, out of view of the Western powers that had more than anything helped to bring the nation to this far more horrible threshold.

The last unlooted item on the wrecked floor of the embassy residence in Mogadishu was the green binding of the Modern Library edition of the Isak Dinesen novel *Out of Africa*. The words burned angrily upward like graffiti. The pages were gone, charred and flaked away. It was as if only these words by themselves had any meaning.

After a few hours of rolling around the embassy grounds littered with heat-sharpened fragments of shrapnel and jagged glass, my tires began to go flat. The security boys with Boss insisted that we all go downtown to the warren of bullet and weapons shops, where one could also get a tire repaired. I removed the tool kit from my bag and unbolted my wheels from the chair frame. Our security detail grabbed the wheels triumphantly and off we went to the Bukhari market. In October 1992 there were no crews and certainly no U.S. soldiers in Mogadishu's Bukhari market. In October 1993 two American army helicopters were downed there, the soldiers pinned down for sixteen hours, and twelve of them killed. One could always buy arms in Bukhari, one could always get a tire patched. A year after we went there to fix a wheelchair tire, the body parts of U.S. servicemen were on display, along with the wreckage of their attack helicopters.

The nation was starving. There was no civic life but this infrastructure of chaos. Tire repair, weapons supplies, and fuel. All three operated even when there was no food. Fuel was available night and day, siphoned from large tanks into smaller tanks into 55-gallon drums, then often just poured, one bucket at a time, into the tanks of waiting vehicles. Mogadishu was hell on earth. It was one of the easiest places on the planet to get a wheelchair tire repaired.

As a solitary crew working in Somalia, arranging even the simplest permission to film places or interview people was a complicated war of nerves, wagering our need for pictures against the whims of the boys with guns we encountered everywhere. As long as people were smiling, we would work. When the smiles vanished, we would leave. At the palace of the exiled dictator, Mohammed Ziad Barre, we walked and rolled through an empty mansion trimmed with expensive marble beneath giant glass chandeliers that tinkled gently in the hot coastal breezes. No one lived here. The boys who guarded it stayed outside in a tattered canvas tent in what was once Ziad Barre's private zoo. The cages were all empty.

Around the palace, the government buildings had sustained massive damage. The walls sagged around car-sized holes, and twisted office furniture protruded from the wreckage. The parking lots were full of spent and live ordinance. A representative of Mohammed Farah Aideed, the south Mogadishu warlord, could not gain us entry to the palace area. As we filmed, a loud argument ensued. This place belonged to these boys. No one could remember who had given it to them. Their leader, who might recognize the representative of Aideed, was not around nor expected back any time soon. We would have to leave.

In each case our request was met by a stern dismissal, which became a challenge to our security detail, who answered by challenging the people from whom we were requesting cooperation. We spent as much time keeping our security detail from firing on people as we watched for people who might fire on us. Mogadishu was a sandlot. The boys in their Toyotas and with their heavy weapons, or "technicals," roamed the streets firing, chewing *qat,* selling their services to people who still had possessions to guard. Each vehicle was armed with an ingenious array of howitzers and grenade-toting boys. "I am the Boss," the T-shirts said. Who could argue?

Each vehicle was bristling with firepower and had its own 55-gallon drum of reserve fuel. Some were truly comical, the welded conglomerations of a Third World auto-mechanics class on acid. In one part of Mogadishu a yellow International Scout four-wheel-drive vehicle had its cab sawn off and in its place, sitting directly over the rear axle, was an air-to-air missile in its launcher taken from under the wing of a Soviet MIG fighter. Khaled laughed as he pointed it out to me. "It will only fire once," he said. "The wheels cannot hold this." He fumbled and could not say clearly what he meant. But looking at the vehicle, it was clear. The rear wheels sagged low from the weight of the missile. If it ever fired, the recoil would shoot the frame clear off the transmission. There was no way the weight of the vehicle could support the force of the missile, let alone aim it properly. The missile's jet would also clearly ignite the drum of fuel the boys had placed directly underneath it. That they were sitting on a doomsday weapon didn't seem to matter to these boys. They drove around scraping their overloaded axle on the ground, smoking, chewing *qat,* and looking important.

The whole business of clan warfare and technicals in Mogadishu was a frantic standoff: underage warriors racing around the city getting high and screaming at terrorized pedestrians. But few shots were fired other than into the air. If any of the technicals had engaged in battle, it would have been over quickly. One bullet or grenade could stop the civilian Toyotas and Isuzus devoid of armor or bulletproof glass. A single bullet would ignite the fuel drums in the back. That on every corner you didn't find burned-out wreckage, melted weapons, and charred bodies was a testimony to how conscious everyone was of the cold war's old doctrine of "mutual assured destruction," Somali-style.

When the U.S. and United Nations–armored attack helicopters and infantry jeeps arrived in Mogadishu months later to keep the peace, this street-corner deterrence broke down. For months the boys had had nothing to shoot at aside from the clouds. Finally, they had found something.

After being chased away from the ruined Somali parliament building by some boys with bazookas, we found an unguarded, apparently unclaimed place near a radio tower. Up a long flight of spiral stairs the tower opened onto a wide view of the city. The camera crew went up to the top. I stayed outside on the street talking with Khaled.

Two boys with machine guns came up to us and began to talk to Khaled. I made my acquaintance by doing some chair tricks. The nice pavement next to the tower allowed me to coast at top speed on two wheels down the hill. Coming back up was strenuous, but with no potholes, live ordinance, or open pit of human waste, it was possible, which was saying a lot for Mogadishu.

Suddenly one of the boys pointed his gun directly at my chest and began to yell. He was still smiling. I smiled back and put my hand on the barrel of his rifle, gently moving it out of the way of my sternum, rib cage, and shoulder. He laughed and quickly moved it back. He was still smiling. I continued to smile back. The other boy went around to the back of the chair and began to lift it. He was looking carefully at the metal tubes, and he ran his fingers along the rubber treads.

The boy with the gun pointed at me and yelled again. He was not smiling this time. He was not going to remove his gun from my chest.

There was no question that this was a moment in which a bullet might just come out of that gun and end my life on this rare, smooth, but unclaimed pavement in south Mogadishu. It was one of those senselessly violent moments in a foreign land that are the stuff of true nightmares: nameless death over something you never understand. Your life bleeds out of you on a dirty street thousands of miles from home, you stare, blinking up at people talking idly about the weather in a foreign language as if you aren't there, and then you aren't.

But I looked at these boys and did understand something. The look was familiar. I had not had an AK-47 pointed at my chest very many times, but something else about this incident made sense. I could tell that the anger of these boys had nothing to do with the money in my pockets, or the color of my skin, or the fact that a crew was up in the tower filming Mogadishu for an American television network.

I put on as angry and severe a face as I could and yelled back at him. "No, this is mine. I'm very sorry." I said to Khaled, "Tell them that they will have to find their own chair. This one won't work for them." Khaled said something to them and gave me a look that said it was time to leave. I smiled and waved. The boy smiled and shook his gun at me. His companion made little motions as though he were riding in a wheelchair. They looked at each other and laughed. Khaled and I went slowly but deliberately back to the Land Cruiser around the corner from the two boys. "They said they had a friend who could not walk," Khaled said. "They were very serious. How did you understand them?" For the first time, Khaled looked scared.

"I just knew it had to be something like that."

I thought of their disabled friend. Hidden away behind the ruined houses, he waits for his friends to return. His body, inert and helpless, ignites anger in those around him. With so much about Somalia impossible and out of control, the possibility of any problem being addressed must have come as a revelation. For an instant the armed boys connected their friend to my wheelchair. Their guns had the power to take it from me and deliver it to someone close to them. Someone who rarely goes out anymore. Where is this boy without a wheelchair? Somewhere in the city with no electricity and endless sun he blinks and looks out from a darkened room, waiting for his friends.

One feeding center in Somalia, near the road between Baidoa and Bardera, stood apart from the others. It was filled with children. At the time the feeding center was set up, no food had come to the ten villages around it for weeks. About 300 children who had all watched their parents die sat waiting while a man walked slowly up and down the rows distributing a bowl of brown-grain mash. Another man with a box of sugar-wafer cookies handed them out one by one. In tents away from the main crowd, people near death lay motionless. Their lips moved slowly as they attempted to swallow a special mixture for those whose bodies were nearly shut down from lack of nutrition. Their eyes bulged beneath their bony foreheads. Their hair was matted and without texture.

The shock of the filth and the ugliness of the starving, wasted bodies passes after a few moments. The sweet pungence of death lingers on each breath, climbing its way down your throat, but you quickly get used to it. It was the silence among these hundreds of children that was the most disturbing thing about them. One could have walked by this feeding center without knowing it existed. At another time, any ten of the same children would have filled the air over a playground with the din of their squeals.

The children did not notice me. They watched as the man with the mash and the other man following him with the wafers slowly made their way through the crowd. Up one row and down another they went. A single scoop of mash and a single wafer for each child. One boy watched me. He was different than the children around him. He was taller and thinner. His eyes stood out. He had no fat on his flesh. He looked like a little old man, but he could not have been more than five years old. The children around him also looked sick, but their bodies still had a layer of fat that gave shape to their arms and cheeks.

The boy tried to stand up, but he was pushed down by the younger but stronger boys next to him. They laughed at him quietly, treating him with a familiar childish contempt that comes with fatness, ugliness, being too smart, or being too dumb. In the middle of a crowd of famine-plagued Somali children, one boy still had to have the cooties, had to be "it." The face of the thin boy understood, as did the faces of the impatient boys around him. The thin boy knew that he was going to die. The other boys only knew that they might still live.

I was drawn to the thin boy. He was the underdog. I identified with him. In an irrelevant gesture, I asked the man with the wafers to give me a handful to pass out. I felt uncomfortable just staring at the children without doing anything for them. The thin boy looked into my eyes and tried to stand. He was staring at me as though I was the last human being on earth. His attempt to stand jostled some of the boys around him. They taunted him and pushed him back down, impatient with the little odd-duck playmate wearing the death mask. He never took his eyes off me as he fell back to the ground and tried to get up again.

I rolled toward him and picked up a wafer from my lap. He and all of the children began to come toward me in a wave. I tried to put the wafer in the little thin boy's hand but each time it was grabbed by other, stronger boys. The wafer crumbled, and the little boys dove for crumbs in the dirt. I grabbed another wafer, and another, but the same thing happened. The thin boy stared at me. The little boys around me stared. The other children in the crowd, too weak to join in this game of wafer toss, also stared. All eyes were on me.

For almost all of my life in a wheelchair I have been stared at, especially by children. The eyes take in my chair and its imagined implications. The chair is embossed, made more visible by the staring of others as I am rendered more invisible. The chair becomes the event while I recede into the background as "occupant." John Doe on wheels. Reporter in a wheelchair, man in a wheelchair, paraplegic in space, handicapped patron, carry-on passenger, injured person. In the feeding center, my wheelchair vanished entirely without my having to leave it. The starving children stared only at the wafers in my hand.

In the center of the reaching, silent children was the thin boy. He was unable to get even one wafer from me. I could not get to him in the center of the crowd. He could not get to me. The men who had been moving at an orderly pace through the crowd now yelled angrily at the slow-motion riot being created as I tried to hand out the wafers. One man grabbed them from me and gave them back to the person distributing them. The children looked away. I didn't exist at all. But the thin boy continued to look. I showed him my hands, which were empty. He looked at them, and then deep into my eyes. He knew he was dead. He knew he would not get the wafers. He knew he was the object of teasing, the one selected, fated; his condemnation at the age of five fit him badly, like his wrinkled, malnourished skin. He did not look sublime or radiant as he gazed at me. He looked childlike. He knew what was to happen next. It was as true an understanding of death as I have ever witnessed.

The thin boy could not have survived for long after I left the village. Or perhaps he is living now. I can still see him watching me. When he looks into my eyes, he sees no wheelchair.

Acknowledgments

I originally imagined calling this book *Incomplete Coincidences* because it began as a way of explaining what have been, in my life, odd and powerful coincidences, coincidences of time and place, theme and circumstance. It's a lousy title but the idea still has meaning when I think about the events and ideas put down here, each linked only by my own unbelieving, and very often terrified, eyes. That one could tell a story in which the history of race relations and the space program meets under someone's vibrating bed and collides head-on with my personal experiences in a wheelchair, along with Middle East war and peace and the darkest secret of my own family, was pushing credulity, even for me. I cannot know if I succeeded, but the coincidences in my life remain incomplete as this book is put aside and I move on to other things..

I owe the greatest debt of gratitude to my friend Bill McKibben, my agent Gloria Loomis, and my editor Pat Mulcahy, who all believed in this book from the moment they heard my first rambling descriptions of it. Their belief and steadfast support helped transform a cauldron of ideas into a coherent narrative. To them I will always be grateful.

Many people contributed to this project in ways they may not even be aware of. The best of these stories were originally told around the warm and generous dinner table of Peter and Esther Brooks of Dublin,

New Hampshire; there is no sharper literary salon between Manhattan and the North Pole. My friend Dorit Peled, on a Tel Aviv beach, first convinced me that these stories were worth putting down on paper. Howard Berkes and Adrienne Ciuffo taught me how to tell stories long ago. The late Timothy Mayer taught me the meaning and responsibilies of fearlessness. Susan Nussbaum taught me not to be ashamed and how to truly learn from my own mistakes.

My grandfather John Slagle taught me that the world was an endless wonder and after he died, taught me how cruel it could be, as well. My fondest wish is that he could have lived to read this book. My parents, brothers, and sister have always been generous and supportive through the good and bad times and their suggestions and advice have always been a part of my work.

My co-workers at ABC News were always eager to make accommodations for my "other job" and their cooperation and indulgence allowed me to complete a book in the middle of jumping headlong into network television, having never done either one before. My ABC colleague Nancy Bergmann read every version of this manuscript and her encouragement and suggestions were crucial to the project. Jim and Barb Mackraz offered a welcome refuge to an insecure writer. Helen Winternitz offered her unrelenting antidote to fuzzy writing, and Alison Craiglow always gave her faith and in the end made a believer out of me.

The story of Charlie Slagle is in this book because of the candor and courage of the three women who agreed to tell his story and their own. My grandmother, mother, and aunt never for a moment hesitated over any of the hard questions I asked. Clearly my questions were not as difficult as the ones they have asked themselves over the years. The staff of the New York State Intermediate Care Facility at Phelps welcomed me when I came as a stranger to visit my Uncle Charlie. They were always cooperative and enthusiastic about this book and my efforts to make contact with their longtime ward. I thank them all and hope that in some small way the story set down here makes the motivations and consequences of the past more understandable.

In my career as a journalist I have been inspired by the work of Deborah Amos, Margo Adler, Noah Adams, Susan Stamberg, John Kifner, Maggie O'Kane, Mark Duvoisen, Steven Franklin, Robert Krulwich, Michael Sullivan, Marika Partridge, Adi Malul, Hugh Pope, Robert Cutler, Timothy Phelps, Alex Chadwick, Geraldine Brooks, Leslie Cockburn, Cecilia Vaisman, Sean Collins, and Ira Glass, among many others. During my years at NPR I had the privilege of working with editor Cadi Simon, who experienced my trials, tribulations, and close calls as her own.

Wherever I went, her spirit, knowledge, and her vision of truth and fairness went with me. In all my travels I have kept my wheelchairs rolling with my own tools and mechanical expertise but it was Ian Chafee in Chicago who put things back together when I came home in pieces. Ian always kept me well supplied with wheels, tubes, bearings, spokes, and bushings anywhere in the world. To this day, when I call him up he invariably asks, "Where are you now, John?"

"Ian, I'm home."